MRI of the Whole Body

An Illustrated Guide to Common Pathologies

MRI of the Whole Body
An Illustrated Guide to Common Pathologies

Edited by

Kshitij Mankad

Edward TD Hoey

Amit Lakkaraju

Nikhil Bhuskute

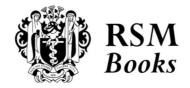

RSM
Books

First published in Great Britain in 2011 by
Hodder Arnold, an imprint of Hodder Education, a division of Hachette UK
338 Euston Road, London NW1 3BH

http://www.hodderarnold.com

© 2011 Hodder & Stoughton Ltd

Hachette UK's policy is to use papers that are natural, renewable and recyclable products and made from wood grown in sustainable forests. The logging and manufacturing processes are expected to conform to the environmental regulations of the country of origin.

Whilst the advice and information in this book are believed to be true and accurate at the date of going to press, neither the author[s] nor the publisher can accept any legal responsibility or liability for any errors or omissions that may be made. In particular, (but without limiting the generality of the preceding disclaimer) every effort has been made to check drug dosages; however, it is still possible that errors have been missed. Furthermore, dosage schedules are constantly being revised and new side-effects recognized. For these reasons the reader is strongly urged to consult the drug companies' printed instructions, and their websites, before administering any of the drugs recommended in this book.

British Library Cataloguing in Publication Data
A catalogue record for this book is available from the British Library

Library of Congress Cataloging-in-Publication Data
A catalog record for this book is available from the Library of Congress

ISBN-13   978-1-853-15776-9

1 2 3 4 5 6 7 8 9 10

Commissioning Editor: Francesca Naish
Project Editor: Stephen Clausard
Production Controller: Joanna Walker
Cover Design: Helen Townson

© *Simon Fraser/Science Photo Library*

The logo of the Royal Society of Medicine is a registered trade mark, which it has licensed to Hodder Arnold.

Typeset in 10pt Palatino LT Std by Phoenix Photosetting, Chatham, Kent
Printed and bound in the UK by CPI Group (UK) Ltd., Croydon, CR0 4YY

What do you think about this book? Or any other Hodder Arnold title?
Please visit our website: www.hodderarnold.com

Contents

Contributors

Unit I   Musculoskeletal MRI
Amit Lakkaraju FRCR PG MED ED Consultant Musculoskeletal Radiologist, Goulburn Valley Base Hospital, Shepparton, Australia
Ram KP Vijay MS MRCS FRCR Consultant Musculoskeletal Radiologist, Barnsley District General Hospital, Barnsley, UK

Special acknowledgement
R Hodgson PHD MRCP FRCR Senior Lecturer in Radiology and Consultant Musculoskeletal Radiologist, Chapel Allerton Hospital, Leeds, UK

Unit II   Neuro MRI
Kshitij Mankad MRCP FRCR Neuroradiology Fellow, Barts and the London NHS Trust, London, UK
Sanjoy Nagaraja MRCS(LON) MRCS(EDIN) FRCR MD Consultant Interventional Neuroradiologist, Coventry, UK
Anthony JP Goddard MRCP FRCR Consultant Interventional and Diagnostic Neuroradiologist, Leeds Teaching Hospitals NHS Trust, Leeds, UK
Omid Nikoubashman Assistenzartz, Klinik fur Diagnostische und Interventionelle Neuroradiologie, Aachen, Germany

Unit III   Body MRI
Nikhil Bhuskute MS FRCS FRCR Consultant Radiologist, Calderdale and Huddersfield NHS Foundation Trust, UK

Hepatobiliary sections edited by:
Ashley Guthrie FRCR Consultant Radiologist, St James' University Hospital, Leeds, UK

Unit IV   Cardiothoracic MRI
Edward TD Hoey BAO MRCP FRCR Consultant Cardiothoracic Radiologist, Heart of England Foundation Trust; Honorary Senior Clinical Lecturer, University of Birmingham Medical School, Birmingham, UK
SK Bobby Agrawal MRCS FRCR Consultant Cardiothoracic Radiologist, Papworth Hospital, Cambridge, UK

Unit V   Vascular MRI
Sapna Puppala MRCS FRCS(ED) FRCR CBCCT Consultant Cardiovascular and Interventional Radiologist, Vascular MRA lead, Leeds Teaching Hospitals NHS Trust, Leeds, UK

Unit VI   Breast MRI
Nisha Sharma BSC(HONS) MRCP FRCR Consultant Breast Radiologist and Director of Breast Screening Services, Leeds Teaching Hospitals NHS Trust, Leeds, UK
Barbara JG Dall FRCP(GLAS) FRCR Consultant Breast Radiologist, Leeds Teaching Hospitals NHS Trust, Leeds, UK

Unit VII   Head and Neck MRI
Amit Roy MRCS DOHNS FRCR Specialist Registrar in Clinical Radiology, Barts and the London NHS Trust, London, UK
Kshitij Mankad MRCP FRCR Neuroradiology Fellow, Barts and the London NHS Trust, London, UK

Preface

MRI of the Whole Body: An Illustrated Guide to Common Pathologies was envisioned as a book to help and guide junior radiologists contriving to learn the basics of clinically applied magnetic resonance imaging. As trainees, the authors often felt the need for a manual that could provide an overview of the modality as applicable to common diseases. Apprentice-modelled MRI teaching continues to be, by and large, *ad hoc*, and voluminous textbooks rarely leave their respective shelves. It is hoped that this illustrated guide will fill the gap and provide the first steps in dispelling the myths of MRI that often cloud the impressionable minds of trainees, residents, fellows, radiographers and general radiologists.

The guide covers all subspecialties and is written in a simplified manner with limited but vital textual matter and greater emphasis on key sequences and protocols, with hints and tips to typical imaging features of common pathologies and their close differential diagnoses.

We are extremely grateful to all our contributing authors and editors and the Royal Society of Medicine Press for having accepted the initial manuscript and for their patience and support throughout this project.

K Mankad
ETD Hoey
A Lakkaraju
N Bhuskute

Dedication

To our families with love and gratitude for their unflinching support.

UNIT I

MRI of the Musculoskeletal System

Amit Lakkaraju, Ram KP Vijay

1 MUSCULOSKELETAL IMAGING

MRI PROTOCOLS

Introduction

MRI protocols for imaging in musculoskeletal conditions vary depending on the part to be imaged, the specific tissues that need to be imaged, and the type of pathology. There is a need to standardize protocols to provide uniformity of imaging and to replicate previous scans.

Scanning of the extremities requires dedicated coils to allow better resolution compared with body coils. The use of phased array coils has become standard, since they are able to obtain maximum signal from each segment of tissue covered.

The sequences commonly used in musculoskeletal imaging are listed in Table 1.1.

Fat-suppression techniques

Fat suppression is a commonly used technique in musculoskeletal MRI. Unsuppressed fat is relatively high signal on both T1- and T2-weighted imaging. The technique is used to delineate oedema from the fat signal.

Two main methods are used to suppress fat: frequency-selective fat saturation and STIR imaging.

Frequency-selective fat saturation

This uses a pulse to cancel out the signal from fat without affecting the signal from water.

In T1-weighted imaging, this technique is used to confirm the nature of fatty tissues and also when gadolinium enhancement is employed.

T2-weighted fast spin echo (FSE) imaging is combined with frequency-selective fat suppression to visualize soft tissue and bone marrow oedema. A major problem with this technique is that it is susceptible to inhomogeneities in the magnetic field and to magnetic susceptibility artefact.

Short-tau inversion recovery (STIR) imaging

This uses an inversion recovery technique to suppress fat. There is an initial inversion pulse at 180° to the longitudinal axis, followed by an excitation pulse at 90° when the recovery of the fat signal reaches zero, thereby removing the signal.

STIR is used when imaging larger fields of view, since the sequence is less susceptible to field inhomogeneities.

STIR is not used with gadolinium enhancement, since the relaxation properties of gadolinium and fat are very similar and so the enhancement would be suppressed along with fat.

Gadolinium enhancement

Gadolinium (Gd) is a rare earth element, whose ion Gd^{3+} contains seven unpaired electrons. The contrast agent Gd-DTPA is a paramagnetic stable compound that demonstrates high signal on T1-weighted imaging. It can be administered by either intravenous or intra-articular injection.

Table 1.1 Sequences used in musculoskeletal MRI[a]

Sequence	TR (ms)	TE (ms)	TI (ms)/flip angle	Strengths/weaknesses
T1-weighted	<1000	≤30		Good anatomic detail and meniscal pathology
Proton density (PD)-weighted	>1000	30–60		Marrow pathology and anatomic detail
T2-weighted	>2000	≥60		Good for oedema, but there is a potential blurring artefact Tissue oedema needs fat saturation for better delineation
T2-weighted gradient echo (GRE)	Variable	≤ 30	5–20°	Good for imaging tendons and ligaments, but poor for marrow pathology and there is a susceptibility artefact
Short-tau inversion recovery (STIR)	≥2000	≥60	120–150 ms with 180°→90°	Marrow and tissue pathology, but not good for using with gadolinium
T1-weighted fat saturation (FS) with Gd				Good for removing the signal from fat so that gadolinium enhancement is seen better

[a]Adapted from Kaplan P, Dussault R, Helms CA, Anderson MW. *Musculoskeletal MRI*, 1st edn. Philadelphia: WB Saunders, 2001.

Contrast enhancement is best seen on T1-weighted fat saturation sequences, where there is enhancement of only those tissues that take up the Gd.

Gd enhancement is used in very specific cases in musculoskeletal MRI, principally the following:

- **Cystic versus solid lesions:** a true cyst will demonstrate only wall enhancement, while a solid lesion will show diffuse enhancement.
- **Tumour:** Gd is used to differentiate solid from cystic tumours and may help in targeting biopsies.
- **Infection:** Gd enhancement is useful in differentiating solid areas from phlegmon and abscess. Abscess shows a thick enhancing wall. Sinus tracts can be better detected by this technique. However, Gd is of no use for differentiating osteomyelitis from marrow oedema, both of which present as marrow enhancement.
- **Spine:** a recurrent disc does not enhance following Gd, while postoperative fibrosis does. This is a useful discriminator in postoperative spinal imaging, although the management of these conditions is similar.
- **MR arthography:** this technique is used to locate pathology within the shoulder and the hip. It can be used to look at labral tears. A 1% Gd solution is injected into the joint (concentrated solutions result in loss of signal from the fluid and render images non-diagnostic). T1-weighted imaging with fat saturation is used to distinguish Gd from fat, along with a T2-weighted sequence in at least one plane to detect oedema or cysts.

TIPS ON INTERPRETING MUSCULOSKELETAL MRI

Interpretation of musculoskeletal MRI needs a combination of skills.

First and foremost is the clinical history, which points fairly accurately to the site of pathology. The site of the symptoms often corresponds to the site of pathology, unlike in other systems such as the abdomen. For example, medial joint tenderness after a twisting injury to the knee consistently localizes the site of pathology to the medial meniscus or the medial collateral ligament of the knee. Similarly, sciatica with paraesthesia in a left L5 nerve root distribution indicates a left L5 disc protrusion.

The sequences used must be appropriate to visualize the pathology that is suspected (and that is mentioned on the request form). When examining the images, it is essential to know the normal anatomy of the site that is being imaged.

An area with high T2 signal on a fat-suppressed sequence is often a marker for the site of the primary pathology. High T2 signal in an area that is normally intermediate to low signal is a sign of oedema and haemorrhage. This signal will be centred on the site of pathology or adjacent to it. For example, in axial fat-saturated T2-weighted images of the knee, high T2 signal in the medial retinaculum indicates oedema and haemorrhage in this ligament and implies a patellar dislocation.

High T2 signal within the bone marrow on fat-suppressed sequences is also a sign of oedema, haemorrhage and microfractures. This occurs as a result of direct or repetitive injury to the area. The pattern of bone oedema can be indicative of the injury process. For example, anterior cruciate ligament tears are associated with bone marrow oedema at the anterior part of the femoral condyles and the posterior part of the tibial plateau. Similarly, patellar dislocation has a typical marrow oedema pattern at the medial facet of the patella and the lateral surface of the lateral femoral condyle that is caused as the patella dislocates, impinging laterally on the lateral femoral condyle.

Correlation of high signal on fat-suppressed T2-weighted sequences with low signal on T1-weighted sequences is important to remove the influence of artefact.

As a general rule, pathology should also be seen on at least two slices, as well as in two orthogonal planes.

ARTEFACTS IN MUSCULOSKELETAL MRI

Magic angle effect

This is seen in structures containing ordered fibres of collagen, such as tendons. There is an artefactual increase in T2 signal within the tendon when it passes 55° to the magnetic field. This artefact is seen for example in the extensor pollicis longus tendon of the wrist and the peroneus longus tendon of the ankle.

Chemical shift artefact

This is seen in gradient echo (GRE) sequences. Fat and water go in and out of phase with one another, depending on the echo time (TE). At a magnetic field of 1.5 T, the period of this alteration is about 4.4 s. Tissues containing both fat and water at the boundaries of structures are prone to this artefact, which manifests itself as a dark rim around the structures (Figure 1.1). GRE techniques are used in imaging of the cervical spine or in the knee, and the chemical shift artefact is seen around muscle fascicles.

Magnetic susceptibility artefact

This occurs at the interface between structures with different magnetic characteristics. There is low signal at the interface. Susceptibility artefact is especially evident when ferromagnetic materials are present, resulting in field distortions. Although susceptibility artefact can occur in any type of sequence, GRE sequences are most prone and are therefore used for its identification. This is especially important in identifying haemorrhage. From

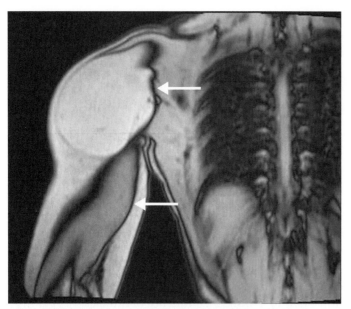

Figure 1.1 Chemical shift artefact at the interface between fat and muscle (predominantly water) in a GRE scout image of the shoulder.

the signal characteristics, the types of blood breakdown products can be identified (Figure 1.2) and the age of the haemorrhage can be estimated. This technique is used extensively in neuroimaging for assessing the age of cerebral haemorrhage. In musculoskeletal MRI, the use of susceptibility artefact is limited to identifying haemorrhage versus oedema.

Metal artefact

Misregistration is the main artefact from metal in sites such as total hip and knee replacements (Figure 1.3) and spinal metal work. This artefact is represented by geometric signal alteration in the frequency encoding direction. The dimensions of the artefact depend on the field strength, the direction in which the metal implant lies in relation to the magnetic field, the magnetic field strength and the bandwidth. Higher field strengths, smaller bandwidths and implants lying perpendicular to the magnetic field tend to worsen the artefact.

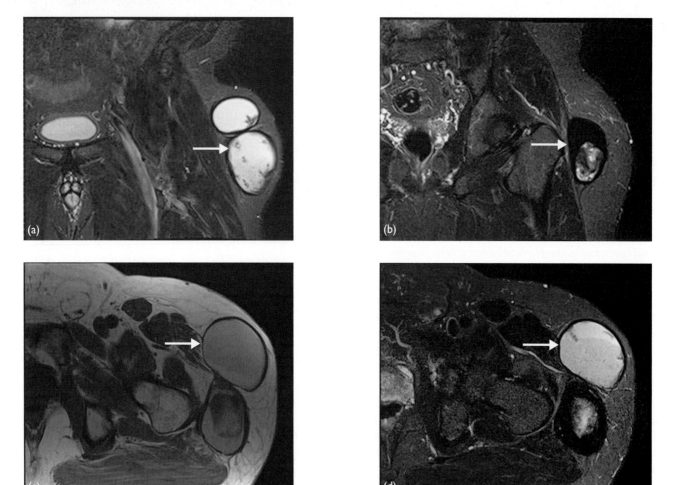

Figure 1.2 Magnetic susceptibility artefact in a resolving left thigh haematoma. In the PD-weighted fat-saturated (FS) image (a) and the T2*-weighted FS image (b), the black rim is consistent with haemosiderin deposition and the high signal is consistent with the presence of other blood products. In the axial T1- and T2*-weighted FS images (c, d), the low-signal rim is consistent with haemosiderin and the high-signal fluid is consistent with extracellular methaemoglobin. The axial T2*-weighted image (d) shows layering of blood products.

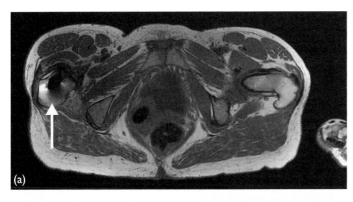

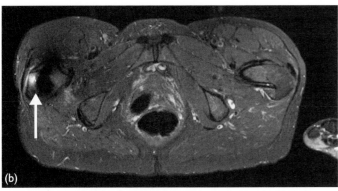

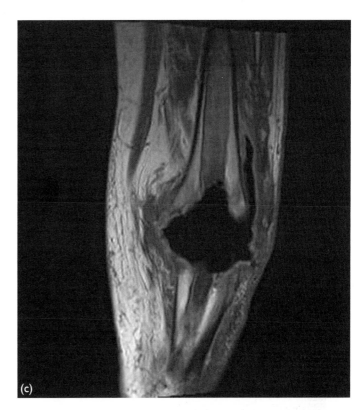

Figure 1.3 (a, b) T1-weighted and fat-saturated T2-weighted sections showing metal artefact from a total hip replacement. (c) Coronal T1-weighted image of a total knee replacement showing complete signal loss.

A number of approaches can be adopted to reduce metal artefact. These include lowering the field strength, broadening the receiver bandwidth, increasing the frequency encoding strength and orientating the implant so that it lies parallel to the main magnetic field.

Some sequences are more prone to metal artefact than others. Using STIR for fat suppression and FSE with short TE have been found to reduce artefact due to metal.

With the advent of the new metallic artefact reduction sequence (MARS), MRI has come to have a very important role in evaluating prosthetic joints, enabling a comprehensive assessment of articular and non-articular pathologies.

FURTHER READING

Stoller D. *Magnetic Resonance Imaging in Orthopaedics and Sports Medicine*, 3rd edn. Philadelphia: Lippincott, William & Wilkins, 2006.

Elster AD, Burdette JH. *Questions and Answers in Magnetic Resonance Imaging*, 2nd edn. St Louis: Mosby, 2001.

Naraghi AM, White LM. Magnetic resonance imaging of joint replacements. *Semin Musculoskelet Radiol* 2006; **10**: 98–106.

2 THE SPINE

SPINAL IMAGING

Protocols

The spine is imaged in segments depending on the site of the symptoms.

Phased array coils help to improve both spatial resolution and signal-to-noise ratio. The drawback to this is the need for smaller fields of view, and hence multiple coil placements are necessary for imaging the whole spine.

Whole-spine imaging is used in:

- trauma
- metastatic infiltrates
- seronegative spondyloarthropathies such as ankylosing spondylitis
- spinal malformations

Key sequences

- T1-weighted fast spin echo (FSE) sagittal and axial (Figure 2.1a, c)
- T2-weighted FSE sagittal and axial (Figure 2.1b, d)
- Short-tau inversion recovery (STIR) sagittal and axial

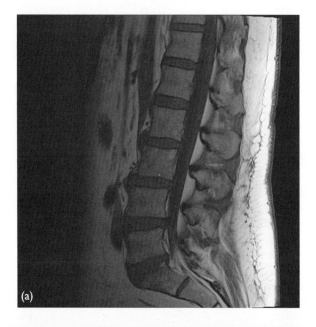

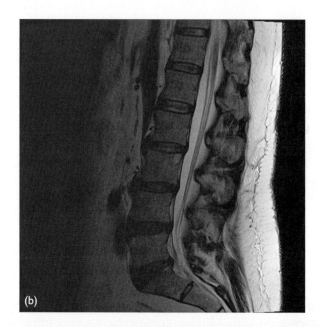

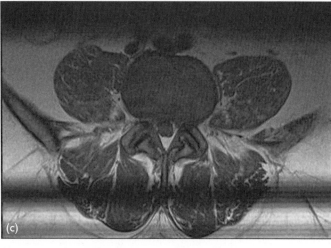

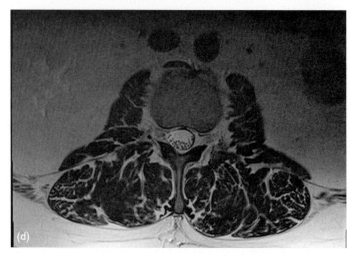

Figure 2.1 Normal lumbar spine sequences: (a) T1-weighted sagittal; (b) T2-weighted sagittal; (c) T1-weighted axial; (d) T2-weighted axial.

Gadolinium

If infection, a spinal cord mass or syrinx is suspected, gadolinium (Gd) is administered and images are obtained using a T1-weighted sequence with fat saturation.

SPINAL ANATOMY

See Figure 2.2.

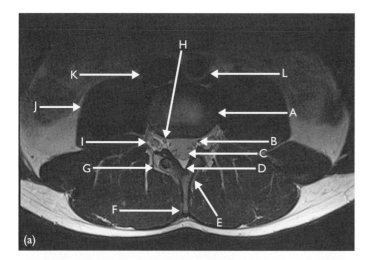

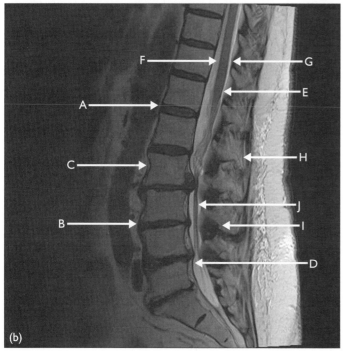

Figure 2.2 (a) T2-weighted axial section through the lumbar spine: A, intervertebral disc; B lateral recess; C, spinal canal; D, epidural fat; E, lamina; F, spinous process; G, facet joint; H, traversing nerve roots; I, exiting nerve roots; J, psoas muscle; K, inferior vena cava; L, aorta.
(b) T2-weighted sagittal section through the lumbar spine: A, intervertebral disc with high signal indicating a hydrated disc; B, dehydrated disc with uniform low signal; C, anterior longitudinal ligament; D, posterior longitudinal ligament; E, conus medullaris; F; spinal canal; G, epidural fat; H, spinous process; I, facet joint; J, cauda equina.

Vertebrae

The vertebral column is made up of 33 vertebrae that differ depending on the anatomic area.

There are seven cervical vertebrae, each with a body and a posterior arch consisting of two pedicles. Each pedicle has superior and inferior facets that articulate with corresponding superior and inferior vertebrae. The facet joints are synovial joints. In addition, there are lateral ridges of bone called the uncinate processes that articulate with the inferior aspect of the vertebral body above to form the uncovertebral joints. These are not true joints.

The C1 and C2 vertebral bodies are unique in their anatomy and provide the main support and pivot for the skull. The atlanto-occipital joints and atlanto-dens joints are both synovial in nature and are important sites in imaging of inflammatory arthropathies.

The thoracic vertebrae are anatomically typical. They have additional attachments to the ribs. The lumbar vertebrae are square-shaped with inferiorly angled spinal processes and, more importantly, neural foramina. This anatomic variation in the vertebrae results from the incongruent growth of the vertebrae and the spinal column. The spinal cord is fully formed at birth and grows at a slower rate than the vertebral column.

Nerves

There are eight cervical nerve roots, which exit the foramina above their respective vertebral bodies; thus the C1 nerve root exits between the occiput and the C1 vertebra and the C8 nerve root exits through the C7/T1 neural foramen.

The T1 and subsequent thoracic nerve roots exit inferior to the corresponding vertebral body; thus the T4 nerve root exits below the T4 pedicle, and so on. Because of the growth of the spinal cord and the vertebral column, the nerve roots become progressively more vertical through the thoracic and lumbar regions. The spinal cord typically ends at T12 and L1 as the conus medullaris, from which descend the filum terminale and the cauda equina. If the conus is seen to extend beyond this point then the question of a tethered cord arises. Ideally, every spinal MR examination should comment on the level of the conus.

The lumbar nerve roots also exit below their corresponding vertebrae.

The dural coverings of the spinal cord and nerve roots are in continuity with the dura in the cranial cavity. The dura and arachnoid are closely adherent to one another, while the pia mater is adherent to the spinal cord. The epidural space is a potential space between the dural and arachnoid membranes and is important to assess when imaging in the context of infection or tumour spread. The cerebrospinal fluid (CSF) circulates within the spinal canal and is in continuity with the circulating CSF in the cranial cavity.

In addition, the spinal canal has a specific configuration in the lumbar region. The lumbar and sacral nerves run parallel within the canal. The exiting nerve root runs down diagonally and through the corresponding neural foramen. The nerve is outlined by fat as it exits the foramen. The subsequent nerve root lies within the most lateral part of the dural sac. This part is known as the lateral recess and the nerve root is termed the traversing root.

Bone marrow

The MRI appearance of vertebral marrow depends on the pulse sequence and the relative amount of cellularity, protein, water and fat within the marrow. In an adult on a T1-weighted image, the yellow (fatty) marrow is isointense to subcutaneous fat. On a T2-weighted image, fatty marrow is usually higher signal than muscle and slightly lower signal than subcutaneous fat.

Changes with age may render bone marrow patchy. Uniform bone marrow change affecting multiple vertebrae is a subtle sign that may indicate marrow pathology and is case-specific. The endplates are made up of cortical bone and are low signal. With aging and changes in axial loading, the endplate signal can change. This appears as differences on T1- and T2-weighted imaging and is graded into three types according to the Modic classification (Table 2.1).

Table 2.1 Modic classification of vertebral body bone marrow changes

Modic type	T1-weighted imaging	T2-weighted imaging	Type of change
1	↓	↑	Oedema
2	↑	↓	Fatty change
3	↓	↓	Sclerosis

Discs and ligaments

The intervertebral discs are intermediate to high signal on T2-weighted imaging and low to intermediate signal on T1-weighted imaging. This is dependent on their degree of hydration and is an important sign to look for, since dehydration is an indicator of degeneration. The vertebral bodies are bounded by the anterior and posterior spinal ligaments, which are low signal on both T1- and T2-weighted imaging. These are best seen on sagittal images. The interspinous ligament is patchy in signal, with striations; this is due to its plane being parallel to the scan plane. The supraspinous ligament is also low signal on both T1- imaging and T2-weighted imaging. Finally, the ligamentum flavum is best seen on axial images and is the thickest ligament. This is seen as intermediate signal on T1- and T2-weighted imaging, owing to differences in chemical composition.

PRACTICAL POINTS

Artefacts

Motion artefact is responsible for many of the technical errors: patient and physiological artefacts from lung, cardiovascular and bowel motion, as well as artefacts due to CSF flow. CSF pulsation artefact is particularly seen on T2-weighted imaging.

A second type of artefact is the truncation or Gibb artefact seen at interfaces of high contrast (e.g. CSF and spinal cord). Seen on sagittal imaging, this may simulate a syrinx. Syrinx may be differentiated from tumour and Gibb artefact by enhancement characteristics.

With increasing use of spinal instrumentation, there is an added problem of susceptibility artefact from the metal. This may obscure the spinal cord and render images non-diagnostic.

Review areas

On cervical spine MRI, review areas include the cerebral contents and the cervical lymph node chains in the field of view. Comment should be made about the craniocervical junction and level of the tonsils (Chiari malformations may be associated with cervical pathology).

The common review areas in the lumbar and thoracic spine are:
- the paravertebral soft tissues
- the aorta for aortic aneurysms
- soft tissues of the back for soft tissue masses

SPINAL TRAUMA

Introduction

MRI of the spine is used to look at soft tissue injuries associated with spinal fractures. In addition, some fractures are also seen well on MRI. The MRI scan is done after conventional radiography of the cervical spine and CT scans for vertebral fractures.

MRI is useful to look for ligamentous injury and traumatic disc protrusions and to examine the cord itself. This examination should ideally be performed within 3 days of the trauma, since the initially high signal from oedema and blood products will decrease over time.

Key sequences

- Whole-spine (non-contiguous spinal trauma is seen in 10–15% of cases)
- T1-weighted axial and sagittal
- STIR axial and sagittal
- GRE (which may identify blood products within the cord)

Key features

Bone oedema is especially well seen on T2-weighted imaging and is an indicator of fracture. Fractures through cortical bone are not visualized on MRI, which is why radiography and CT are used as first-line investigations. Fractures through the cancellous bone of the vertebral bodies appear on T2-weighted imaging as areas of high signal intensity with amorphous outlines and on T1-weighted imaging as low- or intermediate-signal areas. Linear fractures, when seen, are low-signal areas. Uniform high signal within the vertebral body may indicate an axial compression injury, but may also indicate a wedge compression fracture if there is associated loss of vertebral body height and buckling of the anterior cortex.

The anterior and posterior spinous ligaments, the ligamentum flavum, the interspinous ligaments and the supraspinous ligaments can be visualized on MRI. Ligaments are seen as low-signal bands on all sequences, except for the interspinous ligament, which tends to be patchy or striated. Ligamentous injury is seen as high signal on T2-weighted imaging, with disruption of the bands and susceptibility artefacts when associated with blood. There are two forms of ligamentous disruption: full-thickness disruption of the fibres and partial tears.

Traumatic disc disruption is seen in 10–15% of patients presenting with associated neurological compromise. Disc extrusion with facet joint dislocation will need careful consideration for open reduction. Acute disc extrusion is also associated with traumatic cord injuries, including spinal cord haematomas.

Epidural haematoma and pseudo-meningocoele are recognized complications of trauma to the spine.

Vertebral artery dissection is associated with fractures of the foramen transversarium, a review area. Any asymmetry in signal intensity from the vertebral arteries on T2-weighted (STIR) axial images may indicate a traumatic dissection and will need further investigation.

Cord trauma is associated with three major abnormalities:
• cord contusion
• cord oedema
• cord transaction

High signal within the cord on STIR sequences is an indicator of a combination of acute cord contusion and cord oedema, since both of these are high signal on STIR sequences. Cord haemorrhage is a sign of severity of the trauma and can indicate the chronicity or timing of the injury. As blood denatures with time, there are specific changes that can be appreciated on MRI (Table 2.2). Prognosis is poorer with cord haemorrhage than with cord contusion.

Central cord syndrome commonly presents with cord oedema without fractures or haemorrhage. It is seen in hyper-extension injuries, usually secondary to degenerative disease. It appears as low to iso-intense signal on T1-weighted imaging and high signal on STIR.

Muscles, nerves and prevertebral soft tissues are involved in trauma and need to be visualized.

Nerve avulsion or contusion is a well known complication. High T2 signal and thickening of the nerve is an indicator of nerve contusion. With avulsion, there is a loss of continuity with high T2 signal in the adjacent paravertebral soft tissues.

Paraspinal muscle injury is seen as high T2 signal, with areas of low signal indicating blood products, depending on the age of the injury.

Practical points

Spinal trauma is usually part of the spectrum of poly-trauma injuries. These patients often have intensive care issues and so have to have continuous monitoring. This may pose problems in the MRI scanner.

Management decisions are made in two areas:
• **Stability of the spine:** is it stable or unstable? This depends on the number of columns affected and the site of injury.
• **Neurological deficit:** the level and type of the deficit dictate the approach to management.

Whole-spine imaging is mandatory, since in up to 10–15% of cases there is another level involved. The key to imaging is to look for high T2 signal on STIR imaging,

Table 2.2 Blood products and MRI changes

Age	Time period	Blood products	T1-weighted imaging	T2-weighted imaging
Hyperacute	24 h	Oxyhaemoglobin	↔	↑
Acute	24–72 h	Deoxyhaemoglobin	↔	↓
Early subacute	72 h–7 d	Intracellular methaemoglobin	↑	↓
Late subacute	> 7 d	Extracellular methaemoglobin	↑	↑
Chronic	> 2 weeks	Haemosiderin	↓	↓

since this points to the site of injury. Sagittal imaging is useful to look for the site of injury and the ligaments involved. Axial imaging helps to assess the cord injury. The images need to be reviewed carefully in all planes. There is evidence to suggest that GRE sequences are useful to look for blood products, especially with regard to cord injury.

Further reading

Berquist TH, ed. *MRI of the Musculoskeletal System*, 5th edn. Philadelphia: Lippincott Williams &Wilkins, 2006.

Helms CA, Major NM, Anderson MW et al. 2001. *Musculoskeletal MRI*, 2nd edn. Philadelphia: WB Saunders, 2009.

Saifuddin A. MRI of acute spinal trauma. *Skeletal Radiol* 2001; **30**: 237–46.

Case 1: Spinal trauma

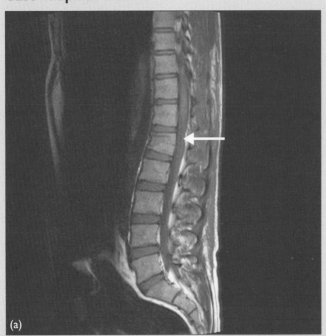

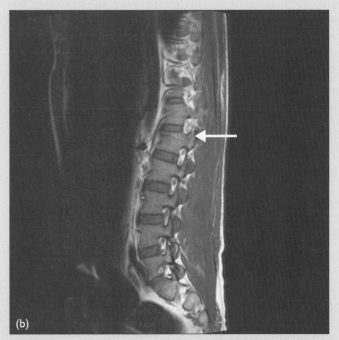

Case 1.1 (a, b) T1-weighted sagittal images of the lumbar spine showing a linear fracture through the L2 vertebral body extending into the pedicle.

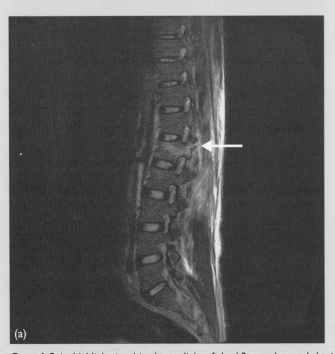

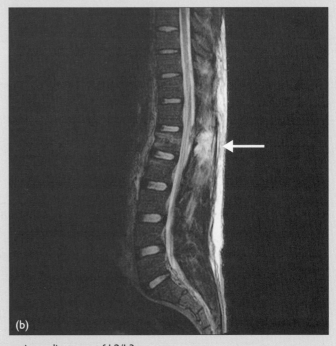

Case 1.2 (a, b) High signal in the pedicle of the L2 vertebra and the interspinous ligament of L2/L3.

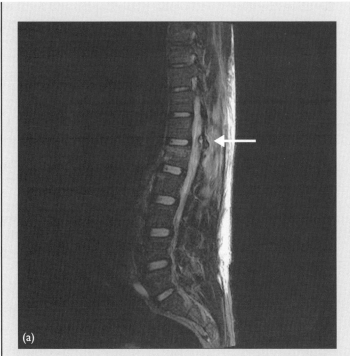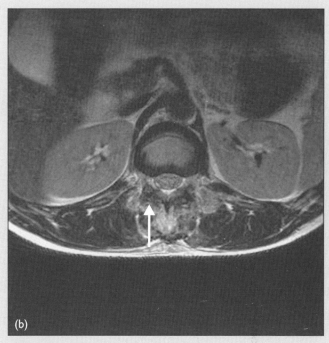

Case 1.3 (a, b) STIR sagittal images showing blood products as susceptibility artefact.

DEGENERATIVE LUMBAR DISC DISEASE

Imaging for chronic back pain forms a large part of the workload for spinal imaging. MRI is a useful tool for imaging significant organic back pain.

Disc degeneration is a spectrum starting initially with loss of hydration from the nucleus of the disc, followed by a radial annular tear and finally disc prolapse.

Lumbar disc prolapse is the most common abnormality, with over 90% occurring at the L4/5 and L5/S1 disc levels.

Key sequences

- T1-weighted sagittal and axial
- T2-weighted sagittal and axial

Imaging findings

Disc degeneration is associated with dehydration of the disc. This is seen as low signal from the disc on T2-weighted imaging.

Annular tears of the disc may be seen as high signal on T2-weighted imaging. Radial annular tears are painful, and are seen on sagittal T2-weighted imaging in the posterior part of the disc, associated with a disc bulge.

Nomenclature

Disc abnormalities are described using a standardized nomenclature set out by the North American Spine Society in 2001 (Box 2.1).

> **Box 2.1 Nomenclature for disc abnormalities**
>
> **Bulge:** A disc bulge is a generalized displacement of disc material. 'Generalized' here implies a bulge that involves at least 50% of the circumference of the disc, but may involve up to 100%. Disc bulge is not considered to be a herniation, which is localized (see below), and the terms should not be used interchangeably.
>
> **Herniation:** A disc herniation is a localized displacement of disc material beyond the limits of the intervertebral disc space. 'Localized' here implies a displacement of less than 50% of the circumference of the disc, in contrast to the generalized displacement in a disc bulge (see above). The disc space is confined by the vertebral endplates and peripherally by the outer edges of the vertebral ring apophyses. Displacement of disc material on MRI is often the only sign. Herniation can be focal or broad-based:
> - **Focal:** This is defined as meaning less than 25% of the disc.
> - **Broad-based:** This signifies between 25% and 50% of the disc.
>
> **Extrusion:** A disc is described as **extruded** when its depth in any one plane is greater than its base. An extruded disc may be further classified as **sequestered** if it has lost complete continuity with the parent disc or **migrated** if it is found distant to its parent disc.
>
> **Protrusion:** A disc is described as **protruded** when its depth is less than its base.

The direction of disc herniation has a bearing on the type of neurology, and this has been further classified into five types:

- **Central:** The disc herniates into the central canal.
- **Paracentral:** The disc herniates off-centre and may impinge on the lateral recess. Depending on the size of the herniated segment, the disc has the potential to impinge on both the exiting and the traversing nerve roots.
- **Foraminal:** The disc is herniated within the neural foramen. This type of disc herniation is associated with exiting nerve root impingement
- **Lateral:** The disc herniates lateral to the neural foramen.
- **Far-lateral:** This type of herniation extends laterally into the paravertebral fat and may not be seen on sagittal images. The disc may impinge upon the exiting nerve root, but this is seen only on axial images and is diagnosed on these images.

About 90% of focal disc bulges are central or paracentral and impinge on the spinal canal.

Effects on ligaments and joints

Disc degeneration is associated with ligamentous and facet joint degeneration.

The ligaments maintain the stability of the spine. Hence, a loss of height of the disc leads to ligamentous laxity with subsequent deterioration.

The facet joints are subjected to increased stress and on imaging appear as low-signal areas owing to sclerosis with osteophytes. The facet joints are synovial in nature. On T2-weighted imaging, the joints may show increased fluid and the appearance of synovial cysts. Synovial cysts may be responsible for impingement upon the exiting nerve root.

The ligamentum flavum is approximately 5 mm thick and any increase in thickness is a sign of degeneration.

Spinal canal stenosis is a well-recognized condition of the spinal canal and is caused by a combination of ligamentum flavum hypertrophy, facet joint hypertrophy, and focal or broad-based disc displacement that narrows the spinal canal. The narrowing may be worsened by spinal instability or a spondylolisthesis.

Hints and tips

Sagittal T2-weighted imaging is a good starting point to assess the level of the degenerated discs.

Lateral images show a 'pork chop' appearance, with the exiting nerve roots surrounded by a rim of fat. The 'pork chop' may be obliterated by the prolapsing disc.

Axial T2-weighted imaging shows disc displacement and this plane helps to further assess any impingement of the traversing nerve roots in the lateral recess or exiting nerve roots in the neural foramen.

Far-lateral discs may impinge upon the exiting nerve root in the paravertebral tissues. Axial imaging is used to diagnose a far-lateral disc prolapse.

Facet joint hypertrophy and fluid within the joint are typically seen with disc degeneration.

Finally, look for evidence of spinal stenosis.

Review areas in the lumbar spine include the aorta, paravertebral soft tissues and sacrum.

Further reading

Fardon DF, Milette PC. Nomenclature and classification of lumbar disc pathology: recommendations of the Combined Task Forces of the North American Spine Society, American Society of Spine Radiology, and American Society of Neuroradiology. *Spine* 2001; **26**: E93–E113.

Helms CA, Major NM, Anderson MW et al. 2001. *Musculoskeletal MRI*, 2nd edn. Philadelphia: WB Saunders, 2009.

Modic MT, Ross JS. Lumbar degenerative disc disease. *Radiology* 2007; **245**: 43–61.

Case 2: Lumbar disc disease

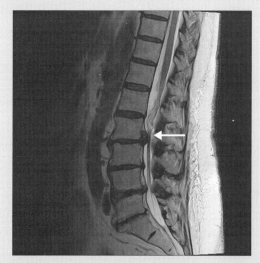

Case 2.1 T2-weighted sagittal image of the lumbar spine showing multiple dehydrated discs and disc protrusion at L2/3.

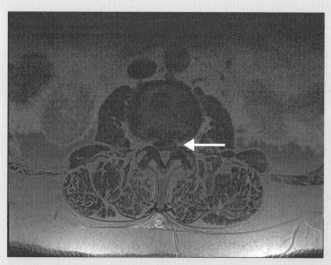

Case 2.2 T2-weighted axial image showing a central disc prolapse with spinal canal stenosis.

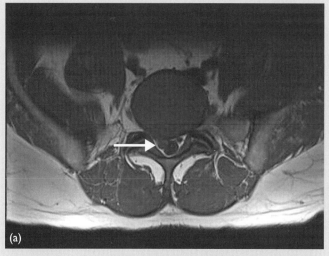

(a)

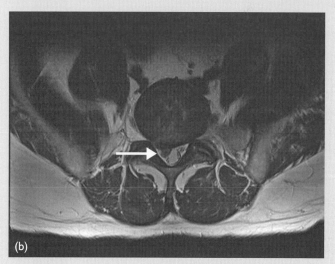

(b)

Case 2.3 (a, b) T1- and T2-weighted axial images showing a right paracentral disc protrusion.

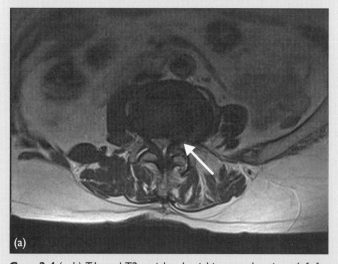

(a)

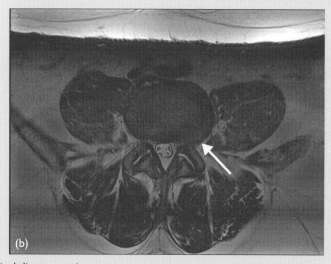

(b)

Case 2.4 (a, b) T1- and T2-weighted axial images showing a left foraminal disc protrusion.

CAUDA EQUINA SYNDROME

Cauda equina syndrome is a complex of neuromuscular and urogenital symptoms and signs resulting from narrowing of the spinal cord and compression of the lumbosacral nerve roots below the level of the conus. The condition is multi-factorial and may be secondary to trauma, disc herniation, neoplasms and inflammatory/infective conditions, among others. Cauda equina syndrome is a neurosurgical emergency. MRI is the best way of determining the level of obstruction and the type of disease process – both crucial factors to assist therapy planning.

Key sequences

- T1-weighted axial and sagittal
- STIR axial and sagittal

Imaging findings

Sagittal T1-weighted and STIR images show significant or complete stenosis of the spinal canal at the level of the cauda equina due to a stenosing lesion. The most common cause is a prolapsed central disc.

Hints and tips

Always start with the sagittal STIR images first and identify the level.

The axial images give information regarding the disc and the paravertebral soft tissues.

Further reading

Helms CA, Major NM, Anderson MW et al. 2001. *Musculoskeletal MRI*, 2nd edn. Philadelphia: WB Saunders, 2009.

Case 3: Cauda equina syndrome

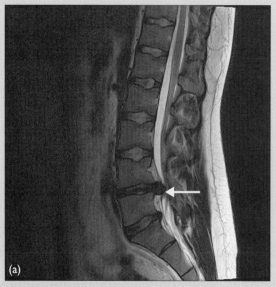
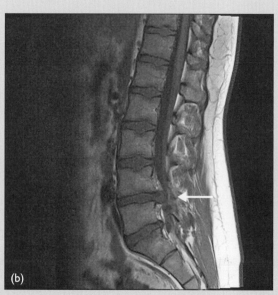

Case 3.1 (a, b) T1- and T2-weighted sagittal images showing an acute disc prolapse producing cauda equina syndrome.

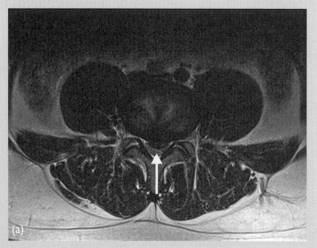
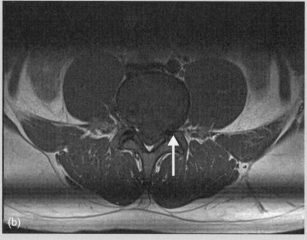

Case 3.2 (a, b) T1- and T2-weighted axial images showing severe spinal stenosis.

SPONDYLODISCITIS

Discitis is inflammation of the intervertebral discs.

Disc space infection may be confined to one space or may be at multiple levels. The most common pathogen is *Staphylococcus aureus*.

Key sequences

- T1-weighted sagittal and axial
- STIR sagittal and axial
- T1-weighted plus fat saturation (FS), with Gd enhancement

Imaging findings

There is an intermediate- to low-signal disc on T1-weighted imaging.

There is intermediate-to high signal on T2-weighted imaging (STIR), with loss of the low-signal intranuclear cleft.

The majority of cases show normal disc height. An apparent increase or decrease in disc height is possible. There is poor delineation of the disc–endplate interface.

There is endplate destruction of the bone with marrow signal loss on T1-weighted imaging, with a corresponding high T2 signal on STIR.

There is Gd rim enhancement of the disc on T1-weighted FS images.

Epidural abscess is best seen on axial images and may cause a mass effect.

Homogeneous enhancement of the epidural mass is consistent with phlegmon, while rim enhancement is associated with an epidural abscess.

Paraspinal abscess is seen in up to 50% of cases and these often track up the iliopsoas muscle.

Hints and tips

Whole-spine imaging is warranted to assess multiple levels.

Vertebral osteomyelitis with relative sparing of the disc on MRI, with large paraspinal collections and iliopsoas abscesses, should raise the possibility of tuberculosis.

Further reading

Ledermann HP, Schweitzer ME, Morrison WB et al. MR imaging of findings in spinal infections: rules or myths? *Radiology* 2003; **228**: 506–14.

The J, Imam A, Watts C. Imaging of back pain. *Imaging* 2005; **17**: 171–207.

Case 4: Spondylodiscitis

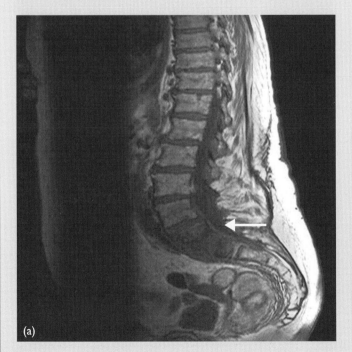
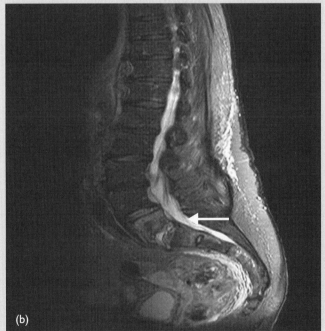

Case 4.1 (a, b) T1-weighted and STIR sagittal images showing pyogenic discitis.

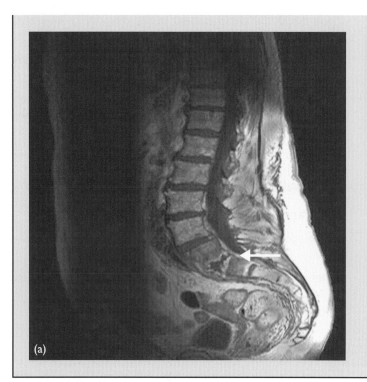

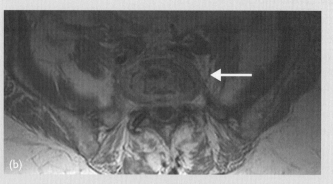

Case 4.2 (a, b) Post-Gd T1-weighted sagittal and axial images showing enhancement of discitis.

Case 5: Spondylodiscitis

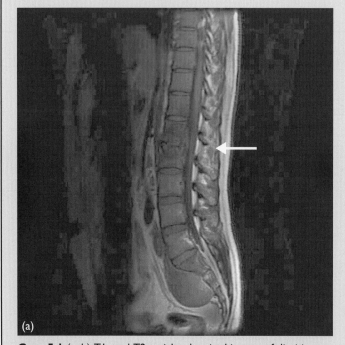

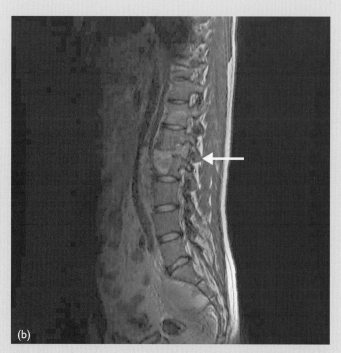

Case 5.1 (a, b) T1- and T2-weighted sagittal images of discitis.

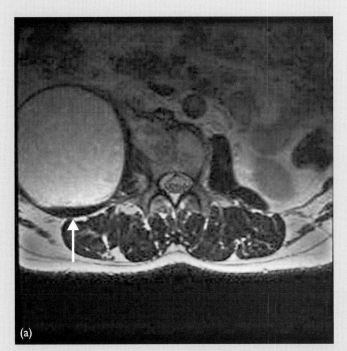 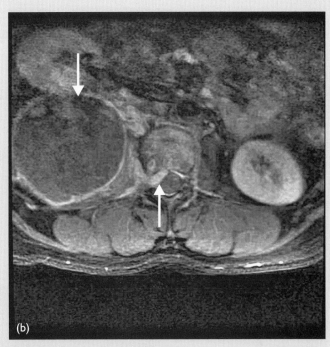

Case 5.2 (a, b) T2-weighted and post-Gd FS T1-weighted axial images showing discitis with extension to psoas abscess and epidural abscess.

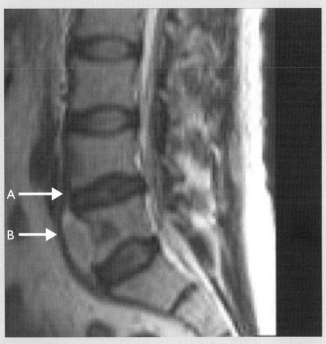

Case 5.3 Potts spine. T2-weighted sagittal image of the lumbar spine showing (A) typical spread deep to the anterior longitudinal ligament and (B) sparing of the disc.

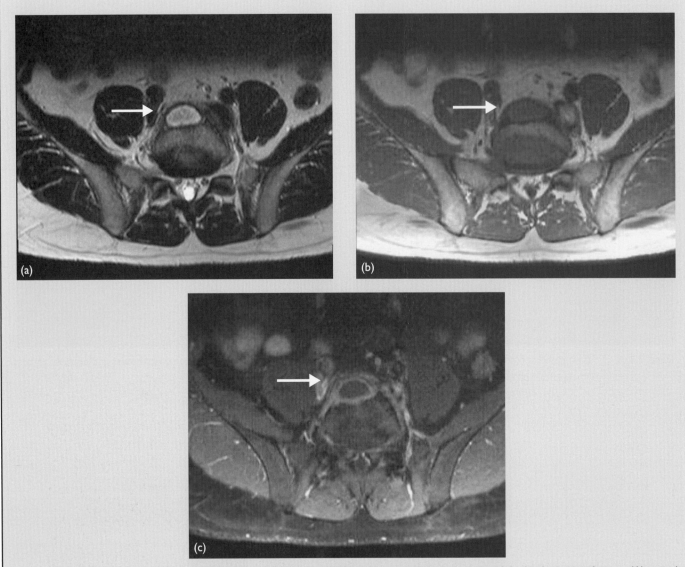

Case 5.4 Potts spine. T2-weighted (a), T1-weighted (b) and post-Gd FS T1-weighted (c) axial images of the lumbar spine showing (A) typical spread deep to the anterior longitudinal ligament and (B) sparing of the disc.

3 THE KNEE

KNEE IMAGING

Protocols

MRI of the knee provides a comprehensive non-invasive examination. The sensitivity and specificity are very high, reaching 90–95% for meniscal injuries and close to 100% for anterior cruciate ligament (ACL) injuries.

Imaging is with a dedicated surface coil. A small field of view is used to optimize resolution. Slice thickness is between 2 and 4 mm, 3 mm being standard.

The knee is rotated in approximately 5° of external rotation to allow imaging of the ACL in a sagittal plane.

The knee has a complex structure with components aligned in many planes, and so multiplanar imaging is required.

Pathology in the knee is both varied and complex, with multiple processes occurring at the same time in different components of the joint. Thus, both T1- and T2-weighted imaging are required in multiple planes.

Key sequences (Figure 3.1)

- Fast spin echo (FSE) proton density (PD)-weighted sagittal and coronal
- Short-tau inversion recovery (STIR)/T2-weighted axial, sagittal and coronal

In general, there is no routine role for Gd enhancement in knee MRI.

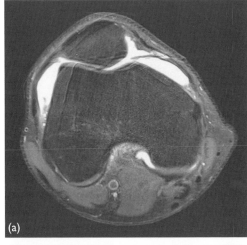

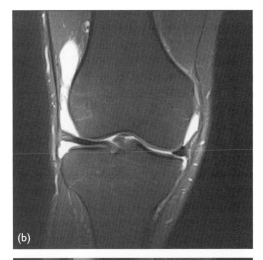

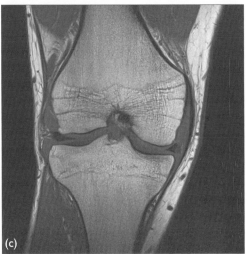

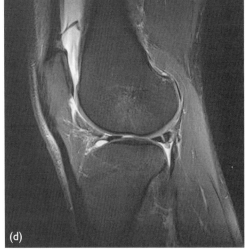

Figure 3.1 Normal knee sequences: (a) fat-saturated (FS) proton density (PD)-weighted axial; (b) FS PD-weighted coronal; (c) T1-weighted coronal; (d) FS PD-weighted sagittal.

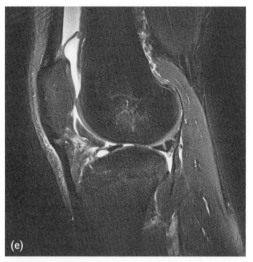

Figure 3.1 *continued* (e) T2*-weighted gradient echo (GRE) sagittal.

ANATOMY (FIGURE 3.2)

The knee is a complex synovial joint that provides flexibility during motion and stability when standing.

Articulation in the knee takes place between the femoral condyles and the tibial plateau. The menisci deepen the flat tibial plateau and improve the congruency of the joint surfaces. The cruciate ligaments help to stabilize the knee during dynamic motion. The collateral ligaments provide lateral stability and the patella and associated tendons provide smoothness of motion during flexion and extension.

Table 3.1 lists the structures of the knee and their optimal viewing planes.

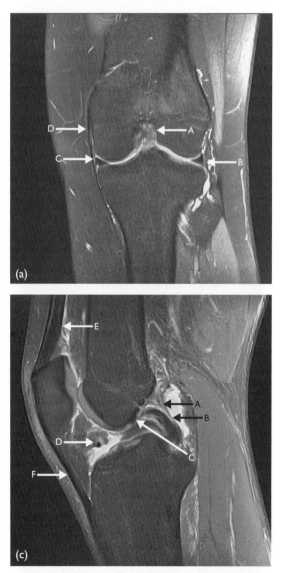

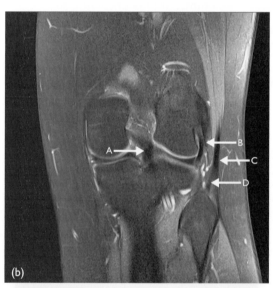

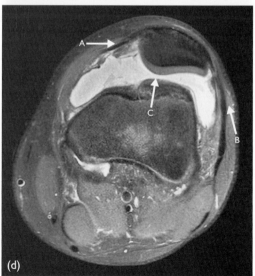

Figure 3.2 Anatomy of the knee: coronal, sagittal and axial sections. (a) Coronal: A, anterior cruciate ligament (ACL); B, lateral meniscus; C, medial meniscus; D, medial collateral ligament (MCL). (b) Coronal: A, posterior cruciate ligament (PCL); B, popliteus tendon; C, biceps femoris tendon; D, lateral collateral ligament (LCL). (c) Sagittal: A, meniscofemoral ligament; B, PCL; C, ACL; D, meniscomeniscal ligament; E, quadriceps tendon; F, patellar tendon. (d) Axial: A, medial retinaculum; B, quadriceps tendon; C, patellar articular surface.

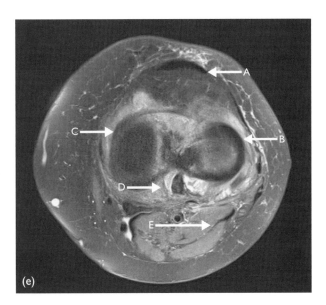

Figure 3.2 (e) Axial: A, patellar tendon; B, lateral meniscus; C, medial meniscus; D, PCL; E, popliteus.

Table 3.1 Structures in the knee and optimal viewing planes

Structure	Optimal planes	Additional planes
Patella and patellofemoral joint	Axial	Sagittal
Menisci	Sagittal	Coronal
Anterior and posterior cruciate ligaments (ACL and PCL)	Sagittal	Coronal and axial
Medial and lateral collateral ligaments (MCL and LCL)	Axial and coronal	Sagittal rarely
Femoral condyle cartilage	Axial and coronal	Sagittal
Posterolateral corner structures	Axial	Coronal

Menisci

The medial and lateral menisci are fibro-cartilaginous structures attached to the tibial plateau. The lateral meniscus is nearly circular, while the medial meniscus is semi-circular and more elongated anteroposteriorly. The roots of the ligaments attach at the tibial spine region. The menisci are concave superiorly, conforming to the shapes of the respective femoral condyles.

Cruciate ligaments

The anterior cruciate ligament (ACL) is a thick tissue responsible for preventing anterior glide of the tibia. It originates from the medial surface of the lateral femoral condyle and attaches to the anteromedial portion of the intercondyloid notch onto the tibial spine. The ACL is extra-articular and has a layer of synovium wrapping around it.

The posterior cruciate ligament (PCL) prevents posterior glide of the tibia on the femur. It arises from the lateral surface of the medial femoral condyle and inserts posteriorly onto the posterolateral part of the intercondyloid notch.

Collateral ligaments

The collateral ligaments prevent lateral sliding and tilt of the knee joint.

The medial collateral ligament (MCL) is a broad, flat ligament that arises from the medial femoral condyle just inferior to the adductor tubercle and attaches to the medial surface of the medial tibial plateau. It has a superficial part that runs vertically in a coronal plane and deep fibres that attach to the capsule and the medial meniscus. Hence, the MCL follows closely the surface of the knee. Crossing over the ligament is the pes anserinus, the joined tendon of the sartorius, gracilis and semitendinosus muscles. Between the pes and the medial collateral ligament is the anserine bursa.

The lateral collateral ligament (LCL) arises from the lateral condyle of the femur and runs posterior to anterior in an oblique fashion. It is never seen on a single slice in coronal images of the knee. The LCL combines with the tendon of the biceps femoris distally to form the conjoint tendon of the knee, which attaches to the fibular head. The LCL is one of the ligaments making up the posterolateral corner structures. It is seen to run deep to the iliotibial band, a thick fascia running from the iliac crest and inserting onto the lateral tibial condyle.

Other ligaments

The transverse meniscal ligament runs in a horizontal plane between the anterior parts of the menisci.

The meniscofemoral ligament runs from the posterior part of the lateral meniscus in an oblique plane to attach to the posterior part of the medial femoral condyle. Its relationship with the PCL can vary. If it runs anterior to the PCL, it is named the ligament of Humphrey. More commonly, it runs posterior to the PCL and is then named the ligament of Wrisberg.

Patella and extensor mechanism

The patella is a triangular bone that articulates with the anterior portion of the femoral condyles.

The patella has two facets articulating with the femoral condyles: the medial facet and a smaller and steeply angulated lateral facet. The lateral facet conforms to the articular surface of the lateral femoral condyle. The angle made by the respective surfaces is responsible for preventing subluxation of the patella laterally during knee flexion.

The patella is held in position by both bony and ligamentous structures. The medial retinaculum is a thick fascia that is attached to the distal fibres of the vastus medialis and attaches to the medial rim of the patella. This prevents lateral displacement of the patella.

The quadriceps tendon is a flat thick tendon that originates from the quadriceps muscles and inserts onto the patella.

The patella tendon arises from the inferior pole of the patella and inserts onto the tibial tubercle. The prepatellar bursa is positioned superficial to the patellar tendon.

There is a large fat pad in the anterior part of the knee joint that lies deep to the patellar tendon and is known as the patellar fat pad or Hoffa's fat pad.

PATELLAR DISLOCATION

Patellar dislocation is a common condition, but clinically often unrecognized because the dislocated patella promptly reverts to its original position.

Key sequences

- PD-weighted axial
- FS T2-weighted axial

Imaging findings

These include:

- lateral femoral condyle bruise due to impaction of the displacing medial facet of the patella – the contusion is more lateral and superior to the bone contusions seen in an ACL tear
- medial patellar facet fracture or bruise

- medial retinaculum injury, ranging from a sprain (thickening and high T2 signal within these fibres) to a tear with extension into the fibres of the vastus medialis
- osteochondral injury of the medial patellar facet, most often at the inferior part of the medial facet
- patella tilted laterally or subluxed
- moderate suprapatellar effusion with haemarthrosis

Hints and tips

Axial PD- and T2-weighted images provide the most information, since the patellar facets are best seen on axial images and the fibres of the medial retinaculum run in an oblique plane.

Occasionally, osteochondral fragments may be seen on axial and sagittal images or may be seen as loose bodies.

Medial collateral and medial meniscal injuries may be associated with lateral patellar dislocation, since the mechanism of injury may be a blow to the outside of the knee.

Further reading

Ellas DA, White LM, Fithlan DC. Acute lateral patellar dislocation at MR imaging: injury patterns of medial patellar soft tissue restraints and osteochondral injuries of the inferomedial patella. *Radiology* 2002; **225**: 736–43.

Kisch MD, Fitzgerald SW, Friedman H, Rogers LF. Transient lateral patellar dislocation: diagnosis with MR imaging. AJR *Am J Roentgenol* 1993; **161**: 109–13.

Sanders TG, Medynski MA, Feller JF et al. Bone contusion patterns of the knee at MR imaging: footprint for mechanism of injury. *Radiographics* 2000; **20**: S135–51.

Case 6: Patellar dislocation

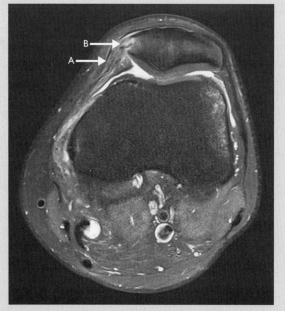

Case 6.1 T2-weighted axial image showing medial retinacular detachment (A) with osteochondral fragment (B).

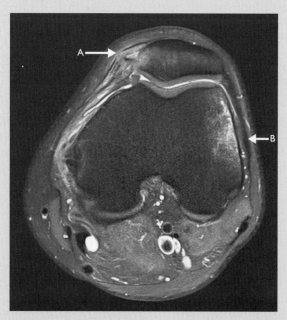

Case 6.2 Oedema pattern of patellar dislocation: A, medial pole of patella; B, lateral condyle of femur.

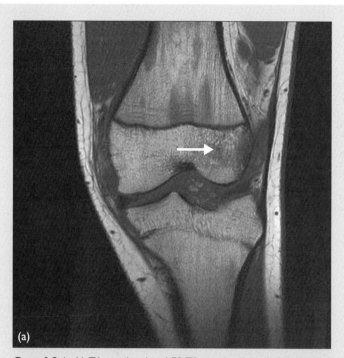
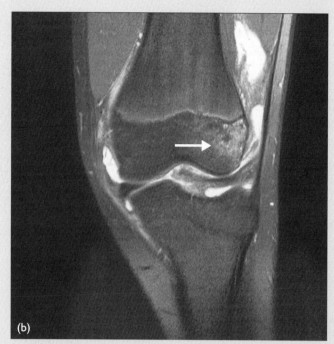

Case 6.3 (a, b) T1-weighted and FS T2-weighted images showing oedema in the lateral femoral condyle.

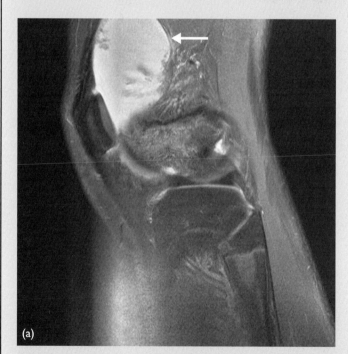
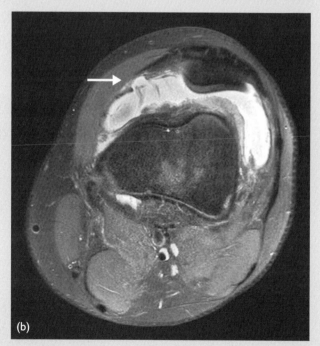

Case 6.4 (a) Large effusion with fluid–fluid level. (b) Vastus medialis and medial retinaculum rupture.

ANTERIOR CRUCIATE LIGAMENT (ACL) TEARS

The ACL is the most commonly disrupted ligament in the knee. This injury is often seen in soccer, rugby, American football and tennis players and skiers. It is eight times more common in females.

Key sequences

- Imaging should be performed in the sagittal, coronal and axial planes. The common mechanisms of injury include forward translation of the tibia with external rotation of the femur and valgus stress.

- Fluid-sensitive sequences, including T2- and PD-weighted sequences, are the most sensitive for evaluation of injury to the ACL and surrounding soft tissues.
- T1-weighted and gradient echo sequences are useful to assess additional injuries to the bones and cartilage.

Imaging findings

Tears are full-thickness, and are located more commonly in the mid to proximal aspect of the ligament.

Torn fibre displays increased T2 signal with an abnormal contour and discontinuity and an abnormal slope.

Hints and tips

ACL injuries should be described as proximal, mid-substance, distal, or involving the femoral or tibial attachment.

ACL injuries are typically associated with other injuries, especially posterolateral corner injury, lateral femoral condylar injury, collateral ligament injuries and meniscal tears. Segond fractures are also associated with ACL tears (avulsion of the lateral tibial cortex at the attachment of the lateral capsular ligament).

The typical contusion pattern with traumatic ACL tears is of bone oedema in the lateral femoral condyle and the posterolateral corner of the tibia.

In children, the equivalent injury is a tibial spine avulsion fracture involving the root of the ACL. The avulsed fragment may also contain the roots of the menisci, and this should be mentioned in the report.

Further reading

Moore SL. Imaging the anterior cruciate ligament. *Orthop Clin North Am* 2002; **33**: 663–74.

Remer EM, Fitzgerald SW, Friedman H et al. Anterior cruciate ligament injury: MR imaging diagnosis and patterns of injury. *Radiographics* 1992; **12**: 901–15.

Roberts CC, Towers JD, Spangehl MJ et al. Advanced MR imaging of the cruciate ligaments. *Radiol Clin North Am* 2007; **45**: 1003–16.

Robertson PL, Schweitzer ME, Bartolozzi AR et al. Anterior cruciate ligament tears: evaluation of multiple signs with MR imaging. *Radiology* 1994; **193**: 829–34.

Case 7: Anterior cruciate ligament tear

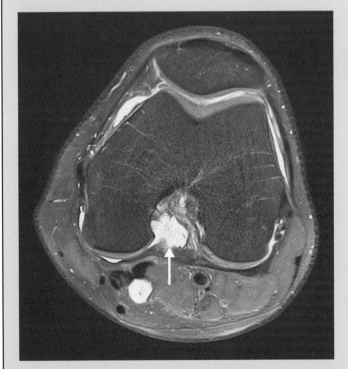

Case 7.1 FS PD-weighted axial image showing an empty intercondylar notch.

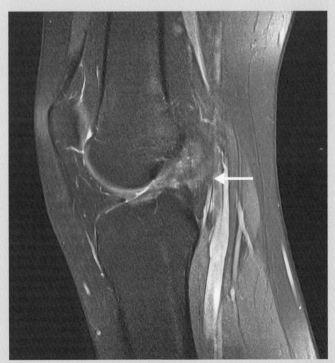

Case 7.2 FS PD-weighted sagittal image showing complete rupture of the ACL.

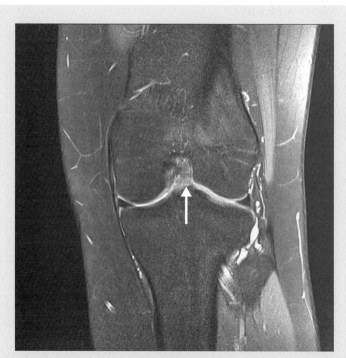

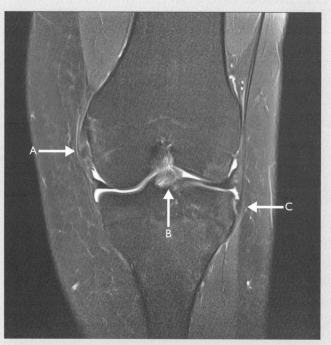

Case 7.3 FS PD-weighted coronal image showing high signal in the intercondylar notch with poorly defined ACL fibres.

Case 7.4 FS PD-weighted coronal image showing an MCL tear (A), an ACL tear (B) and a Segond fracture (C).

Case 8: Tibial spine avulsion in a child

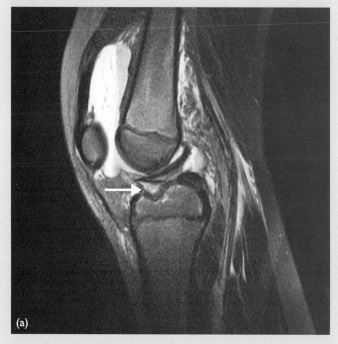

(a)

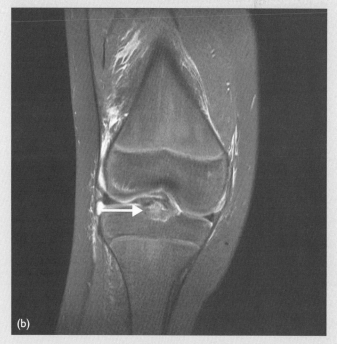

(b)

Case 8.1 (a, b) FS PD-weighted FSE sagittal and coronal images showing a spinous process avulsion fracture in a child.

POSTERIOR CRUCIATE LIGAMENT (PCL) TEARS

The PCL most commonly tears at its mid portion, secondary to direct trauma with displacement of the knee posteriorly (dashboard-type injury).

Key sequences

- PCL tears are best evaluated in the sagittal plane using PD-weighted and STIR sequences.

Imaging findings

A normal PCL appears as decreased signal on all pulse sequences.

There may be associated avulsion fractures of the posterior tibia.

Torn sites appear as high signal on fluid-sensitive sequences.

There is a loss of 'hockey-stick' appearance on sagittal cuts.

Hints and tips

Consider PCL injury when there is anterior tibial trabecular oedema.

A peel-off PCL tear refers to a full-thickness tear along the femoral attachment without an avulsion fracture.

Magic angle artefact can cause diagnostic difficulties.

A ruptured PCL rarely maintains a normal contour.

The 'double-PCL' sign is caused by a displaced bucket handle tear of the medial meniscus.

MCL tears and medial meniscal injuries are common.

Anterior tibial fractures or oedema are seen in association with anterolateral femoral condyle injuries.

Further reading

Sonin AH, Fitzgerald SW, Hoff Fl et al. Posterior cruciate ligament: normal, abnormal and associated injury patterns. *Radiographics* 1995; **15**: 551–61.

Case 9: Posterior cruciate ligament tear

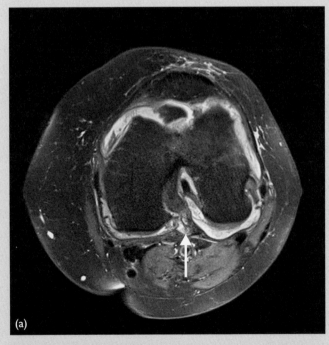 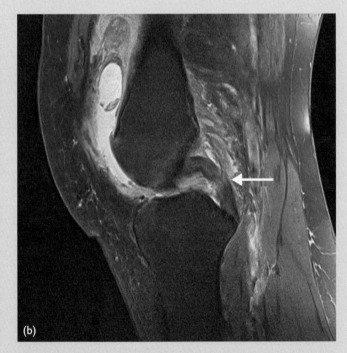

Case 9.1 (a, b) FS T2-weighted axial and sagittal images showing a PCL tear.

MENISCAL TEARS

The menisci make the knee congruous. They are the main cushions of the knee and transfer forces within it. The outer third of the meniscus is vascular while the inner two-thirds is avascular. The medial meniscus is attached to the MCL and is relatively fixed at the posterior horn, resulting in more injury to the medial meniscus as a whole, with the posterior horn being most commonly affected. The lateral meniscus is attached to the joint capsule less intimately than the medial meniscus. This increased mobility results in less injury to the lateral meniscus. The anterior and posterior horns of the lateral meniscus are equal in size. Parameniscal cysts are more common with lateral meniscus tears. In the lateral meniscus, additional meniscofemoral ligaments can variably be found, extending from the posterior horn of the lateral meniscus to the medial femoral condyle. If, on sagittal images, the ligament is anterior to the PCL then it is termed the ligament of Humphrey; if it is posterior to the PCL, it is termed the ligament of Wrisberg.

Key sequences

- PD- or T1-weighted coronal and sagittal images are the most accurate way of evaluating the menisci.
- Fluid-sensitive sequences are sensitive for tears.

Imaging findings

The normal meniscus is devoid of signal (black) on all sequences and looks like a bow tie on sagittal images, measuring approximately 7–8 mm.

A tear is diagnosed when there is increased signal within the meniscus that extends to the articular surface. If there is increased signal within the meniscus that almost, but not quite, extends to the articular surface, this is intrasubstance degeneration.

There should be at least three 'bow ties' when looking at the body of the meniscus on 3 mm sagittal sections of a knee image. The presence of less than three 'bow ties' points to tears of the meniscus.

The medial meniscus is most commonly torn, with 60% of tears occurring in the posterior horn of the meniscus itself. The body and the anterior horn are less affected, and tears do not occur without an extension to the posterior horn.

Lateral meniscus tears are seen in up to 25% of acutely injured knees. The posterior horn is affected in up to 86% of tears.

The classification of meniscal tears is shown in Box 3.1.

Box 3.1 Classification of meniscal tears

- Linear tears
  - Vertical
  - Horizontal
  - Radial
- Displaced fragment tears
  - Bucket handle tears
  - Flap tears
- Complex tears

Bucket handle tears of the medial meniscus give rise to distinct appearances:

- There is a small meniscus with less than three bow ties on sagittal slices.
- The fragment may be within the intercondylar notch and seen as increased soft tissue in this area.
- The 'double–PCL' sign with two parallel PCLs is seen on sagittal scans.
- The 'absent meniscus' sign is seen when the whole of the meniscus is flipped into the intercondylar notch.
- The 'flipped meniscus' or 'fast forward' sign is seen when the fragment becomes juxtaposed with the anterior third of the meniscus.

Hints and tips

The meniscofemoral and transverse ligaments may give rise to false positives on sagittal scans.

The popliteus tendon separates the lateral meniscus from the joint capsule.

Meniscal injuries are often associated with tears of other soft tissue within the knee joint. There are well-defined combinations of injury, including the following:

- Acute meniscal tears with acute ACL injury are usually bucket-handle-type tears. It is important to be aware of associated capsular separation. This is seen as a high-signal cleft between the meniscus and the capsule, with associated collateral ligament injury or avulsion of the attachment (Segond fracture or reverse Segond fracture).
- Chronic ACL injury is usually associated with medial meniscus injury.
- ACL and MCL tears occur most often with a lateral meniscus tear. O'Donoghue's triad – a combination of ACL, MCL and medial meniscus tears – is rare.
- In children, meniscal tears are associated with ACL disruption or there may be a lateral discoid meniscus, a congenital anomaly.

Further reading

Aiello MR. *Knee, Meniscal Tears (MRI)*. eMedicine article. Available at: http://emedicine.medscape.com/article/399552-overview.

Helms CA, Major NM, Anderson MW et al. 2001. *Musculoskeletal MRI*, 2nd edn. Philadelphia: WB Saunders, 2009.

Mesgarzadeh M, Leder D, Russoniello A et al. MR imaging of the knee: expanded classification and pitfalls to interpretation of meniscal tears. *Radiographics* 1993; **13**: 489–500.

Ostlere S. Imaging of the knee. *Imaging* 2003; **15**: 217–41.

Case 10: Meniscal tears

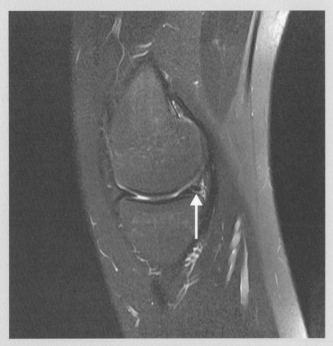

Case 10.1 T2*-weighted sagittal image showing the meniscofemoral ligament. In this case, this ligament runs anterior to the PCL, making it the ligament of Humphrey.

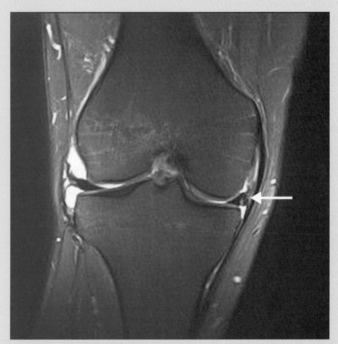

Case 10.2 FS PD-weighted coronal image showing a tear in the body of the lateral meniscus.

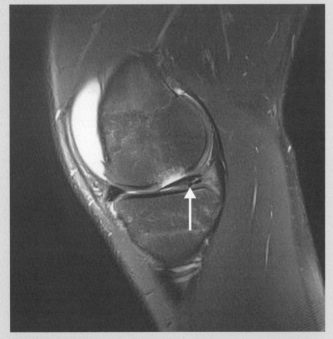

Case 10.3 FS PD-weighted sagittal image showing a tear in the posterior horn of the medial meniscus.

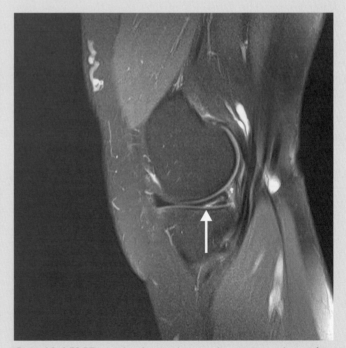

Case 10.4 FS PD-weighted sagittal image showing an under-surface tear.

Case 11: Flipped fragment

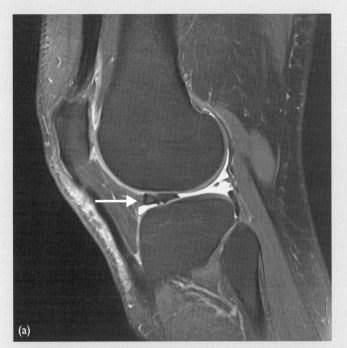
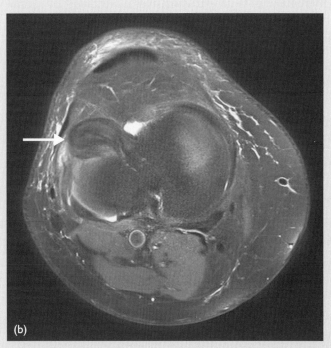

Case 11.1 (a, b) Anterior flipped lateral meniscal fragment. Note the 'fast forward' sign, with the two triangular meniscal fragments juxtaposed in the anterior part of the knee.

Case 12: Bucket handle tear of the medial meniscus

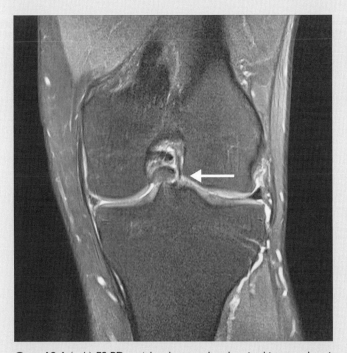
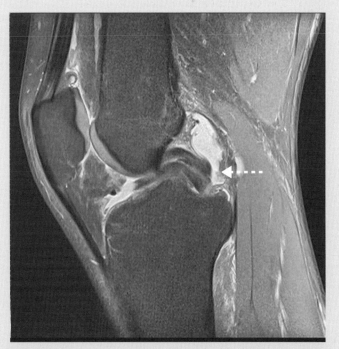

Case 12.1 (a, b) FS PD-weighted coronal and sagittal images showing a bucket handle tear of the medial meniscus. In (a), note the extra soft tissue in the intercondylar notch (arrow) representing the medially displaced fragment of the medial meniscus. The sagittal image (b) shows the 'double–PCL' sign (dotted arrow).

MENISCAL CYSTS

A meniscal cyst is an extrusion from a meniscus. By definition, the underlying meniscus is degenerate. The synovial fluid initially accumulates within the degenerate meniscus. Once the meniscus is torn, the fluid extrudes from the meniscus into the surrounding soft tissues. Intrameniscal cysts are far less commonly seen than parameniscal cysts.

Key sequences

- Fluid-sensitive sequences in axial, sagittal and coronal planes.

Imaging findings

Between 90% and 98% of meniscal cysts are in direct contact with an adjacent meniscal tear.

Parameniscal cysts are septate, complex, fluid-filled cysts associated with a horizontal cleavage tear or a complex meniscal tear.

Medial cysts arise from the posterior third of the medial meniscus, corresponding to the most common site of medial meniscus tears. Owing to the intimate relationship with the medial collateral ligament, they tend to be found posteromedially and are relatively further away from the meniscus. Medial cysts are also asymptomatic and larger.

Lateral cysts arise from the anterior and mid portions of the lateral meniscus. As the lateral capsule is not adherent to the lateral meniscus, lateral cysts tend to be deeper and smaller and produce symptoms.

All meniscal cysts are associated with a meniscal tear.

High T2 signal may not always be present if the fluid has become resorbed.

Rarely, meniscal cysts may become apparent on T1-weighted sequences if they have a high protein content that results in high T1 signal.

Hints and tips

Most cysts can be visualized on T2-weighted and PD-weighted FS FSE sequences.

Always look for the meniscal tear associated with a cyst. However, meniscal cysts occasionally may not be associated with a classical meniscal tear that extends to the articular surface. Hence, without the presence of a tear, the meniscal cyst can be missed at arthroscopy.

Look for direct extension between the cyst and the meniscus

The differential diagnosis includes bursae around the medial meniscus (e.g. a pes anserine bursa) or lateral meniscus (e.g. a MCL bursa) and acpopliteus bursa.

Further reading

McCarthy CL, McNally EG. The MRI appearance of cystic lesions around the knee. *Skeletal Radiol* 2004; **33**: 187–209

Case 13: Parameniscal cyst

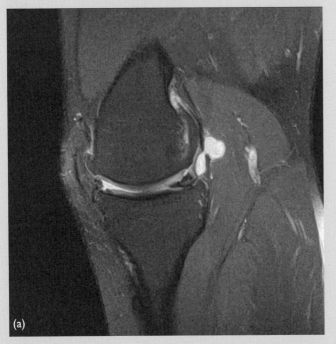 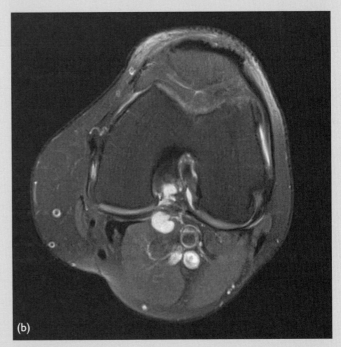

Case 13.1 (a, b) FS PD-weighted sagittal and axial images showing a posteromedial meniscal cyst.

COLLATERAL LIGAMENT INJURIES

The knee is stabilized by the LCL and MCL when locked. Injuries to these ligaments are often seen in association with other soft tissue and cartilage injuries owing to their intimate relationship with these structures and the biomechanics of the injury.

The MCL arises from the medial femoral epicondyle and inserts into the medial metaphysis of the tibia. It has a superficial layer and a deep layer that attaches to the medial meniscus and capsule. The MCL is commonly injured when there is a valgus strain applied to the knee. The MCL can also be injured when there has been injury to other soft tissues, such as the medial meniscus or the ACL or both (O'Donoghue's triad).

The LCL arises from the lateral femoral epicondyle and inserts conjointly with the biceps femoris tendon onto the fibular head. The LCL is completely extracapsular. Injuries to the LCL occur as a result of varus strain applied to the knee. It is more commonly injured together with the structures in the posterolateral complex, such as the popliteus and the biceps femoris tendon.

Collateral ligament injuries are graded as follows:
• grade 1: microscopic tears of the ligament
• grade 2: partial tears of the ligament
• grade 3: complete tears of the ligament

Key sequences

• PD-weighted FS coronal and axial
• T1-weighted FSE coronal

Imaging findings

In grade 1 injuries, the MCL is seen to be intact and closely applied to the medial femoral condyle. On fluid-sensitive sequences, there is a high T2 signal surrounding the MCL.

In grade 2 tears, the fibres are seen to be separate from the femoral condyle. The deep portion is more often affected. There is high T2 signal in the region of the MCL. Grade 2 MCL tears are associated with ACL and medial meniscus pathology as previously noted.

Grade 3 tears show complete discontinuity of the fibres, with haemorrhage and oedema in the adjacent soft tissues.

Differentiating between grade 2 and grade 3 tears can be difficult.

Chronicity of the injury is indicated by a thickened MCL with a relative lack of oedema.

LCL injuries appear different from MCL tears, since the LCL is extracapsular. Isolated LCL tears are uncommon, most LCL tears being seen to be associated with posterolateral corner injuries.

The LCL is rarely seen completely on a single coronal slice. Hence, tears of the LCL are identified when there is a serpiginous LCL or LCL that does not appear taut and is seen on a single slice. Because of its extracapsular nature, there is little oedema associated with it.

Hints and tips

Coronal fluid-sensitive sequences show MCL tears well.

Always look for associated injuries to the MCL and ACL. Isolated LCL injuries are rare. Always assess the posterolateral corner structures such as the biceps femoris tendon and the popliteus.

Further reading

Ostlere S. Imaging of the knee. *Imaging* 2003; **15**: 217–41.

Recondo JA, Salvador E, Villanua JA. Lateral stabilizing structures of the knee: functional anatomy and injuries assessed with MR imaging. *Radiographics* 2000; **20**: S91–102.

Stoller DW, Cannon WD, Anderson LJ. The knee. In: *Magnetic Resonance Imaging in Orthopaedics and Sports Medicine,* 2nd edn. Philadelphia: Lippincott Williams & Wilkins, 2006.

Case 14: Collateral ligament injury

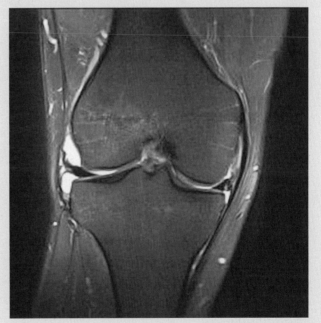

Case 14.1 Full-thickness (grade 3) tears of the MCL. Note the lateral meniscal tear.

CHONDROMALACIA PATELLAE

This is a condition characterized by softening, fraying and ulceration of the patellar articular cartilage. There are two forms of chondromalacia patellae: traumatic and non-traumatic.

The condition has been graded on the basis of arthroscopic findings into four groups. MRI is able to visualize the condition in moderate and severe forms.

Key sequences

- PD-weighted FS coronal and axial
- T2*-weighted GRE

Imaging findings

Normal articular cartilage has uniformly homogeneous high signal on T2*-weighted and FS PD-weighted imaging. The underlying bone is of uniform intensity, with no sclerosis. Signs of chondromalacia include:

- abnormal signal of cartilage
- irregularity of the patellar articular cartilage
- fissuring of the cartilage
- ulceration of the cartilage
- underlying bone marrow oedema
- sclerosis of the bone
- osteochondral fragments

Hints and tips

Always start with the axial PD-weighted FS images of the patella.

T2*-weighted images may show bone marrow oedema in the trochlear region better.

Grading of chondromalacia patella is by arthroscopy.

Further reading

Conway WF, Hayes CW, Loughran T et al. Cross-sectional imaging of the patellofemoral joint and surrounding structures. *Radiographics* 1991; **11**: 195–217.

McCauley TR, Kier R, Lynch KJ, Joki P. Chondromalacia patellae: diagnosis with MRI. *AJR Am J Roentgenol* 1992; **158**: 101–5.

Case 15: Chondromalacia patellae

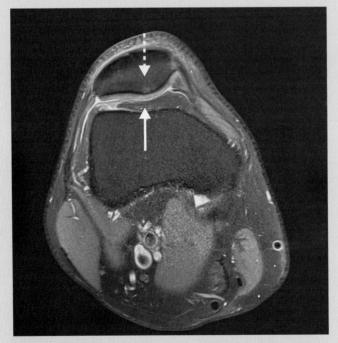 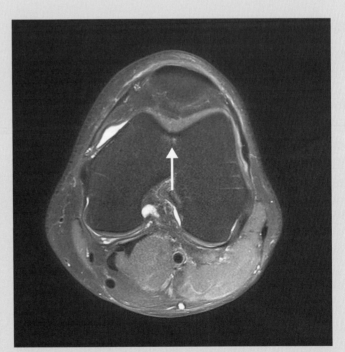

Case 15.1 FS PD-weighted FSE axial image showing medial facet articular cartilage irregularity (full arrow) and bone oedema (dotted arrow).

Case 15.2 FS PD-weighted FSE axial image showing the corresponding subchondral oedema in the trochlear groove.

DISCOID LATERAL MENISCUS

This is the most common cause of meniscal injury in children. Discoid lateral meniscus is more common in the Oriental population, with an incidence of 0.4–16.6%. Patients usually present with joint line tenderness, 'snapping' or locking of the knee. In comparison, discoid medial menisci are much less frequent. Discoid menisci have an increased risk of tear and degeneration.

Key sequences

- PD-weighted
- STIR

Imaging findings

Meniscal tissue identified on at least three continuous sagittal 5 mm thick slices, or a meniscal body on coronal images greater than 15 mm is diagnostic. Normal meniscal tissue is hypointense.

'Tears' are seen as hyperintense signal on T1-weighted, PD-weighted and GRE T2*-weighted images.

Hints and tips

There are three types of discoid meniscus: complete, incomplete and the Wrisberg variant. The complete and incomplete types have a firm, normal posterior tibial attachment and, when symptomatic, are treated with partial meniscectomy. The Wrisberg variant does not have a posterior capsular attachment.

Further reading

Fox MG. MR imaging of the meniscus: review, current trends, and clinical implications. *Radiol Clin North Am* 2007; **45**: 1033–53.

Samoto N, Kozuma M, Tokuhisa T et al. Diagnosis of discoid lateral meniscus of the knee on MR imaging. *Magn Reson Imaging* 2002; **20**: 59–64.

Silverman JM, Mink JH, Deutsch AL. Discoid menisci of the knee: MR imaging appearance. *Radiology* 1989; **173**: 351–4.

Case 16: Discoid meniscus

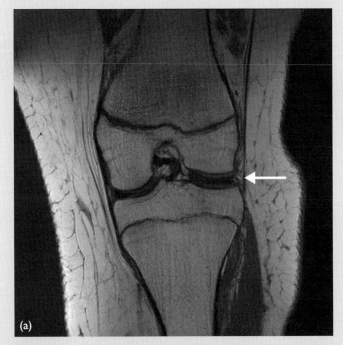 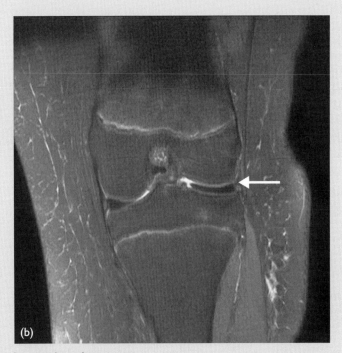

Case 16.1 (a, b) T1-weighted and FS PD-weighted FSE coronal images showing discoid meniscus.

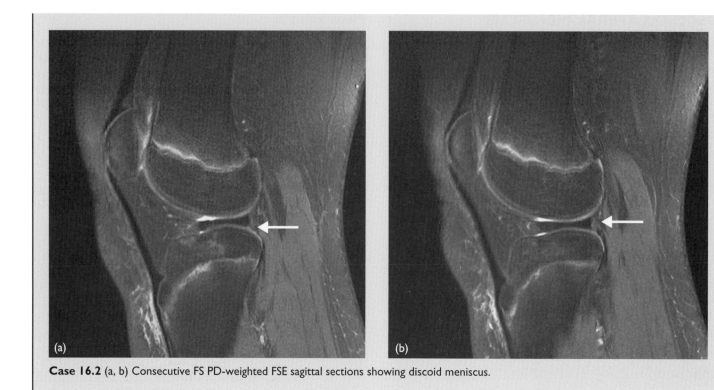

Case 16.2 (a, b) Consecutive FS PD-weighted FSE sagittal sections showing discoid meniscus.

POSTEROLATERAL COMPLEX INJURY

This is a complex set of structures that provide both static and dynamic stability. It consists of the popliteus tendon, the PCL, the LCL and the arcuate complex, which is made up of fascia and ligaments. The only ligament of the arcuate complex that is consistently visualized on MRI is the popliteofibular ligament, also called the fibular attachment of the popliteus, which extends from the lateral aspect of the popliteus and inserts into the styloid process of the fibula. Injuries occur owing to external rotation of the flexed knee or hyperextension injury to the lateral structures of the knee, and result in rotational instability.

Key sequences

- PD-weighted FS and STIR/T2-weighted FS

Imaging findings

Bone bruising is seen anteromedially on the medial femoral condyle. It is seen best on STIR sequences.

There may be vulsion, tear or rupture of the LCL, popliteus myotendinous junction, popliteofibular ligament or PCL.

These injuries can be graded depending on the degree of injury:
- grade 1: minimal injury
- grade 2: partial tears
- grade 3: complete tears

Grade 3 tears need emergent surgical management.

Posterolateral complex injury is often associated with ACL injuries.

Fractures associated with this type of injury include:
- Segond fractures
- avulsion fracture of the proximal fibula: the 'arcuate fracture'
- fracture of the insertion of the ilio-tibial band: 'Gerdy's tubercle'.

Hints and tips

Injuries of the posterolateral corner are often missed. Any fluid signal in or around tendons should alert to its possibility.

ACL or PCL tears are often associated with posterolateral corner injuries.

Fluid seen posterior to the popliteus tendon is an indicator of this injury

Bone oedema in the proximal fibula or the anterior part of the medial femoral condyle is another sign of this type of injury

Further reading

Beall DP, Googe JD, Moss JT et al. Magnetic resonance imaging of the collateral ligaments and the anatomic quadrants of the knee. *Magn Reson Imaging Clin N Am* 2007; **15**: 53–72.

Harish S, O'Donnell P, Connell D, Saifuddin A. Imaging of the posterolateral corner of the knee. Clin Rad 2006; **61**: 457–66.
Ostlere S. Imaging of the knee. *Imaging* 2003; **15**: 217–41.

Recondo JA, Salvador E, Villanua JA. Lateral stabilizing structures of the knee: functional anatomy and injuries assessed with MR imaging. *Radiographics* 2000; **20**: S91–102.

Case 17: Posterolateral corner injury

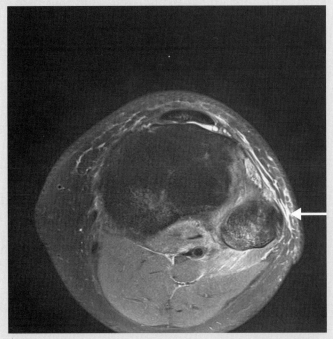

Case 17.1 FS PD-weighted FSE image showing extensive oedema in the posterolateral corner and irregularity of the fibres of the LCL.

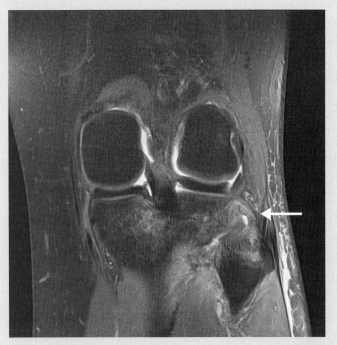

Case 17.2 FS PD-weighted FSE coronal image showing oedema within the fibres of the tibiofibular ligament, insertion of the biceps femoris and the head of the fibula.

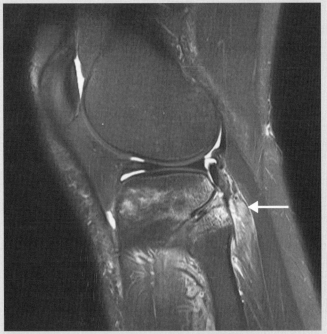

Case 17.3 FS PD-weighted FSE sagittal image showing oedema within the posterolateral corner structures and the head of the fibula.

OSTEOCHONDRAL DEFECT (OCD)

This term is used to describe osteochondral defects of any form. OCD is most commonly seen in the knee, although the condition is known to occur in all major synovial joints, including the ankle, elbow, shoulder and hip joints. In the knee, OCD classically involves the non-weight-bearing part of the lateral aspect of the medial femoral condyle in 75% of cases. Other areas include the weight-bearing areas of the knee, such as the medial and lateral femoral condyles and the patella.

Key sequences

- FS T2*-weighted GRE or STIR coronal and sagittal
- FS PD-weighted FSE

Imaging findings

There is a semi-oval shaped lesion with heterogeneous low T2 signal surrounded by a high-T2-signal rim at the site of demarcation.

Subchondral oedema may be seen.

Fluid within the space between the fragment and underlying bone is a sign of instability of the fragment.

Continuity of cartilage cover over the fragment indicates stability of the lesion. Irregularity of the cartilage cover and discontinuity at the margins indicate an unstable fragment.

The **Anderson MRI classification** of osteochondral lesions is as follows:

- Stage I: bone marrow oedema (subchondral trabecular compression; radiographic results are negative with positive bone-scan findings)
- Stage IIa: subchondral cyst
- Stage IIb: incomplete separation of the osteochondral fragment
- Stage III: fluid around an undetached, undisplaced osteochondral fragment
- Stage IV: displaced osteochondral fragment

Hints and tips

Coronal images localize the lesion.

High signal at the interface between the osteochondral fragment and the underlying bone is a good indicator of instability of the fragment.

Further reading

Bohndorf K. Osteochondritis dessicans: a review and MRI classification. *Eur Radiol* 1998; **8**: 103–12.

De Smet AA, Fisher DR, Graf BK et al. Osteochondritis dessicans of the knee: value of MR imaging in determining lesion stability and the presence of articular cartilage defects. *AJR Am J Roentgenol* 1990; **155**: 549–53.

Anderson IF, Crichton KJ, Grattan-Smith T, Cooper RA, Brazier D. Osteochondral fractures of the dome of the talus. *J Bone Joint Surg [Am]* 1989; **71-A**: 1143–52.

Case 18: Osteochondral defect

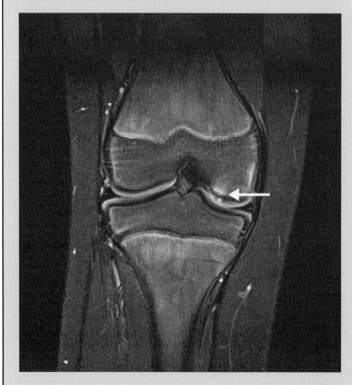

Case 18.1 FS PD-weighted coronal image showing an osteochondral fragment with overlying cartilage irregularity and underlying bone oedema.

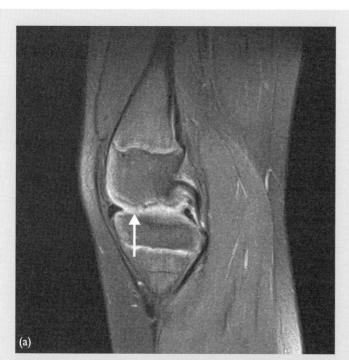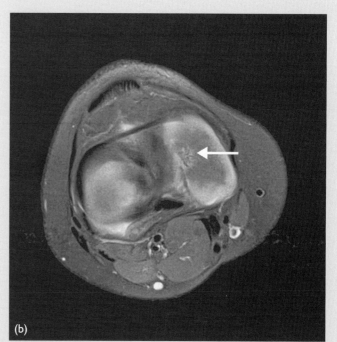

Case 18.2 (a, b) FS PD-weighted sagittal and axial sections showing an osteochondral fragment.

BAKER'S CYST

Baker's cyst is a sign of degenerative disease of the knee. It is the most common mass in the back of the knee. Baker's cyst is caused by distension of the semimembranosus gastrocnemius bursa with fluid, and is characteristically located in the medial portion of the popliteal fossa. The cyst communicates with the knee joint through a narrow opening posteromedially. The fluid from the knee joint is pumped into the cyst, but fibrin in the walls of the opening produces a ball-valve mechanism imposing one-way flow of the fluid. Hence, Baker's cysts generally expand. Baker's cysts have a high incidence of rupture (approximately 10%), resulting in a pseudo-thrombophlebitis syndrome mimicking a deep-vein thrombosis.

Key sequences

- FS PD-weighted FSE and T2*-weighted GRE sagittal and axial

Imaging findings

Cysts of variable size are seen in the posteromedial portion of the popliteal fossa.

There is a thin low-signal wall.

The cyst may contain loose bodies or synovium.

The neck of the cyst is characteristically seen to be between the medial head of the gastrocnemius and the semimembranosus tendon sheath.

Baker's cysts are associated with meniscal tears and degenerative arthropathy.

Hints and tips

Sagittal images reveal the extent of a Baker's cyst.

Axial images are useful to identify the neck of the cyst.

Additional review of the menisci is necessary to look for meniscal tears.

Further reading

Guerra J Jr, Newell JD, Resnick D. Pictorial essay: gastrocnemio-semimembranosus bursal region of the knee. *AJR Am J Roentgenol* 1981; **136**: 593–6.

Fielding JR, Franklin PD, Kustan J. Popliteal cysts: a reassessment using magnetic resonance imaging. *Skeletal Radiol* 1991; **20**: 433–5.

Case 19: Baker's cyst

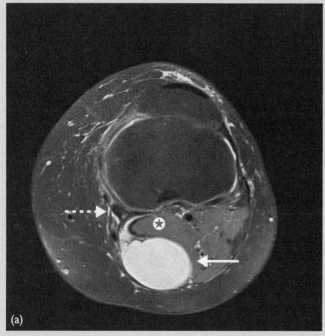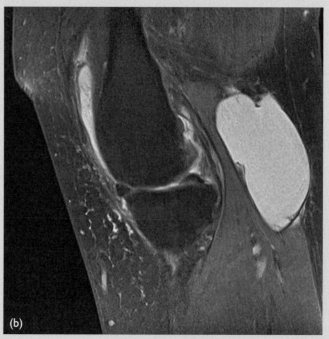

(a)

(b)

Case 19.1 (a, b) T2-weighted axial and sagittal images showing a Baker's cyst (full arrow) arising from the joint between the medial head of the gastrocnemius (star) and the semimembranosus tendon (dotted arrow).

HOFFA'S SYNDROME

Hoffa's fat pad is intracapsular but extrasynovial. Hoffa's syndrome is caused by inflammation of the pad. There is impingement of the fat pad between the femoral condyles and the patella. Recurrent impingement results in chronic anterior knee pain.

Key sequences

- FS PD-weighted FSE axial and sagittal
- T2-weighted sagittal

Imaging findings

High T2 signal and low T1 signal in the infrapatellar fat pad is characteristic.

Bowing of the patellar tendon due to mass effect is often seen.

Joint effusion may be seen.

Recurrent inflammation results in fibrosis and haemosiderin deposition, causing low signal on both T1- and T2-weighted images.

Ossification of the fat pad is a known sequela that may manifest as a low-signal area in the pad. Plain-film correlation may be needed.

Hints and tips

HIV/AIDS is known to be associated with infrapatellar fat pad inflammation.

Intracapsular chondromas is a known entity that is seen to arise in the fat pad. Some believe this to be the end-stage of Hoffa's syndrome.

T2-weighted imaging is the key to diagnosis.

Further reading

Jacobson JA, Lenchik L, Ruhoy MK et al. MR imaging of the infrapatellar fat pad of Hoffa. *Radiographics* 1997; **17**: 675–92.

Pluot E, Singh J, James SLJ et al. Abnormality of the infrapatellar fat pad (Hoffa's fat pad) in a patient with HIV: MR findings with histological correlation. *Eur J Radiol* 2008; **68**: 29–32.

Case 20: Hoffa's fat pad syndrome

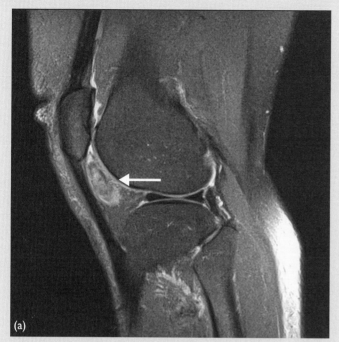 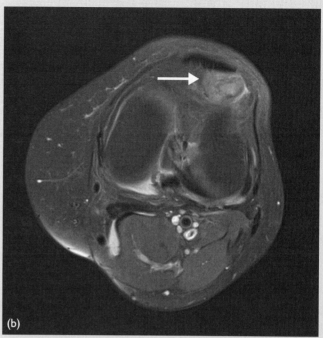

Case 20.1 (a, b) PD-weighted FS axial and sagittal images of the knee showing high signal in Hoffa's fat pad in keeping with Hoffa's syndrome.

4 THE HIP

IMAGING OF THE HIP

MRI of the hip poses many problems, the most important being the ability to assess the joint itself. As with imaging of any joint, the hip is imaged in three planes with a variety of sequences to look at both anatomy and oedema. In addition, hip arthrography is carried out to assess for labral tears.

Key sequences (Figures 4.1 and 4.2)

- T1-weighted fast spin echo (FSE) and STIR coronal imaging to assess the femoral heads and the hip joints
- PD-weighted FSE and fat-saturated (FS) T2-weighted FSE axial
- FS T2-weighted FSE sagittal

The axial and sagittal sequences are used to assess the labrum and the soft tissues around the hip, including the muscles, the bursae and the neuromuscular bundles. Axial images are also useful in visualizing the hernial orifices in the pelvis.

MR arthrography

Arthrography of the hip uses a dilute solution of gadolinium (Gd), usually 2%. The normal approach to injecting the hip joint is either anteriorly, directing the needle to the proximal part of the neck of the femur, or laterally along the femoral neck. The procedure may be carried out under fluoroscopic or ultrasound guidance. Arthrography is predominantly used to assess the labrum.

ANATOMY

The anatomy of the hip is illustrated in Figure 4.3.

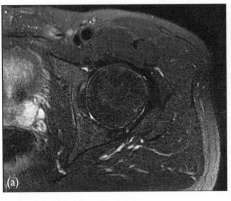

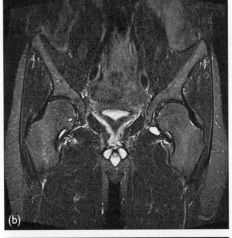

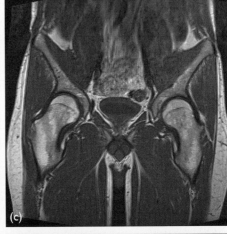

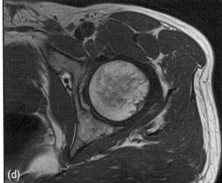

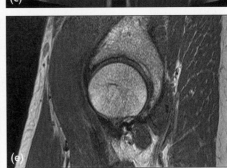

Figure 4.1 Hip sequences: (a) short-tau inversion recovery (STIR) axial; (b) STIR coronal; (c) T1-weighted coronal; (d) T1-weighted axial; (e) T1-weighted sagittal.

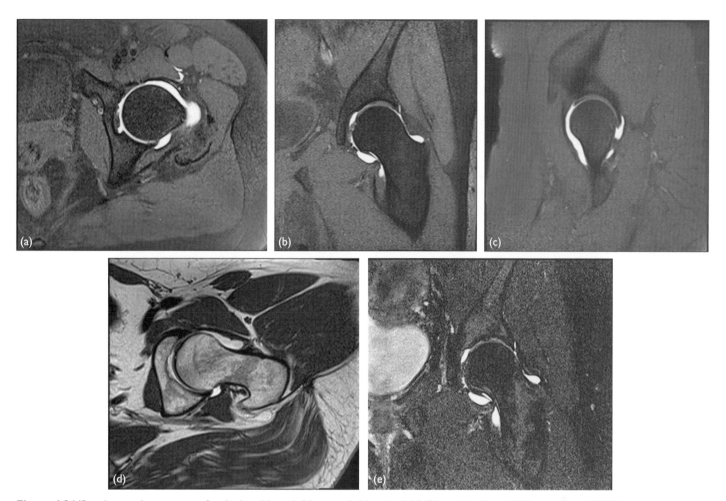

Figure 4.2 MR arthrography sequences for the hip: (a) axial; (b) coronal; (c) sagittal; (d) T1-weighted axial: (e) fat-saturated (FS) T2-weighted coronal.

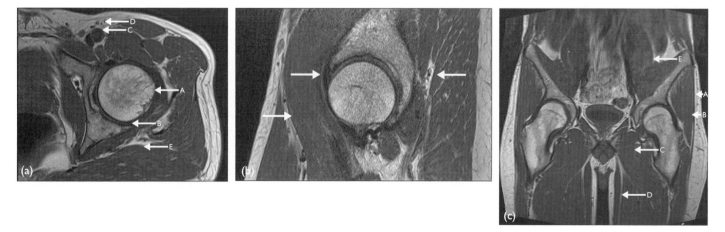

Figure 4.3 Anatomy of the hip: axial, sagittal and coronal sections. (a) T1-weighted axial: A, femoral head; B, labrum; C, femoral vessels; D, inguinal canal; E, gluteal vessels. (b) T1-weighted sagittal: A, anterior labrum; B, psoas; C, gluteal vessels. (c) T1-weighted coronal: A, fascia lata; B, tensor fascia lata; C, adductor origin; D, gracilis; E, iliopsoas.

AVASCULAR NECROSIS (AVN) OF THE HIP

Avascular necrosis of the hip is common. It can be due to a number of causes (Box 4.1), most often prolonged high-dose steroid intake. There is a vascular insult to the blood supply of the femoral head, resulting initially in myeloid cell death in the first 6–12 hours, following which there is osteocyte death at 48 hours. Following this, granulation of the site of avascular necrosis occurs, finally leading to fibrosis.

Box 4.1 Causes of avascular necrosis

- Chronic steroid intake
- Alcohol intake
- Trauma
- Chronic pancreatitis
- Metastasis
- Haemoglobinopathies/haemophilia
- Hypercoagulable states

Key sequences

- T1-weighted FSE
- FS T2-weighted FSE or T2*-weighted

Imaging findings

On T1-weighted images, the necrotic focus within the femoral head appears hypointense.

A hypointense line is typically seen adjacent to the subchondral plate.

On T2-weighted images, there is hyperintense bone marrow oedema.

The ischaemic area remains hypointense.

In the 'double-line' sign, there is a hypointense outer line due to sclerosis and fibrosis and a hyperintense inner line due to granulation tissue.

Hints and tips

It is important to distinguish AVN of the femoral head from migratory osteoporosis. The latter condition is self-limiting and is seen in pregnant women and in young men. Repeat imaging in 6 months shows that it has completely resolved.

Further reading

Aiello MR. Avascular necrosis, femoral head. eMedicine article. Available at: http://emedicine.medscape.com/article/386808-overview.

Fang C, Teh J. Imaging of the hip. *Imaging* 2003; **15**: 205–16.

Vande Berg BE, Malghem JJ, Labaisse MA et al. MR imaging of avascular necrosis and transient marrow edema of the femoral head. *Radiographics* 1993; **13**: 501–20.

Case 21: Avascular necrosis of the hip

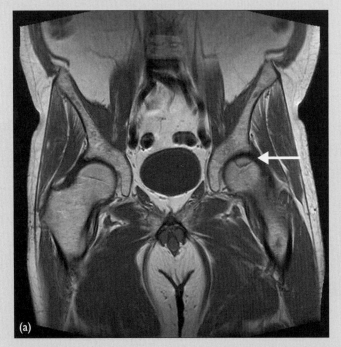
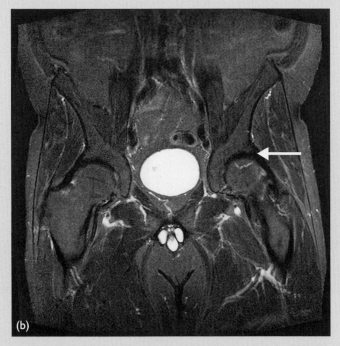

Case 21.1 (a, b) T1-weighted and FS T2-weighted FSE coronal images of the hips and pelvis showing avascular necrosis (AVN) of the left femoral head.

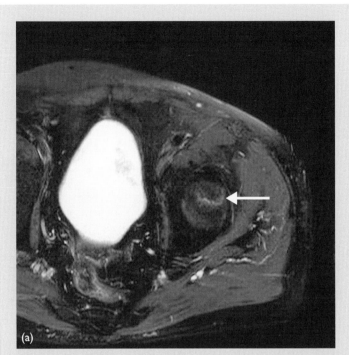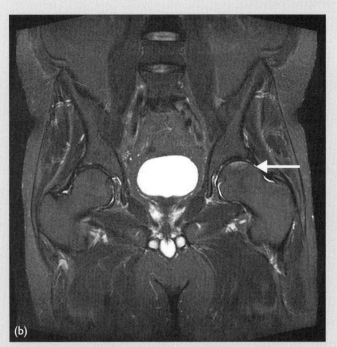

Case 21.2 (a, b) FS T2-weighted FSE axial and coronal images showing AVN and adjacent oedema.

FEMORAL NECK FRACTURES

Fractures of the neck of the femur are a major cause of hip pain after falls in the elderly. These may be either intracapsular or intertrochanteric. Intracapsular fractures of the neck of the femur have a high incidence of AVN and in most instances are treated with a hemiarthroplasty. The great majority of femoral neck fractures are well visualized on anteroposterior plain radiographs of the pelvis and horizontal-beam lateral scans of the hip on the side of the pain.

Occasionally, fractures may not be seen at the initial presentation. There are many ways to identify such occult femoral neck fractures. These include follow-up radiography, bone scintigraphy and MRI. Of these, MRI is the most sensitive.

Key sequences

- T1-weighted and STIR axial and coronal sequences of the pelvis.

Imaging findings

The fracture line is low signal on both T1-weighted and STIR sequences. The thickness of the fracture line is an indicator of sclerosis of the fracture line, reflecting chronicity.

There is bone marrow oedema and haemorrhage in the more acute setting, identified by high signal at the femoral neck on STIR sequences with corresponding low signal on T1-weighted sequences. In more chronic fractures, the degree of oedema settles, completely disappearing at 6 months.

There is associated hip effusion in some cases.

Associated findings include osteonecrosis of the femoral head in intracapsular fractures.

A pathological cause (metastasis or myeloma) should be ruled out by assessing the marrow signal of the pelvis and the proximal femur.

Hints and tips

Bone marrow oedema identifies the site of the fracture and is the initial sign to look for.

Assessment of the pelvis for stress fractures of the sacrum and other causes of hip pain such as pubic rami fractures should be looked for.

High signal within the soft tissues of the hip should be looked for to exclude muscle injury or ligamentous injury. Specifically, avulsions of the muscle origins of the adductors, sartorius and the straight head of the rectus femoris or trochanteric bursitis may produce hip pain.

Further reading

Berger PE, Ofstein RA, Jackson DW et al. MRI demonstration of radiographically occult fractures. What have we been missing? *Radiographics* 1989; **9**: 407–37.

Oka M, Monu JUV. Prevalence and patterns of occult hip fractures and mimics revealed by MRI. *AJR Am J Roentgenol* 2004; **182**: 283–8.

Case 22: Traumatic right femoral neck fracture

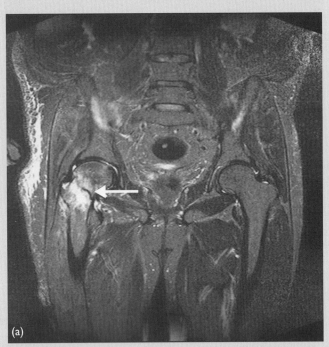

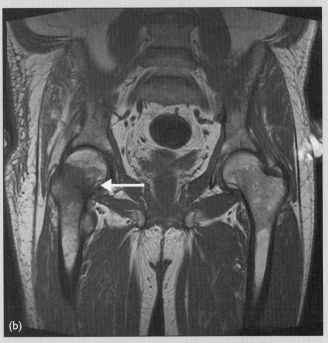

Case 22.1 (a, b) Intracapsular fracture of the neck of the femur. Note the low-signal fracture line with adjacent high T2 signal in the femoral neck.

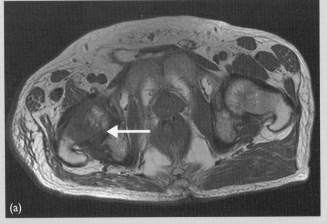

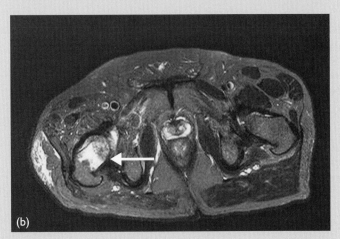

Case 22.2 (a, b) T1-weighted and STIR axial images showing the intracapsular fracture of the neck of the femur.

Case 23: Pathological right intertrochanteric fracture of the neck of the femur

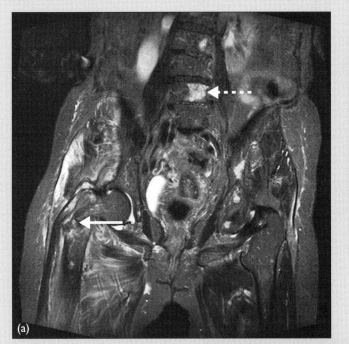

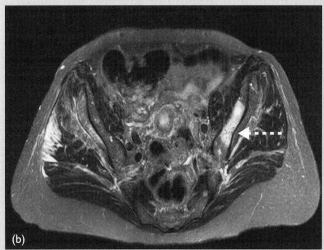

Case 23.1 (a, b) STIR coronal and axial images showing a pathological intertrochanteric fracture of the neck of the femur with multiple high-signal areas in the pelvis and lumbar spine. These were identified as metastatic deposits from breast cancer.

5 THE SHOULDER

IMAGING OF THE SHOULDER

The shoulder joint is the most mobile and unstable of joints. MRI of the shoulder allows accurate assessment of the anatomic structures, including the glenoid, the humeral head and articular cartilage, the labrum, and the rotator cuff.

MR arthrography

MR arthrography is used in glenohumeral instability to assess the labrum. The injection of a 2% solution of gadolinium (Gs) is done under either fluoroscopic or ultrasound guidance, using either an anterior or posterior approach.

ABER position

The ABER (abduction external rotation) position is used to assess the anterior labrum and partial undersurface tears of the rotator cuff. This position places the inferior glenohumeral ligament under tension, resulting in stressing of the antero-inferior labrum. The humeral head also moves away from the undersurface of the rotator cuff, allowing better visualization of this portion of the rotator cuff.

Key sequences (Figures 5.1 and 5.2)

- Imaging in all three planes to assess the shoulder, with a dedicated fluid-sensitive sequence in at least one plane
- FS T1-weighted imaging in true axial, oblique coronal and oblique sagittal planes for MR arthrography

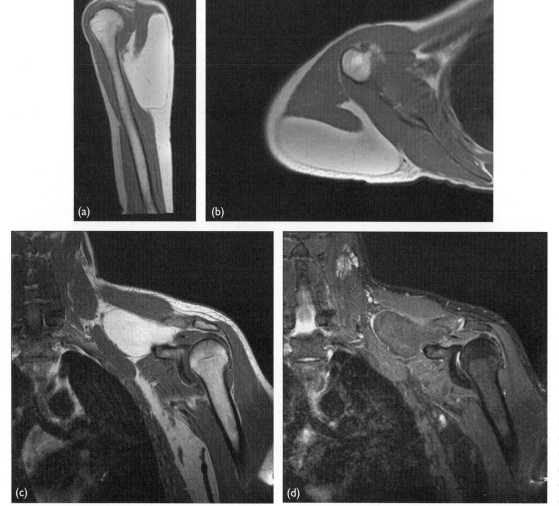

Figure 5.1 Standard shoulder sequences: (a) T1-weighted sagittal oblique; (b) T1-weighted axial; (c) T1-weighted coronal oblique; (d) T2-weighted coronal oblique.

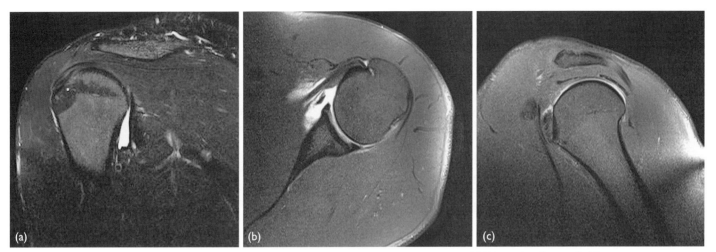

Figure 5.2 MR arthrography sequences: (a) T1-weighted coronal oblique; (b) T1-weighted axial; (c) T1-weighted sagittal oblique.

SHOULDER ANATOMY (FIGURE 5.3)

The shoulder joint is a combination of three joints: the glenohumeral joint, the acromioclavicular joint and the scapulothoracic articulation. The main movement takes place at the glenohumeral joint, which is a ball-and-socket synovial joint. To facilitate a wide range of motion, the glenohumeral joint is shallow.

The glenoid is made deeper by a fibrocartilaginous rim known as the glenoid labrum. The labrum is the site of attachment of the long head of the biceps tendon superiorly and the glenohumeral ligaments, which provide stability to the joint.

The glenohumeral joint has two sets of ligaments: the coracohumeral ligament and the glenohumeral ligaments.

The coracohumeral ligament lies anterosuperiorly, arising from the coracoid and inserting into the greater tuberosity of the humerus. This ligament plays two roles: it strengthens the superior portion of the joint and restrains external rotation.

There are three glenohumeral ligaments:

- The superior glenohumeral ligament (SGHL) runs anteriorly in front of the long head of the biceps tendon between the 12 and 1 o'clock positions in front of the biceps tendon and inserts into the lesser tuberosity. The

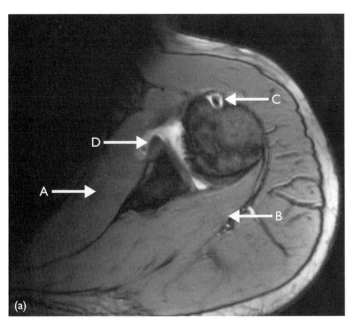

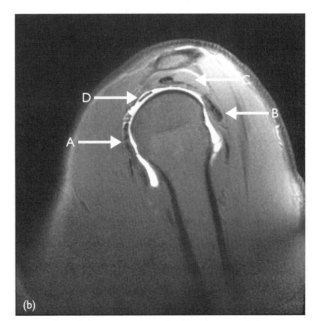

Figure 5.3 Anatomy of the shoulder: axial and sagittal oblique sections. (a) T1-weighted axial: A, subscapularis; B, infraspinatus; C, biceps tendon; D, anterior labrum. (b) T1-weighted sagittal oblique, showing the rotator cuff muscles: A, subscapularis; B, infraspinatus; C, supraspinatus; D, biceps tendon.

SGHL forms a sling with the coracohumeral ligament around the intra-articular portion of the long head of the biceps tendon.

- The middle glenohumeral ligament (MGHL) is the most variable in position and thickness. It runs from the anterosuperior portion of the glenoid rim to blend with the subscapularis tendon. It may be absent.
- The inferior glenohumeral ligament (IGHL) is the most constant. It arises from the inferior portion of the labrum and has two parts: an anterior band that is thicker and a posterior band that tends to be thinner. Both bands insert into the surgical neck of the humerus. The capsule between the two bands is patulous and is called the axillary recess. This portion is dependent and a potential space.

The common anatomic variant seen with the ligaments is the Buford complex. Here the anterosuperior capsule is absent and the MGHL is thickened and cord-like and may be mistaken for an anterior labral tear.

The glenohumeral joint is stabilized by the rotator cuff, a combined tendon formed by the subscapularis anteriorly, the supraspinatus superiorly, and the infraspinatus and teres minor posteriorly. The rotator cuff inserts along the humeral head. The subscapularis portion inserts onto the lesser tuberosity, while the rotator cuff from the supraspinatus, infraspinatus and teres minor inserts onto the greater tuberosity of the humerus.

The bursae associated with the joint are the subacromial bursa and the subscapularis bursa. The subacromial bursa is situated in the space between the capsule and the deltoid and does not communicate with the joint. It is thickened in impingement syndrome. The subscapularis bursa lies between the subscapularis tendon and the capsule. This bursa communicates with the joint.

ROTATOR CUFF TEARS

The normal rotator cuff runs through the subacromial space and inserts onto the greater and lesser tuberosity.

The muscles that constitute the rotator cuff include the subscapularis, inserting onto the lesser tuberosity, and the supraspinatus, infraspinatus and teres minor, which insert onto the greater tuberosity.

Tears of the rotator cuff often occur as a result of chronic impingement syndrome. Chronic inflammation of the supraspinatus tendon results in oedema of the tendon, narrowing of the subacromial space and eventual abrasion of the tendon. Continued abrasion results initially in a partial-thickness tear, which may progress to a full-thickness tear.

Although diagnosis of full-thickness tears can usually be made by ultrasound, diagnosing partial-thickness tears by ultrasound is more operator-dependant. MRI gives a good overview of the shoulder joint and can accurately assess the dimensions of the tear and the quality of the muscles of the rotator cuff. The latter is useful in identifying patients who may be suitable for rotator cuff repair.

Key sequences

- T2-weighted coronal oblique and sagittal oblique
- T1-weighted coronal and sagittal oblique, ABER position with MR arthrography

Imaging findings

MRI is useful in assessing not only the rotator cuff itself but also the subacromial space, the morphology of the acromion and the subacromial bursa.

The rotator cuff tendon is uniformly low signal on all sequences.

Tendinosis is displayed as intermediate signal on T1-weighted imaging and normal signal on T2-weighted imaging.

Partial tears of the cuff appear on T2-weighted imaging as high-signal areas within the tendon that may communicate either with the glenohumeral joint (undersurface tears) or the subacromial bursa (bursal tears) or may remain within the substance of the tendon (intrasubstance tears).

Footprint or rim rent tears arise from the insertion of the supraspinatus on the greater trochanter.

Full-thickness tears are best visualized on coronal oblique images and are identified as high signal running through the full thickness of the tendon (i.e. from the bursal surface to the articular surface). The tears tend to be associated with fluid in the subacromial and subdeltoid bursae.

Large tears produce retraction of the tendon.

Long-standing tears are associated with atrophy of the muscle belly of the involved muscles.

Ancillary signs include fluid in the subacromial–subdeltoid bursa, obliteration of the peribursal fat stripe and atrophy of the muscle belly.

Hints and tips

Impingement is a clinical diagnosis, but imaging has a key role for rotator cuff tears.

High T2 signal traversing the rotator cuff to a surface should raise suspicion of a rotator cuff tear.

Coronal oblique images are the best way to assess for rotator cuff tears.

Further reading

Farber A, Fayad L, Johnson T et al. Magnetic resonance imaging of the shoulder: current techniques and spectrum of disease. *J Bone Jt Surg [Am]* 2006; **88**: 64–79.

Ostlere S. Imaging of the shoulder. *Imaging* 2003; **15**: 162–73.

Case 24: Rotator cuff pathology

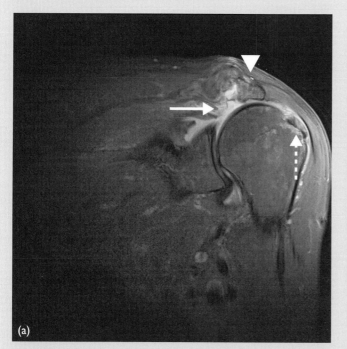 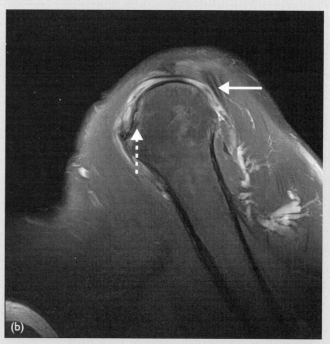

Case 24.1 (a, b) T2-weighted coronal oblique and sagittal oblique images showing a full-thickness rotator cuff tear (full arrow) with irregularity of the greater tuberosity (dotted arrow) from chronic impingement. The arrowhead shows an os acromiale – a normal variant and a cause of rotator cuff tears.

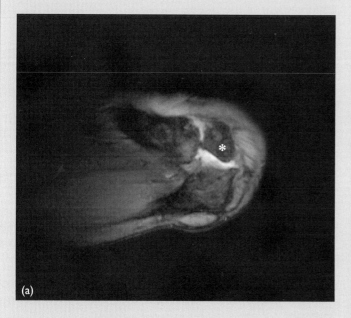 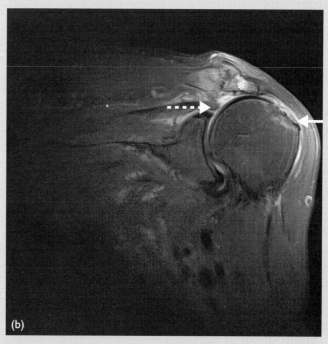

Case 24.2 (a, b) T2-weighted axial and sagittal images showing an os acromiale (asterisk). The full arrow shows bone oedema from impingement. The dotted arrow shows a full-thickness rotator cuff tear with a bare head of the humerus.

LABRAL TEARS

Tears of the labrum are responsible for symptoms of shoulder instability, clicking or pain.

Common lesions of the labroligamentous complex include:
- Bankart/Hill–Sachs lesion
- Bankart variants:
  - anterior ligamentous periosteal sleeve avulsion (ALPSA)
  - Perthes lesion
- superior labrum anteroposterior (SLAP) tears

Bankart/Hill–Sachs lesion

This is a true avulsion of the labrum, occurring at the anterior–inferior portion of the labrum. The scapular periosteum is seen to be torn. The anterior–inferior glenohumeral ligament is intact.

The lesion is part of the anterior dislocation and is associated with a depression fracture of the posterior superior part of the humeral head called the Hill–Sachs lesion.

Bankart variants

Both Bankart variants differ from a true Bankart lesion by remaining attached to the periosteum of the glenoid.

Anterior ligamentous perisoteal sleeve avulsion (ALPSA)

In this lesion, the antero-inferior portion of the labrum is torn but still remains attached to the scapular periosteum. This results in medial displacement of the torn labrum.

Perthes lesion

A Perthes lesion is similar to ALPSA lesions except that, although the torn antero-inferior portion of the labrum remains attached to the scapular periosteum, the torn fragment remains in place. This often heals with fibrous tissue, but is inherently unstable.

Superior labrum anteroposterior (SLAP) tears

These tears take place at the superior portion of the glenoid labrum and extend anterior-to-posterior in direction. They involve the biceps anchor and start posteriorly.

SLAP tears have been classified into six groups depending on the extent of involvement of the labrum and adjacent structures. Surgical treatment, however, is based on the involvement of the biceps anchor. The most common type involves avulsion of the superior labrum and the biceps anchor from the glenoid.

Key sequences

MR arthrography is important to pick this type of lesion up. The key sequences that show Bankart tears are true axial, sagittal oblique and ABER position images.

The ABER position is not useful for SLAP tears, since the labral tear in these is superior whereas the ABER position helps in imaging the inferior portion of the glenoid labrum.

Imaging findings

Bankart lesions are seen in the antero-inferior portion of the labrum and may extend cranially to involve the superior labrum and the biceps anchor.

Associated bony oedema in the glenoid is seen in more acute injuries, which are also associated with joint effusions.

Old and healed Bankart lesions show as intermediate-signal areas between the tear and the glenoid.

The key sign distinguishing between the normal Bankart lesion and the variants is the attachment of the periosteum to the scapula. Tears of this define a true Bankart lesion.

Hill–Sachs lesions may be best seen on axial images of the shoulder at the level of the coracoid process, and range from flattening to a wedge-shaped fracture.

SLAP tears show contrast entering the labral tear laterally.

Involvement of the biceps anchor is an important finding and relates to surgical management.

Hints and tips

MR arthography provides improved sensitivity for identifying tears.

Bankart lesions are associated with Hill–Sachs lesions in 75% of cases.

Hill–Sachs lesions should always be looked for on axial images at the level of the coarcoid process.

SLAP tears need to be differentiated from a known anatomic variant called a sublabral recess. SLAP tears extend posteriorly beyond the biceps tendon. This is not seen in a sublabral recess.

ABER positioning in MR arthrography improves the detection of Perthes lesions and differentiation between other variants.

Further reading

Beltran J, Bencardino J, Mellado J et al. MR arthrography of the shoulder: variants and pitfalls. *Radiographics* 1997; **17**: 1403–12;

Robinson G, Ho Y, Finlay K et al. Normal anatomy and common labral lesions at MR arthrography. *Clin Radiol* 2006; **61**: 805–21.

Case 25: Labral tear

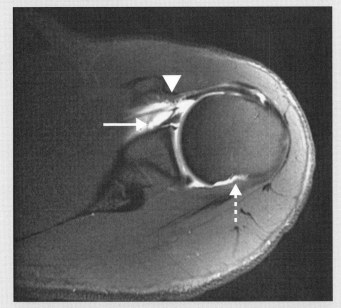

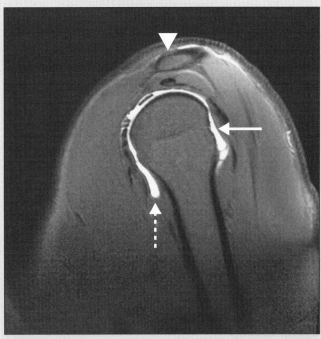

Case 25.1 FS T1-weighted axial MR arthrogram showing a Bankart lesion of the anterior labrum (full arrow) with a Hill–Sachs lesion at the posterior part of the head of the humerus (dotted arrow) and anterior rupture of the capsule (arrowhead).

Case 25.2 FS T1-weighted sagittal oblique MR arthrogram showing the posterior Hill–Sachs lesion (full arrow). The arrowhead indicates the acromion process pointing anteriorly and the dotted arrow shows the axillary recess.

Case 26: SLAP tear

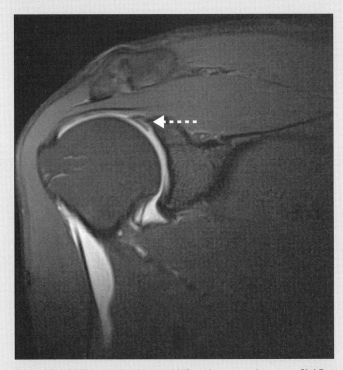

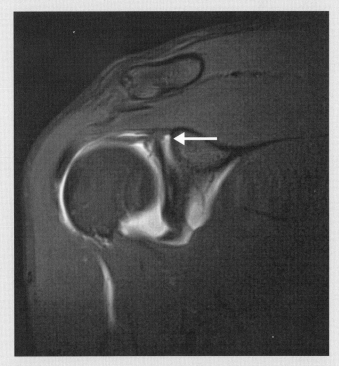

Case 26.1 FS T1-weighted sagittal MR arthrogram showing a SLAP tear with the contrast entering the tear and involving the root of the biceps.

PARALABRAL CYSTS

A paralabral cysts is a degenerative cyst produced in the shoulder. The cyst is associated with a labral tear or SLAP tear and may cause nerve entrapment of the suprascapular nerve in the suprascapular notch.

Paralabral cysts may be unilocular or multilocular and may have a communication to a labral tear. The cyst is within 1 cm of the tear in the same position as the tear.

Nerve entrapment by paralabral cysts is well documented. The suprascapular nerve in the suprascapular notch and the axillary nerve in the quadrilateral space (a space bounded superiorly by the teres minor, inferiorly by the teres major, medially by the triceps and laterally by the humeral shaft).

Key sequences

- T2-weighted axial for the site of the lesion and often the tear
- FS T1-weighted sagittal and axial for arthrography

Imaging findings

A paralabral cyst is usually high signal on fluid-sensitive sequences, although if it contains proteinaceous material, it may be high signal on T1-weighted sequences.

The cyst may be uniloculated or multiloculated, with a tapering end pointing to the joint.

There is usually an associated tear of the labrum of the glenoid. The finding of a paralabral cyst may warrant MR arthrography, which may show the track between the labral tear and the cyst.

The position of the cyst corresponds to the site of the tear.

Fat atrophy of the rotator cuff muscles indicates a nerve entrapment syndrome.

Hints and tips

T2-weighted axial images are useful to visualize both the cyst and the tear.

Cysts are often associated with labral tears. The site of the cyst corresponds to the site of the tear. For example, a cyst in the suprascapular notch may show a SLAP tear.

Further reading

Linker CS, Helms CA, Fritz RC. Quadrilateral space syndrome: findings at MR imaging. *Radiology* 1993; **188**: 675–6.

Mellado JM, Salvado E, Camins A et al. Fluid collections and juxta-articular lesions of the shoulder: spectrum of MRI findings. *Eur Radiol* 2002; **12**: 650–9.

Tung GA, Entzian D, Stern JB et al. MR imaging and MR arthrography of paraglenoid labral cysts. *AJR Am J Roentgenol* 2000; **174**: 1707–15.

Case 27: Paralabral cyst

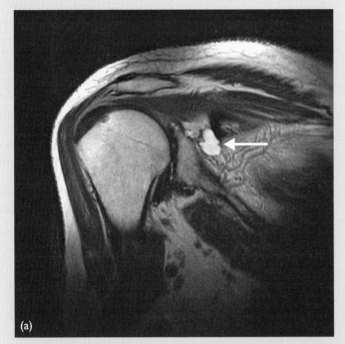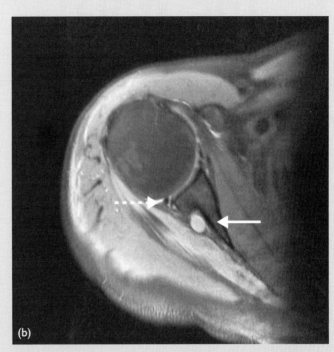

Case 27.1 (a, b) T1-weighted coronal oblique and FS T1-weighted images showing a paralabral cyst (full arrow). Note the high signal indicating high protein content. The dotted arrow indicates an anterior labral tear.

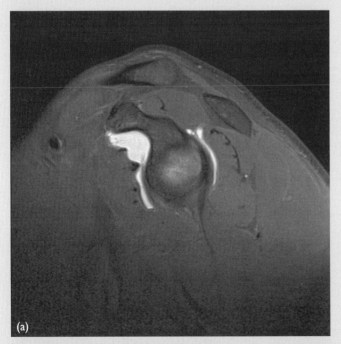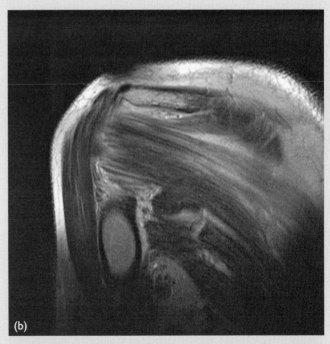

Case 27.2 (a) FS T1-weighted sagittal oblique image showing a paralabral cyst jutting anteriorly and adjacent to the suprascapular notch. (b) T1-weighted coronal image showing fat atrophy of the infraspinatus, a muscle innervated by the suprascapular nerve

6 THE WRIST

IMAGING OF THE WRIST

MRI of the wrist is a well-established method of assessment. Owing to its relative size, the wrist is ideally imaged with dedicated wrist coils. With the wrist placed at the patient's side, in the periphery of the magnetic field, the detail obtained can be distorted owing to field inhomogeneities. However, more recent scanners are able to provide better field homogeneity.

Abnormalities of the tendons and muscles around the wrist are better assessed with ultrasound.

MR arthrography

When there is a question about the intrinsic ligaments of the wrist, MR arthrography is used. Conventional MRI cannot resolve these intrinsic ligaments because of size and other technical factors.

Two techniques are used:
- Direct MR arthrography involves direct instillation of dilute gadolinium (Gd) into the radiocarpal joint. The procedure is done under either fluoroscopic (the preferred method) or ultrasound guidance. Fluoroscopy involves confirming the placement of the Gd with iodinated

contrast. During this process, additional information can be obtained regarding the integrity of the radiocarpal and intercarpal ligaments. Specifically, if iodinated contrast is seen to run into the distal radio-ulnar joint, a triangular fibrocartilage complex (TFCC) tear is confirmed. Direct arthrography carries with it the risk of iatrogenic infection and the added time for injecting the contrast.
- Indirect MR arthrography is seldom practised. In this technique, intravenous Gd diffuses into the joints, usually after exercising the wrist.

Key sequences (Figures 6.1 and 6.2)

- Conventional wrist MRI images the wrist in axial, coronal and sagittal planes and utilizes T1-weighted imaging, proton density (PD)-weighted and fat-saturated (FS) T2-weighted imaging. T1- and PD-weighted images show the anatomy.
- PD-weighted and FS T2-weighted imaging give additional information regarding abnormalities of the bones, ligaments and soft tissues.
- The sequences used for MR arthrography of the wrist are similar to those for shoulder MR arthrography. FS T1-weighted axial and coronal images are used to view the ligaments of the wrist.

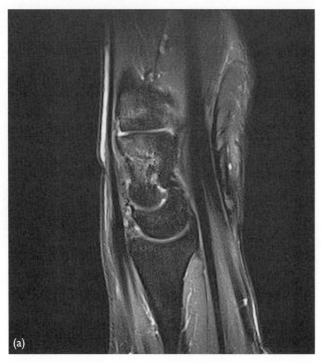 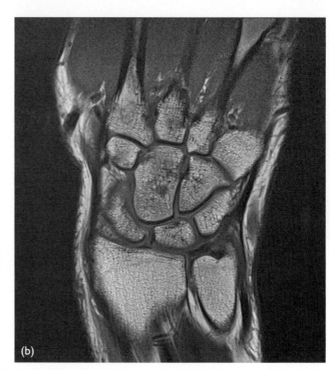

Figure 6.1 Normal wrist sequences: (a) T2-weighted sagittal; (b) T2-weighted coronal (b).

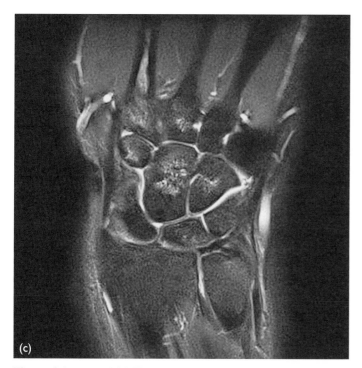

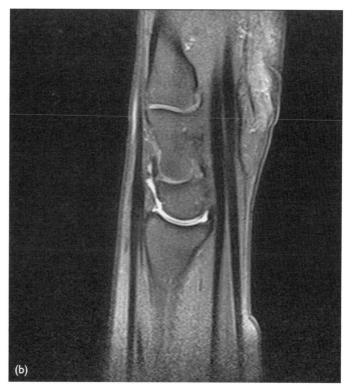

Figure 6.1 *continued* (c) T1-weighted coronal; (d) T1-weighted axial.

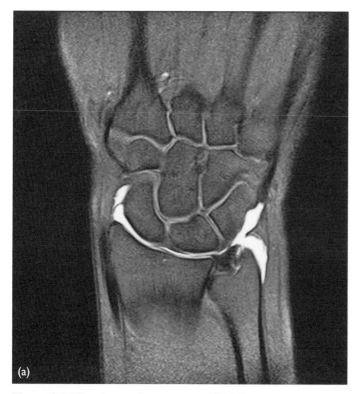

Figure 6.2 MR arthrography sequences: (a) FS T1-weighted coronal; (b) FS T1-weighted sagittal.

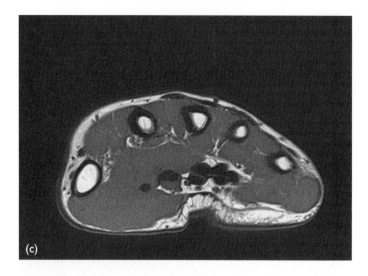

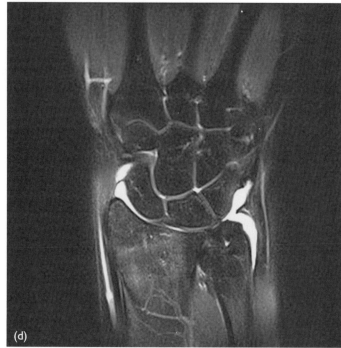

Figure 6.2 *continued* (c) T1-weighted axial; (d) FS T2-weighted coronal.

ANATOMY OF THE WRIST (FIGURE 6.3)

The wrist is a complex synovial hinge joint. The wrist consists of the distal radio-ulnar joint (DRUJ), the radiocarpal joint, the intercarpal joint and the carpometacarpal joint. The important ligaments in the wrist are the scapholunate and the luno-triquetral ligament. The triangular fibrocartilage complex (TFCC) is a fibrocartilagenous structure in the radiocarpal joint and is the main stabilizer of the joint.

The scaphoid articulates with the multiple bones and bridges the two carpal rows. It is the main stabilizer of the carpals and is the primary route for the transmission of force. The main blood supply is through the distal pole; because of this, its proximal portion is prone to avascular necrosis.

The lunate bone is the pivot for the wrist. Flexion and extension take place at this bone. It articulates with the radius proximally and the capitate distally.

The TFCC consists of the articular disc and supporting ligaments that help to stabilize the radiocarpal joint. The TFCC lies adjacent to the ulnar styloid and splits radially into two parts: a horizontal portion that attaches to the radius and a vertical portion that dips into the distal radio-ulnar joint. The TFCC is a barrier between the DRUJ and the radiocarpal joint. Rupture of the TFCC provides a route into the DRUJ. Hence, in arthrography of the wrist, when contrast is instilled into the radiocarpal joint, it is seen to seep into the DRUJ.

The scapholunate ligament is a deep ligament of the wrist and **runs between** the scaphoid and the lunate. The

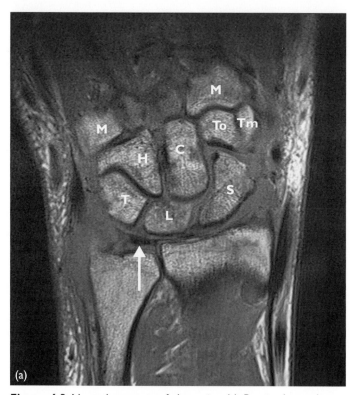

Figure 6.3 Normal anatomy of the wrist. (a) Proximal carpal row: S, scaphoid; L, lunate; T, triquetral; the arrow indicates the triangular fibrocartilage complex (TFCC). Distal carpal row: Tm, trapezium; To, trapezoid; C, capitate; H, hamate; M, metacarpals.

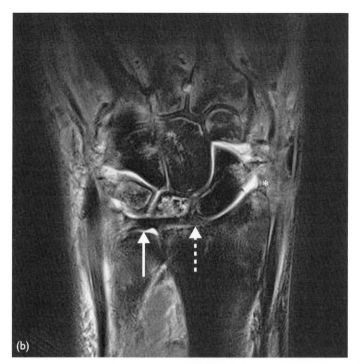
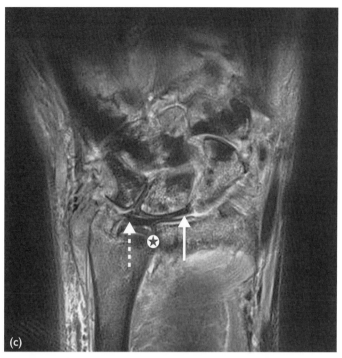

Figure 6.3 *continued* (b) The TFCC (full arrow), scapholunate ligament (dotted arrow) and radial collateral ligament (asterisk). (c) The TFCC (dotted arrow), scapholunate ligament (full arrow) and distal radio-ulnar joint (star).

ligament is delta-shaped and low signal on both T1- and T2-weighted images. It is responsible for the stability of the carpals.

The lunotriquetral ligament is linear and runs between the lunate and the triquetral bone.

TRIANGULAR FIBROCARTILAGE COMPLEX (TFCC) TEARS

The TFCC lies between the distal ulna and the ulnar carpus. The components of the TFCC include the articular disc (the main component), the dorsal and volar radioulnar ligaments, the meniscus homologue, the extensor carpi ulnaris tendon sheath and the ulnocarpal ligaments. It is the major stabilizer of the distal radio-ulnar joint and is prone to injury because of the axial and shear forces that are applied to it as the carpi rotate over the radius and ulna. Tears can therefore be traumatic (in the young population) and degenerative (in the older population).

MRI provides help in the following ways: confirmation of the tear and its location, provision of a good presurgical road map and demonstration of associated wrist pathologies such as positive ulnar variance or chondral lesions.

Key sequences

- FS T1-weighted coronal arthrography, which will also reveal

Imaging findings

Tears appear as low signal areas on T1-weighted images and high signal areas on T2-weighted images, extending from one surface to another.

Fluid in the DRUJ or extravasation of contrast into the DRUJ is an important ancillary sign.

Associated ulnar positive variance and oedema of the lunate are ancillary signs.

Degenerative TFCC tears are associated with chondromalacia (loss of cartilage) of the lunate and triquetral and tears of the lunotriquetral ligament.

MR arthrography of the wrist is the most sensitive method of identifying TFCC tears.

The Palmer classification of TFCC tears depends on the mechanism, location and involved structures and divides the tears into two main groups: traumatic and degenerative. Further subdivisions identify associated abnormalities of adjacent structures such as the ulna, the lunate and the ligaments of the wrist.

Hints and tips

An intact TFCC has low signal intensity on all sequences.

There may be an area of high signal near the ulnar insertion of the TFCC that is due to the presence of loose connective tissue. This is normal. At the junction of the radial insertion, there may be a linear area of intermediate signal. This is also normal.

Central tears of the TFCC are mostly degenerative, and therefore good clinical correlation is advised at the time of reporting.

TFCC tears are associated with positive ulnar variance, since an ulnar-shortening process may be coupled with a primary repair surgery.

On MR arthrography, during fluoroscopic injection of contrast, if contrast is seen to enter the DRUJ, this is a sign of a TFCC tear.

Further reading

Cerezal L, del Pinal F, Abascal F et al. Imaging findings in ulnar sided wrist impaction syndromes. *Radiographics* 2002; **22**: 105–21.

McAlinden PS, Teh J. Imaging of the wrist. *Imaging* 2003; **15**: 180–92.

Palmer AK, Werner FW. The triangular fibrocartilage complex of the wrist – anatomy and function. *J Hand Surg [Am]* 1981; **6**: 153–62.

Sugimoto H, Shinozaki T, Ohsawa T. Triangular fibrocartilage in aymptomatic subjects: investigation of abnormal MR signal intensity. *Radiology* 1994; **191**: 193–7.

Case 28: TFCC tear

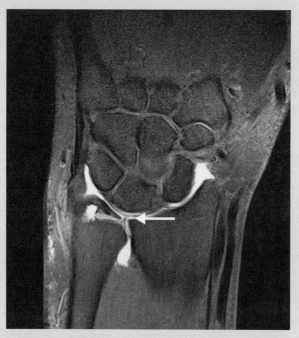 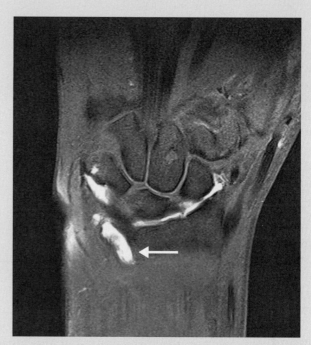

Case 28.1 FS T1-weighted MR arthrogram showing a tear of the TFCC.

Case 28.2 FS T1-weighted MR arthrogram showing extravasation of contrast into the distal radio-ulnar joint (DRUJ).

SCAPHOID FRACTURES

The scaphoid bone is the most common carpal bone to be fractured. The sequelae of scaphoid fractures include avascular necrosis, which can lead to significant functional abnormalities of the wrist.

The scaphoid obtains its blood supply from its distal pole. Fractures of the scaphoid at the waist can disrupt the blood supply and cause non-union and avascular necrosis of the proximal pole. Plain films have a poor sensitivity, even when there is repeat radiography at 2 weeks. Bone scintigraphy is sensitive after 48 hours. MRI is the most sensitive imaging technique, being able to pick up scaphoid injury within 10 hours.

Key sequences

- T1-weighted coronal
- T2-weighted/STIR
- Post-Gd FS T1-weighted FSE coronal

Imaging findings

On T2-weighted images, there is oedema in the scaphoid, centred on the fracture line. This is low signal on all sequences. If the fracture is old, it may show a thick low-signal rim due to sclerosis.

On T1-weighted images, the fracture line is more obvious, with adjacent low signal due to oedema. If the fracture fragments return a normal bone marrow signal, this indicates viability.

Post-contrast images show poor enhancement of the fracture fragment if the blood supply is a compromised. These post-contrast images may be either a single acquisition or dynamically acquired. Dynamic imaging shows a gradual increase in enhancement of the fracture fragment. This highlights asymmetrical enhancement of the fragments.

Hints and tips

Oedema of the scaphoid on T2-weighted coronal images is an indicator of a bony injury to the scaphoid.

Post-contrast images are a sensitive tool in assessing the vascularity of the proximal fracture fragment.

Further reading

Brydie A, Raby N. Early MRI in the management of clinical scaphoid fracture. *Br J Radiol* 2003; **76**: 296–300.

Fowler C, Sullivan B, Williams LA et al. A comparison of bone scintigraphy and MRI in the early diagnosis of the occult scaphoid waist fracture. *Skeletal Radiol* 1998; **27**: 683–7.

Case 29: Scaphoid fracture with non-union and osteonecrosis

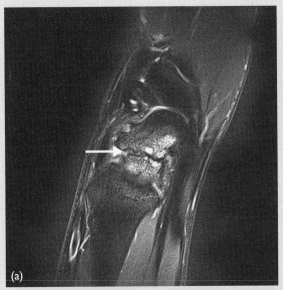
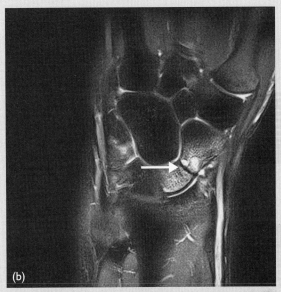

Case 29.1 (a, b) STIR sagittal and coronal images showing scaphoid fracture with sclerotic fracture margins and cystic change. Note the oedema in the fracture fragments.

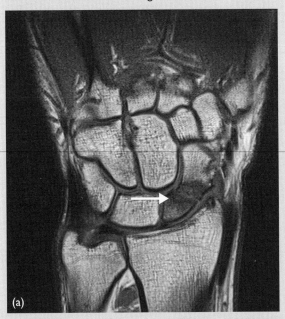
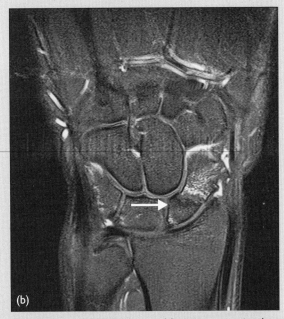

Case 29.2 T1-weighted and post-Gd FS T1-weighted FSE coronal images of the wrist showing an abnormal bone marrow signal on the T1-weighted image (a) and reduced enhancement of the proximal pole on the post-Gd image (b), consistent with osteonecrosis.

7 THE FOOT AND ANKLE

ANKLE IMAGING

The ankle is a peripheral joint that suffers from similar problems to the wrist. To improve resolution, dedicated ankle coils are used. Most ankle pathology can be investigated with ultrasound.

Key sequences (Figure 7.1)

- T1-weighted axial and sagittal and fat-saturated (FS) T2-weighted for bone and ligament pathology
- Proton density (PD)-weighted for cartilage and marrow abnormalities

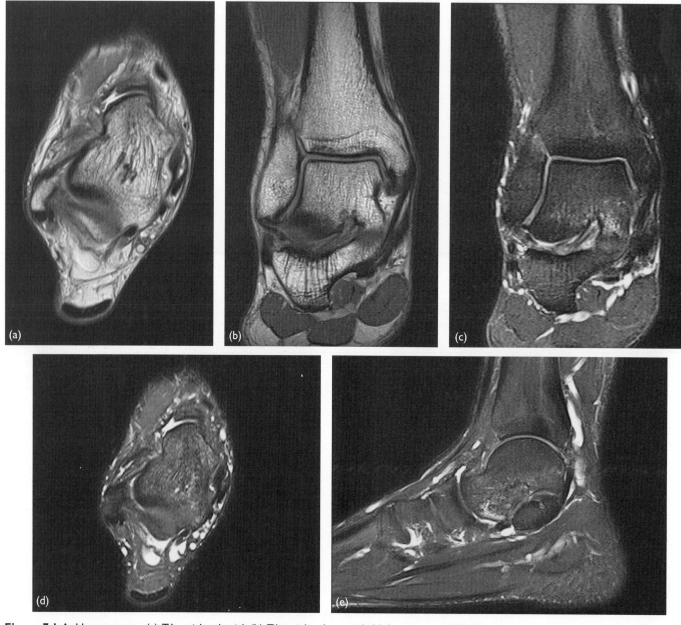

Figure 7.1 Ankle sequences: (a) T1-weighted axial; (b) T1-weighted coronal; (c) fat-saturated (FS) T2-weighted coronal; (d) FS T2-weighted axial; (e) FS T2-weighted sagittal.

- FS PD-weighted coronal to look at the talar dome, foot and tendons
- FS PD-weighted axial to look at medial and lateral ligaments, tendons and foot
- Sagittal to assess Achilles tendon and plantar fascia

ANATOMY (FIGURE 7.2)

The relevant anatomy of the ankle relates ligaments and the tendons around the ankle joint.

Lateral ligaments

The lateral ligament complex of the ankle acts as a lateral stabilizer and prevents inversion. It consists of superior and inferior groups. The superior group, which forms part of a syndesmosis, consists of anterior and posterior tibiofibular ligaments. The more important inferior group has three main ligaments:

- The anterior talofibular ligament (ATFL) is seen best on T2-weighted axial images of the ankle at the level of the tibiotalar joint as a homogeneous low-signal structure running anteriorly from the fibula to the talus.
- The posterior talofibular ligament (PTFL) runs from the posterior part of the distal fibula to the talus as a striated low-signal structure on T2-weighted axial images of the ankle at the level of the tip of the lateral malleolus.
- The calcaneofibular ligament (CFL) runs obliquely from the fibula to the calcaneum. Because of its obliquity, the

CFL is best appreciated in a number of T2-weighted coronal or axial slices as a homogeneous low-signal structure running deep to the peroneal tendons.

Medial ligament

This is also known as the deltoid ligament. It has a deep portion and a superficial portion. It extends deep to the medial flexor tendons from the medial malleolus to the talus and calcaneus. The medial ligament prevents valgus talar tilt.

Tendons around the ankle

Medial tendons

These comprise the tibialis posterior, the flexor digitorum and the flexor hallucis longus from anterior to posterior (mnemonic: 'Tom, Dick and Harry'). Between the flexor digitorum and flexor hallucis longus runs the neurovascular bundle.

Lateral tendons

The two tendons running laterally are the peroneus longus and peroneus brevis. The longus runs in a groove formed by the brevis behind the lateral malleolus before they separate. The brevis inserts on to the base of the fifth metatarsal, while the longus through the sinus tarsi of the calcaneum and enters the sole of the foot.

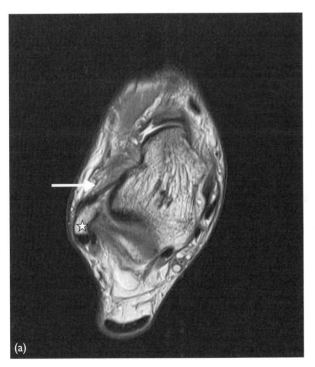

(a)

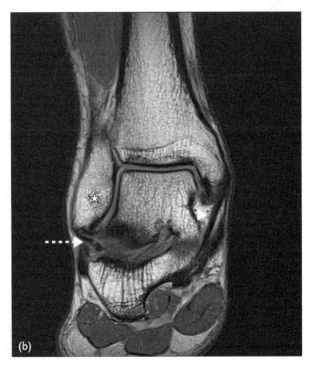

(b)

Figure 7.2 Ankle anatomy: T1-weighted axial and coronal images showing the anterior talofibular ligament (ATFL: full arrow) and the calcaneofibular ligament (CFL: dotted arrow) attached to the lateral malleolus (star). The deltoid ligament is seen to arise from the medial malleolus (arrowhead).

Anterior tendons

The anterior tendons from medial to lateral are the tibialis anterior, extensor hallucis longus and extensor digitorum.

Posterior tendons

The only posterior tendon is the Achilles tendon, a combined tendon formed by the union of the tendons of the gastrocnemius and soleus muscles.

ANKLE LIGAMENT TEARS

Lateral ligament injury

Injuries of the lateral ankle ligaments are seen to occur commonly with inversion injuries. The ATFL is the most commonly ruptured ligament and is classically injured in inversion injuries of the ankle. The next most common ligament to rupture is the CFL. This is injured in combination with the ATFL in the majority of patients. The PTFL is rarely injured.

Anatomic classification depends on the number of ligaments injured. First-degree sprains involve partial- or full-thickness rupture of the ATFL. Involvement of both the ATFL and CFL constitutes a second-degree sprain. Finally, third-degree sprains are defined as rupture of all three ligaments. Third-degree sprains are associated with ankle instability. Full-thickness tears of the ATFL can also be associated with anterolateral impingement syndrome due to synovial hypertrophy impinging in the tibiotalar joint.

Medial ligament injury

Medial ligament injuries occur owing to inversion sprains. The medial ligament is also involved in eversion injuries. The deep portion of the medial ligament is more often injured.

Key sequences

- T1-weighted fast spin echo (FSE) axial and coronal
- FS PD-weighted FSE

Imaging features

High signal within the substance of the ligament is a sign of injury.

Discontinuity, detachment or thinning of the ATFL on axial images are signs of an acute tear.

Talar dome oedema, joint effusion and obliteration of fat planes are ancillary signs.

Chronic tears manifest as thickening or a wavy, irregular contour.

Decreased signal in the fat abutting the ligament on all sequences is indicative of scarring or synovial proliferation.

CFL injuries are diagnosed on coronal images as thickening and heterogeneity.

Fluid within the peroneal tendon sheath is a secondary sign of CFL tears.

Medial ligament contusions manifest as homogeneous, intermediate signal and a thickened ligament. The medial ligament is normally heterogeneous in its signal.

Hints and tips

Axial sequences are best for identifying the lateral and medial ligaments.

Oedema inferior to the malleoli points to injury of the ligaments.

Talar dome oedema and fluid within the tendon sheaths is a secondary sign of ligament sprain.

Further reading

Chiller JC, Peace K, Hulme A et al. Pictorial Review: MRI of foot and ankle injuries in ballet dancers. *Br J Radiol* 2004; **77**: 532–7.

Rosenberg ZS, Beltran J, Bencardino JT. Refresher Course: MR imaging of the ankle and foot. *Radiographics* 2000; **20**: S153–79.

Case 30: ATFL injury

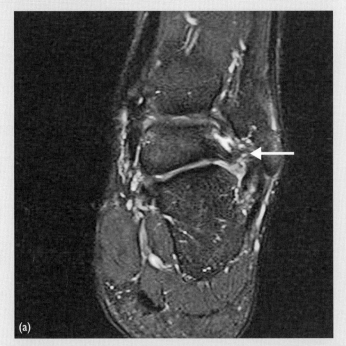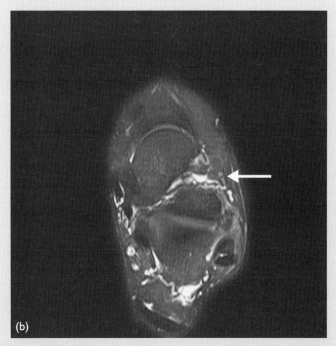

Case 30.1 (a, b) T2-weighted coronal and axial images showing a tear of the ATFL.

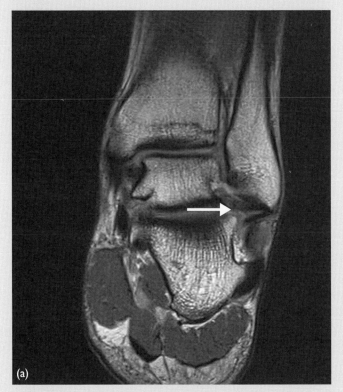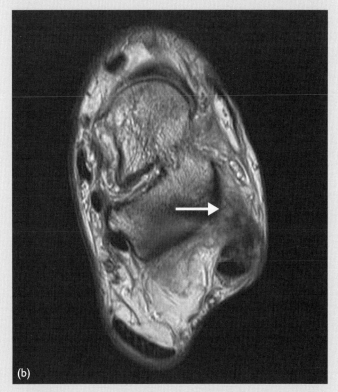

Case 30.2 (a, b) T1-weighted coronal and axial images showing a tear of the ATFL.

ACHILLES TENDON INJURIES AND TENDINOPATHY

The Achilles tendon does not have a tendon sheath and hence tenosynovitis does not occur. Achilles tendon pathology ranges from acute inflammation through chronic inflammation to tears.

Tendinopathy is an umbrella term to describe inflammatory conditions of the tendon. The common causes of tendinopathy include overuse and ischaemia.

The spectrum of Achilles tendinopathy ranges from tendinosis (intrasubstance degeneration and focal swelling), peritendinosis (inflammation of the paritenon, the connective tissue sheath of the Achilles tendon), and partial- and full-thickness rupture.

Most imaging of the Achilles tendon is by ultrasound, although MRI can be useful in assessing for heel pain or postoperative scanning.

Key sequences

- T1-weighted axial and sagittal
- Short-tau inversion recovery (STIR) axial and sagittal

Imaging features

Tendinosis manifests as focal thickening of the Achilles tendon, with intrasubstance high signal.

Paratenon thickening is best seen on axial sections in association with the tendon abnormality.

There is increased signal in the tissues adjacent to the tendon.

High signal in the pre-Achilles tendon fat pad (Kager's fat pad) or retrocalcaneal bursitis adjacent to the insertion of the Achilles tendon on the calcaneum on FS images is an associated finding.

Partial-thickness tears are manifested by high signal within the substance of the tendon on STIR images and by focal thickening. Differentiating partial-thickness tears and tendinosis may be difficult.

Complete rupture is seen as discontinuity of the fibres, fraying of the ends and retraction of the tendon. In acute rupture, there is high T2 signal on fluid-sensitive sequences, while in chronic rupture, there is scarring represented by intermediate T2 signal.

Hints and tips

FS fluid-sensitive sagittal images allow accurate interpretation of Achilles tendinopathy.

Axial images help assess paratenon involvement.

Secondary signs of tendinopathy are seen in the fat pad and as bursitis.

Further reading

Karjalainen PT, Soila K, Aronen HJ et al. MR imaging of overuse injuries of the Achilles tendon. *AJR Am J Roentgenol* 200; **175**: 251–61.

Rosenberg ZS, Beltran J, Bencardino JT. Refresher Course: MR imaging of the ankle and foot. *Radiographics* 2000; **20**: S153–79.

Case 31: Achilles tendinopathy

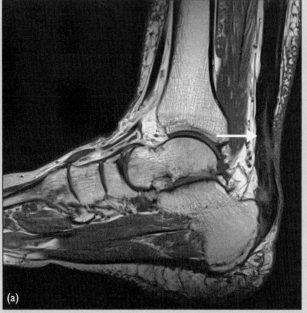 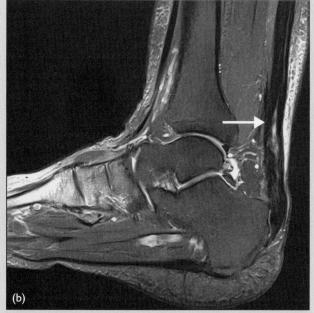

(a)   (b)

Case 31.1 (a, b) T1- and T2-weighted axial images showing altered signal in the Achilles tendon consistent with Achilles tendinopathy.

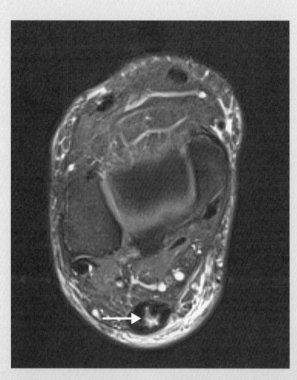

Case 31.2 T2-weighted axial image showing high signal from Achilles tendinopathy.

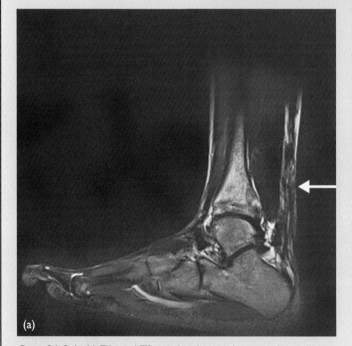

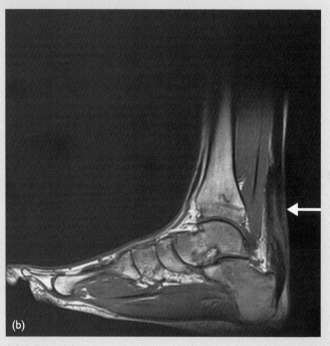

Case 31.3 (a, b) T1- and T2-weighted sagittal images showing a ruptured Achilles tendon.

OSTEOCHONDRAL DEFECTS OF THE TALUS

Osteochondral fractures of the talus originate from trauma. This may be chronic or acute. Over time, it leads to partial or complete detachment with ostoenecrosis. Talar dome

osteochondral fractures are seen in the posterior part of either the medial or lateral portion of the talus.

Osteochondral lesions are classified into four stages:

• Stage 1: osteochondral lesion involving subchondral bone but preservation of the articular cartilage

- Stage 2: osteochondral lesion involving articular cartilage with partial detachment
- Stage 3: complete detachment of the fragment, but situated within the defect
- Stage 4: detached fragment away from the site

Key sequences

- T1-weighted coronal and sagittal
- FS PD-weighted FSE

Imaging features

A subchondral fracture appears as high T2 signal on the talar dome.

A fragment with irregular cartilage cover can be seen.

There is oedema of the underlying bone.

Loose bodies can be seen in the joint.

Hints and tips

Posterior slices on the coronal images are the main site of pathology.

The signal of the osteochondral fragment has an important role. High T1 signal implies viable marrow. Low signal on all sequences implies osteonecrosis.

Further reading

Rosenberg ZS, Beltran J, Bencardino JT. Refresher Course: MR imaging of the ankle and foot. *Radiographics* 2000; **20**: S153–79.

Case 32: Osteochondral defect of the talar dome

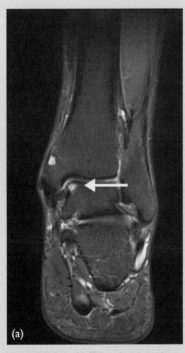 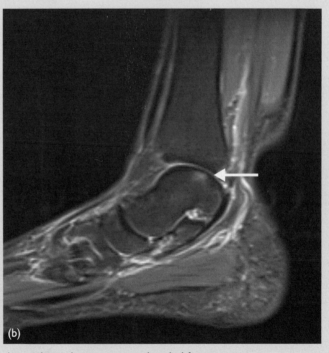

Case 32.1 (a, b) Talar dome oedema and irregularity due to an osteochondral fragment.

DIABETIC FOOT

Peripheral neuropathy, vasculopathy and subsequent infections make imaging of the diabetic foot difficult and challenging. MRI is the imaging modality of choice to evaluate pedal complications related to diabetes.

Key sequences

- T1-weighted images are used to evaluate marrow changes and subcutaneous fat.
- Fat-suppressed sequences (e.g STIR) in the short axis are used to look for osseous and tendinous oedema.
- The short-axis view (in the plane perpendicular to the toes) is the key plane in which the relationship of diabetic ulcers to the underlying bone is best evaluated.
- Sagittal imaging is employed to evaluate the metatarsophalangeal joints, while the axial and coronal planes are useful to evaluate the malleoli and surrounding structures.
- Contrast administration is crucial to distinguish oedema from cellulitis (the latter enhances) and to detect sinus tracts and abscesses.

- When there is considerable metallic artefact due to previous surgery, metal-suppression techniques should be used (e.g. avoid gradient echo sequences and use STIR).

Imaging features

Calluses are low signal on T1-weighted images and low to intermediate signal on T2-weighted images.

In ulcers, the granulation tissue is low signal on T1-weighted images and high signal on T2-weighted images. There is intense enhancement following contrast administration.

Abscesses display low T1 signal and high T2 signal with rim enhancement.

Marked contrast enhancement is characteristic of foreign-body granulomas.

Complex joint effusion is typical of septic arthritis.

Hints and tips

Osteomyelitis should be distinguished from reactive bone oedema. The way to do this is to concentrate on T1-weighted images. Osteomyelitis demonstrates low signal from marrow, whereas reactive changes return a normal T1 signal.

Again the osseous extent of infection is best seen on T1-weighted images, and is often overestimated on T2-weighted images.

It may be difficult to distinguish osteomyelitis from purely neuropathic changes. One practical way of doing this is to focus on the location of the changes that are seen. While osteomyelitis primarily affects interphalangeal joints and metatarsal heads, neuropathic changes are more common in the midfoot.

Further reading

Chatha DS, Cunningham PM, Schweitzer ME. MR Imaging of the diabetic foot: diagnostic challenges. *Radiol Clin North Am* 2005; **43**: 747–59.

Case 33: Diabetic foot

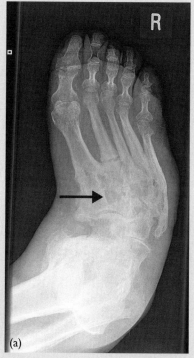
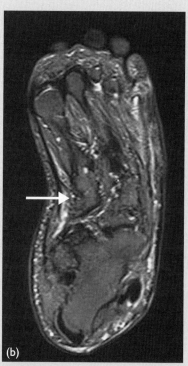

Case 33.1 (a, b) Plain radiograph and STIR coronal MRI of the foot showing a midfoot Charcot joint with extensive disorganization.

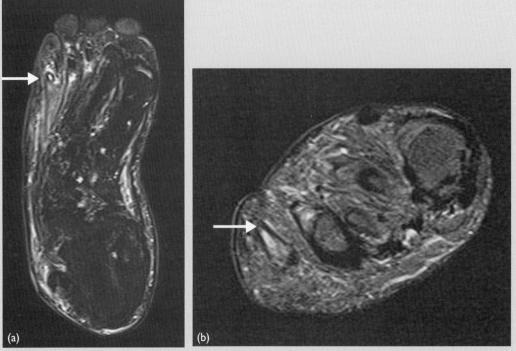

Case 33.2 (a, b) STIR coronal and axial images showing high signal within the neck of the fifth metatarsal and extensive soft tissue oedema. Note the high signal at the metatarsophalangeal joint, in keeping with septic arthritis.

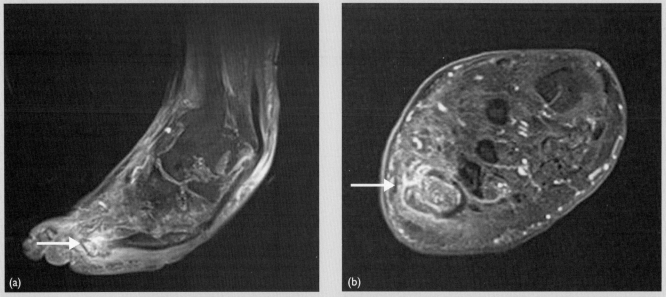

Case 33.3 (a, b) Post-Gd FS T1-weighted FSE sagittal and axial images showing enhancement of the fifth metatarsal shaft with destruction of the metatarsal head and soft tissue, in keeping with osteomyelitis.

MORTON'S NEUROMA

This condition is caused by recurrent trauma to the inter-digital nerve of the foot at the level of the metatarsal heads. The nerve becomes fibrosed and thickened. Morton's neuroma is found between the second and third or the third and fourth interspaces in 90% of cases.

Key sequences

- T1- and T2-weighted axial

Imaging findings

Low-signal rounded lesions are seen on T1- and T2-weighted images at the level of the metatarsal heads.

The neuroma enhances post-contrast.

Morton's neuroma is associated with intermetatarsal bursitis and metatarsophalangeal synovitis.

Further reading

Beggs I. Pictorial Review: Imaging of peripheral nerve tumours. *Clin Radiol* 1997; **52**: 8–17.

Delfault EM, Demondion X, Bieganski A et al. Imaging of the foot and ankle nerve entrapment syndromes: from well demonstrated to unfamiliar sites. *Radiographics* 2003; **23**: 613–23.

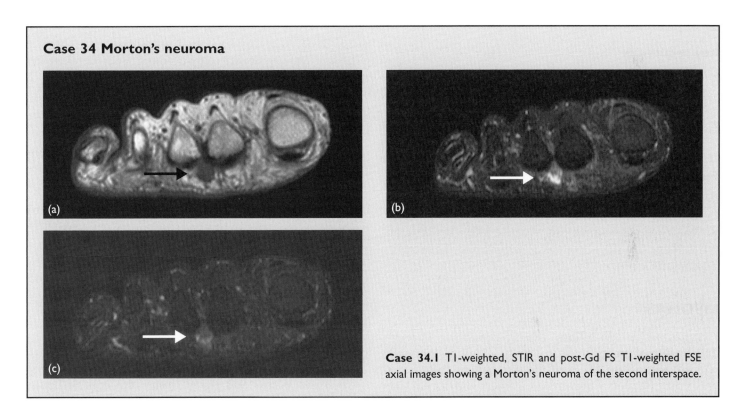

Case 34 Morton's neuroma

Case 34.1 T1-weighted, STIR and post-Gd FS T1-weighted FSE axial images showing a Morton's neuroma of the second interspace.

8 MALIGNANCY AND INFECTION

IMAGING OF MALIGNANCY

Imaging of soft tissue lesions is an important part of musculoskeletal imaging. The vast majority of soft tissue masses can be imaged with ultrasound and need no further imaging. Soft tissue masses that are suspicious on ultrasound need further investigation with MRI.

In the staging of soft tissue sarcomas, MRI provides information on the site and extent of the mass and its spread within muscle compartments and regional nodal metastasis.

Key sequences

- T1-weighted and fat-saturated (FS) T2-weighted fast spin echo (FSE) axial, sagittal and coronal
- Short-tau inversion recovery (STIR) in the best plane
- FS T1-weighted FSE with contrast to cover the lesion and assess its internal configuration

Further reading

Royal College of Radiologists. *Recommendations for Cross-Sectional Imaging in Cancer Management*. London: Royal College of Radiologists, August 2006. Available at: www.rcr.ac.uk/docs/oncology/pdf/Cross_Sectional_Imaging_12.pdf.

LIPOMAS

Lipomas are benign lesions, usually presenting as well-defined homogeneous soft tissue masses. They are common and are seen in up to 1% of the population. They occur with equal frequency in men and women, with a peak age of presentation of 40–60 years.

Key sequences

- T1-weighted
- T2-weighted
- T1-weighted with contrast
- STIR

Imaging findings

Lipomas are high signal on T1-weighted images, intermediate signal on T2-weighted images and low signal on STIR images.

There is no significant enhancement with contrast on T1-weighted imaging.

Hints and tips

Lipomas match the signal intensity of subcutaneous fat on all sequences, and so fat suppression is useful to distinguish them.

Intramuscular and intraosseous lipomas are more complex to characterize. Intramuscular lipomas may not be as well defined and may be seen to infiltrate muscle planes.

Fatty lesions greater than 5 cm in size with enhancement or septae should raise the suspicion of liposarcoma and should be biopsied for histological confirmation.

Further reading

Weiss SW, Goldblum J. Benign lipomatous tumors. In: *Enzinger and Weiss's Soft Tissue Tumors*, 4th edn. St Louis, MO: Mosby, 2001: 571–639.

Case 35: Lipoma

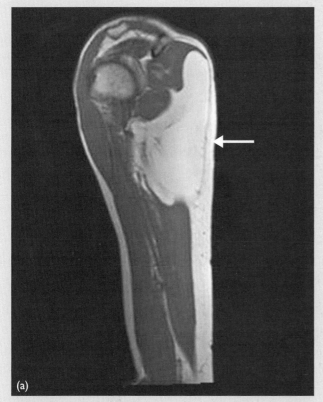

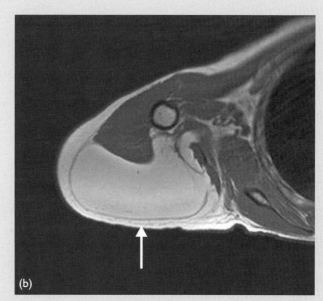

Case 35.1 (a, b) T1-weighted sagittal and axial images showing a subcutaneous lipoma.

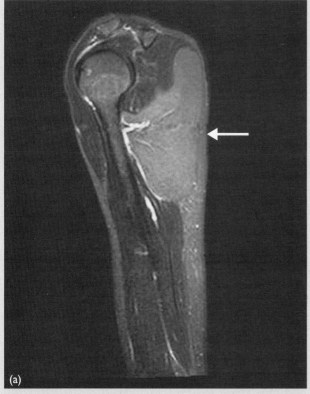

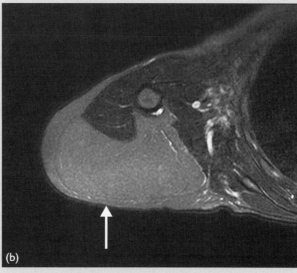

Case 35.2 (a, b) FS T1-weighted sagittal and axial images showing suppression of fat signal, proving that this is a lipoma.

OSTEOSARCOMA

Osteosarcoma is the most common primary malignancy of bone and affects adolescents and young adults. Its estimated incidence is 4–5 per million. Various histological subtypes have been defined, and, based on their location within the bone, they may be described as intramedullary (high-grade, telangiectatic and low-grade), surface (parosteal and periosteal) and extraskeletal. Osteosarcomas are known to affect bones that have pre-existing underlying benign conditions such as cysts or Paget's disease. MRI is the examination of choice for local staging of these tumours and should always precede biopsy, since blood and oedema from the biopsy can be difficult to distinguish from tumour.

Key sequences

- T1-weighted spin echo
- T2-weighted
- STIR
- Proton density (PD)-weighted
- Contrast-enhanced T1-weighted

Imaging findings

Osteosarcoma is typically a metaphyseal tumour in the young. In older individuals and in patients with pre-existing benign pathologies, the tumour more commonly occurs in flat bones and vertebral bodies.

Tumour is seen as areas of intermediate signal intensity on T1-weighted images, and high signal on T2-weighted images. Low-intensity areas within the primary tumour on both T1- and T2-weighted images represent mineralized matrix.

A skip metastasis (i.e. a metastatic deposit within the same bone) may occasionally be seen.

STIR and PD-weighted sequences are useful for assessing the relationship of the tumour to the adjacent neurovascular bundle. The presence of a clear fat plane between the two structures implies non-involvement of the neurovascular bundle.

Hints and tips

Direct epiphyseal extension of osteosarcomas is now known to be considerably more common than previously believed. T1-weighted and STIR sequences can help depict epiphyseal tumour extension.

Patients with skip metastases are more likely to have distant metastases, and further imaging recommendations should be made to the clinicians.

The multiplanar capabilities of MRI should be adopted for accurate anatomic localization and for estimation of epiphyseal, joint and neurovascular involvement. The accuracy of biopsy can be improved by accurate localization of viable tumour.

Dynamic contrast-enhanced MRI has been used in some centres.

Further reading

Murphey MD, Robbin MR, McRae GA et al. The many faces of osteosarcoma. *Radiographics* 1997; **17**: 1205–31.
White LM, Kandel R. Osteoid producing tumors of bone. *Semin Musculoskelet Radiol* 2000; **4**: 25–43

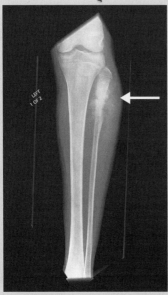

Case 36: Osteosarcoma of the fibula

Case 36.1 Radiographic appearance of proximal fibula osteosarcoma.

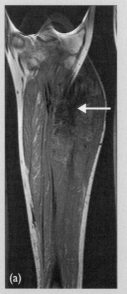 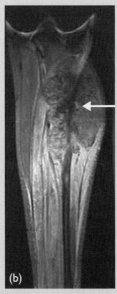

Case 36.2 (a, b) T1-weighted FSE and FS T2-weighted gradient echo (GRE) coronal images showing proximal fibula osteosarcoma. Note the low-signal area from chemical shift artefact due to calcium.

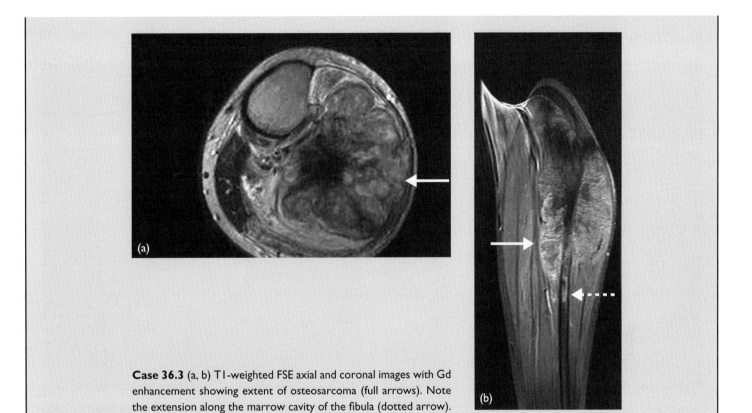

Case 36.3 (a, b) TI-weighted FSE axial and coronal images with Gd enhancement showing extent of osteosarcoma (full arrows). Note the extension along the marrow cavity of the fibula (dotted arrow).

SOFT TISSUE SARCOMA

Soft tissue sarcomas are seen in approximately 1% of the population. Malignant fibrous histiosarcoma (MFH) is the most common soft tissue sarcoma of late adult life, occurring typically in the deep soft tissues of the extremities. It is also the most common tumour of fibrous origin to affect the bone. A third of these lesions occur in pre-existing conditions such as Paget's disease and bone infarction, post-radiotherapy, and with other malignant lesions such as chondrosarcoma. Common sites include the metadiaphyseal regions of long bones, usually around the knee. MRI plays a key role in detection, presurgical planning and postsurgical follow-up for recurrence.

Key sequences

- T1-weighted FSE
- FS T2-weighted FSE
- Gadolinium (Gd)-enhanced T1-weighted FSE

Imaging findings

Intermediate signal intensity on T1-weighted images, heterogeneously increased signal intensity on T2-weighted images and post-contrast enhancement of solid components are typical.

Cortical erosions are characteristic of bony involvement (but computed tomography may be a better imaging modality).

Hints and tips

Although there are no specific diagnostic features of MFH on MRI, it is extremely useful to detect 'skip' metastasis.

Biopsy should be directed towards the non-haemorrhagic and non-myxoid elements of the tumour.

Further reading

Murphey MD, Gross TM, Rosenthal HG. Musculoskeletal malignant fibrous histiocytoma: radiologic–pathologic correlation. *Radiographics* 1994; **14**: 807–26.

Case 37: Soft tissue sarcoma

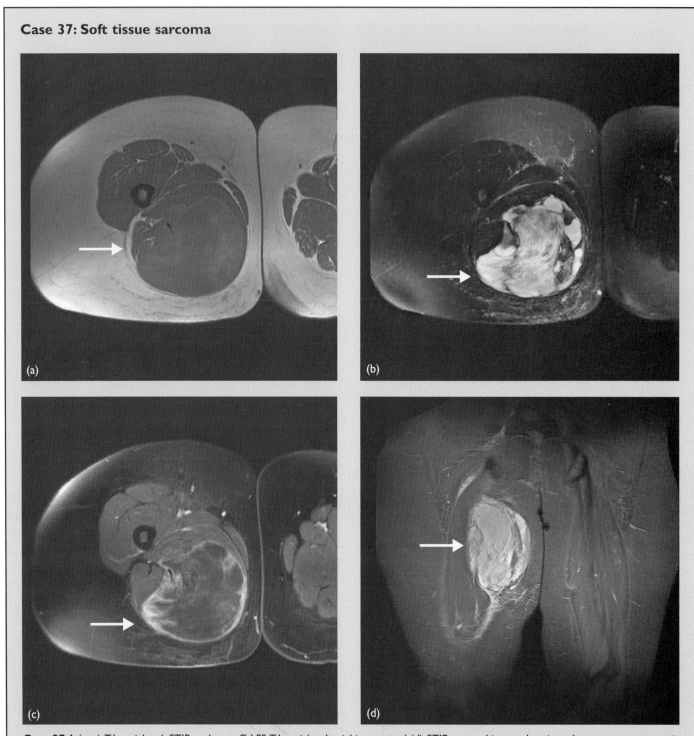

(a)

(b)

(c)

(d)

Case 37.1 (a–c) T1-weighted, STIR and post-Gd FS T1-weighted axial images and (d) STIR coronal image showing a heterogeneous mass in the adductor compartment of the thigh. Note the central necrosis on the post-contrast images. Histologically, this was found to be a malignant fibrous histiosarcoma.

BONE METASTASES

Solitary malignant lesions are more likely to represent a metastatic deposit rather than a primary bone tumour, especially in the middle-aged and elderly. Metastases are most common from primaries within the breast, bronchus, prostate, kidney and thyroid. Whole-body MRI is the most sensitive imaging modality to detect skeletal metastases, since it is the only modality allowing direct visualization of bone marrow.

Key sequences

- T1-weighted spin echo
- Fast STIR

Imaging findings

Metastases usually have low signal on T1-weighted spin echo images compared with fat (yellow marrow as in the elderly). The presence of red marrow in children and younger adults makes this differentiation difficult and a fat-suppressed sequence such as fast STIR is employed as a problem-solving tool.

Hints and tips

The presence of a perilesional high-signal 'halo' on T2-weighted images is a highly specific feature of metastasis.

Further reading

Abrams HL, Sprio R, Goldstein N. Metastasis in carcinoma. Analysis of 1000 autopsied cases. *Cancer* 1950; **3**: 74–85.

Schweitzer ME, Levine C, Mitchell DG et al. Bull's eyes and halos: useful MR discriminators of osseous metastases. *Radiology* 1993; **188**: 249–52.

Vanel D. MRI of bone metastases: the choice of the sequence. *Cancer Imaging* 2004; **4**: 30–5.

Case 38: Metastasis to the femur

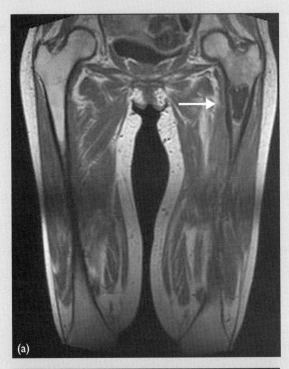
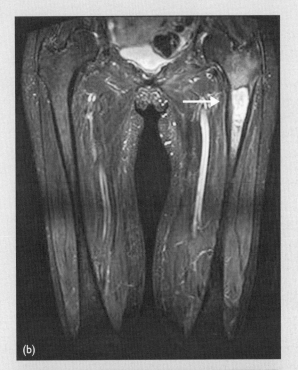
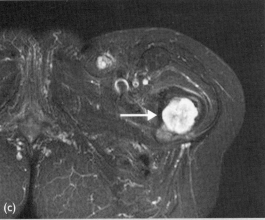
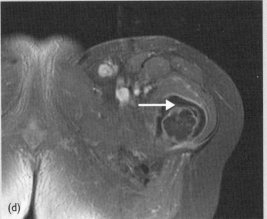

Case 38.1 (a, b) T1-weighted and STIR sagittal images and (c, d) STIR and post-Gd FS T1-weighted FSE axial images showing a metastasis in the proximal femur destroying the cortex posteriorly.

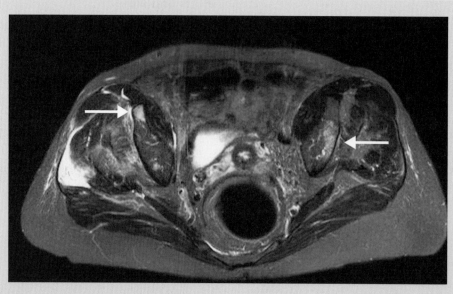

Case 38.2 FS T2-weighted axial image showing areas of high signal in the ischial bones in a different patient with multiple metastasis.

PIGMENTED VILLONODULAR SYNOVITIS (PVNS)

PVNS is a monoarticular proliferation of haemorrhagic synovium occurring in joint, bursa and tendon sheaths.

Key sequences

- FS PD-weighted FSE
- T2*-weighted

Imaging findings

There is a large effusion and subtle erosions.

Synovial masses may be solitary nodular or extensive, extending along juxta-articular ligaments.

On T1-weighted images, PVNS is low signal and homogeneous. On T2-weighted images it is low signal and inhomogeneous, depending on variable contents and blood products.

Blooms appear on gradient echo (GRE) images, due to the presence of haemosiderin.

There is moderate to intense inhomogeneous enhancement.

Hints and tips

Blooming on GRE is not pathognomic – haemophilia does the same.

Further reading

Murphey MD, Rhee JH, Lewis RB et al. Pigmented villonodular synovitis: radiologic–pathologic correlation. *Radiographics* 2008; **28**: 1493–518.

Case 39: PVNS of the knee

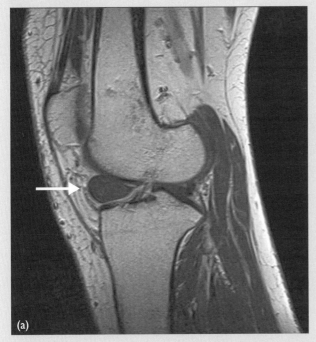
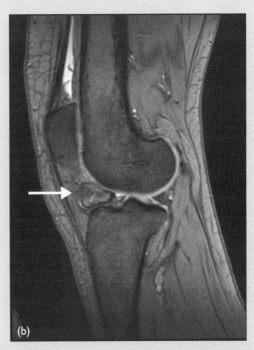

Case 39.1 (a, b) T1-weighted and PD-weighted sagittal images showing an abnormal-signal soft tissue mass in the anterior knee joint.

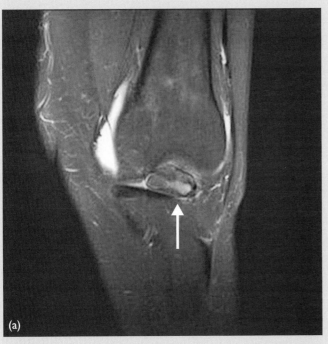
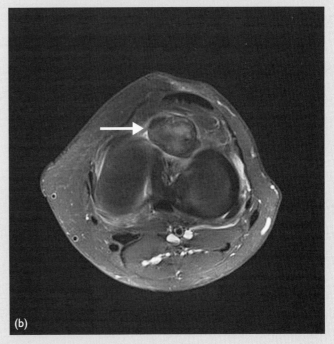

Case 39.2 (a, b) FS PD-weighted FSE images showing the soft tissue mass with heterogeneous signal within the mass.

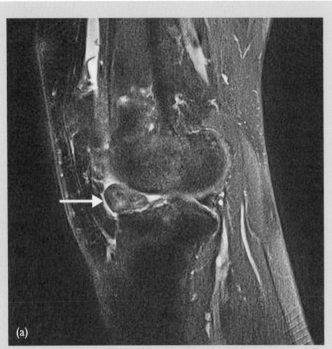 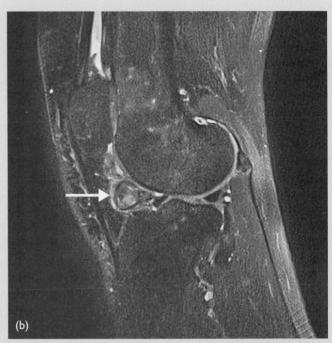

Case 39.3 (a, b) FS T2-weighted GRE images showing the predominantly low-signal soft tissue mass in the anterior knee, indicating paramagnetic material, in keeping with PVNS

OSTEOMYELITIS

Infection of the bone is called osteomyelitis. The most common cause is staphylococci. Other bacteria include streptococci, *Mycobacterium tuberculosis* and *Salmonella*. Osteomyelitis shows age-specific pathogens:
- age < 1 year: group B streptococci and *Staphylococcus aureus*
- age < 1 year: *S. aureus*, *Escherichia coli* and *Haemophilus influenzae*
- adults: *S. aureus* and *Pseudomonas* spp.

In addition, there are pathogens specific to people with certain pre-existing conditions:
- sickle cell disease: *Salmonella* spp.
- diabetes: Gram-positive cocci

A localized form of osteomyelitis is a Brodie abscess. This occurs with a subacute presentation.

MRI reveals the extent of the disease, along with soft tissue components and articular extension. Identifying sequestrated bone may be difficult. Computed tomography is the modality of choice for assessing sequestration.

Key sequences

- T1-weighted sequences show bony destruction and may reveal low-signal sequestered bone. With gadolinium

(Gd) enhancement, the soft tissue component and extent can be better appreciated.
- FS T2-weighted or STIR sequences help identify bony and soft tissue oedema.

Imaging features

On T1-weighted imaging, there is bony destruction with subperiosteal abscess.

Bone oedema is seen as low T1 and high T2 signal.

Secondary signs of osteomyelitis include ulcers, cellulitis, soft tissue collections, sinuses and cortical interruption.

Low signal within collections is identified as either sequestered bone or pockets of gas.

Gd enhancement identifies the extent of soft tissue involvement and defines the wall of the abscess cavity from phlegmon.

As osteomyelitis becomes more chronic, there is increasing heterogeneity of marrow signal. Sclerosis is identified by low T1 and T2 signal of the bone surrounding the abscess cavity.

A Brodie abscess shows a low-signal wall from sclerosed bone, with surrounding bone marrow oedema and a central low-signal sequestrum.

Hints and tips

STIR imaging points to the sight of the pathology.

T1-weighted imaging with Gd enhancement helps to assess the extent of the collections.

Further reading

Sammak B, Abd El Bagi M, Al Shahed M et al. Pictorial Review: Osteomyelitis: a review of currently used imaging techniques. *Eur Radiol* 1999; **9**: 894–900.

Case 40: Osteomyelitis of the femoral stump

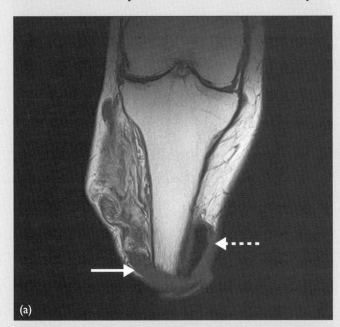 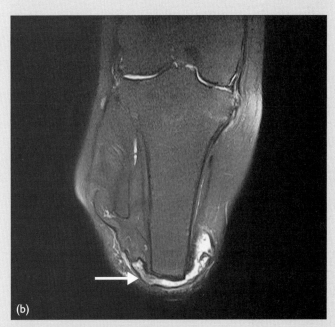

Case 40.1 (a, b) T1-weighted and FS PD-weighted coronal images showing a collection adjacent to the amputation stump of the femur (full arrow), with signal loss in gas (dotted arrow).

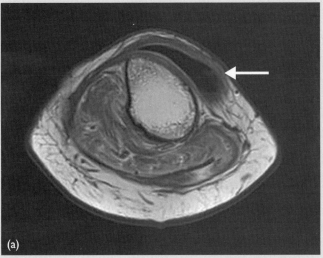 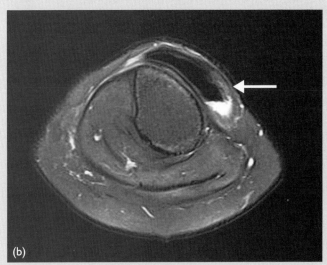

Case 40.2 (a, b) T1-weighted and FS PD-weighted axial images showing an air (signal loss) and fluid (low T1-weighted/high T2-weighted) level.

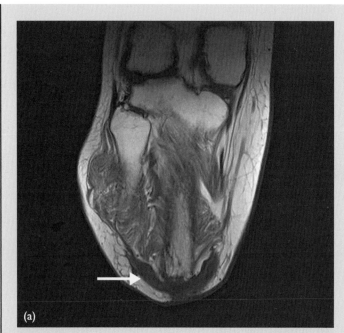
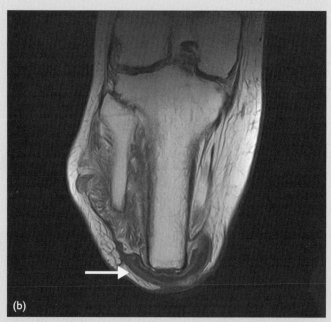

Case 40.3 (a, b) T1-weighted and Gd-enhanced T1-weighted coronal images showing enhancement of the wall of the collection.

Case 41: Brodie abscess of the tibia

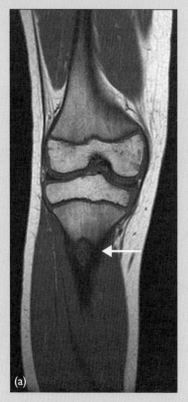
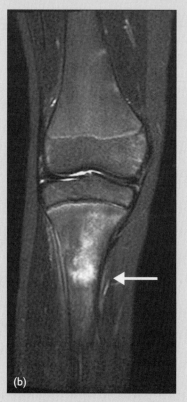

Case 41.1 (a, b) T1- and T2-weighted coronal images showing a Brodie abscess with adjacent bone oedema.

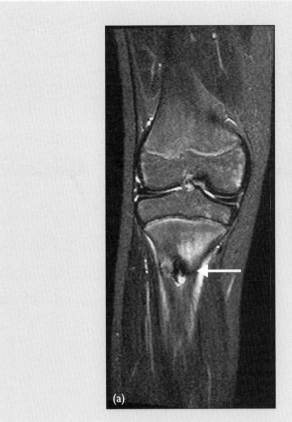

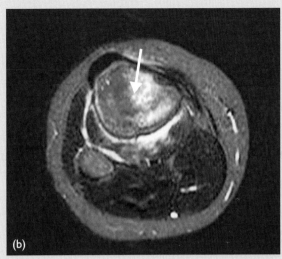

Case 41.2 (a, b) FS T2-weighted coronal and axial images showing the abscess.

Case 42: Osteomyelitis after a total knee replacement

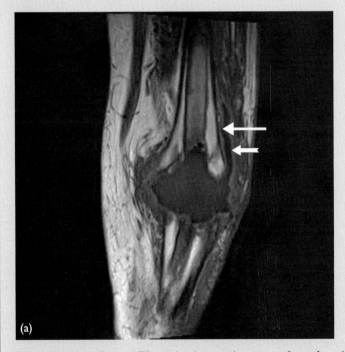

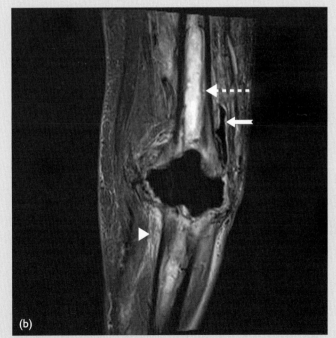

Case 42.1 (a, b) T1- and T2-weighted coronal sections of an infected total knee replacement showing raised periosteal reaction (full arrow) with marked bone marrow (dotted arrow) and soft tissue oedema (arrowhead). There is signal loss from gas in the soft tissues (notched arrow).

UNIT II
Neuro-MRI

Kshitij Mankad, Sanjoy Nagaraja, Anthony JP Goddard,
Omid Nikoubashman

1 SEQUENCES AND PROTOCOLS IN NEURO-MRI

SEQUENCES

From the neuroradiological perspective, the following sequences may be considered as key. A basic understanding of the practical importance of each is described, without delving too much into the physics of MR sequences.

T1 weighting

T1 is the exponential time constant of a tissue during which it recovers its magnetization towards its horizontal equilibrium state (along $\mathbf{B}_0$) after having been subjected to a radiofrequency pulse. Tissues differ in their T1 values, and therefore T1-weighted sequences are good for assessing regional anatomy.

Table 1.1 lists commonly used T1-weighted sequences.

T2 weighting

The relaxation time constant T2 refers to the decay of transverse magnetization due to spins getting out of phase. T2 is affected by pathophysiological changes more easily than T1, and is therefore a good sequence for assessing pathology.

Table 1.2 lists commonly used T2-weighted sequences.

T2* weighting

T2* takes into account local magnetic field homogeneities and is like a T2-weighted sequence but with extra dephasing effects. It is specifically sensitive to the presence of iron in the brain parenchyma and is therefore good for estimating the age of blood products.

DWI/ADC

Diffusion-weighted imaging (DWI) probes the Brownian motion of water molecules. The greater the displacement, the greater the signal attenuation. It is most widely used in acute stroke imaging, where the diffusion of water molecules is restricted, returning a high signal. The apparent diffusion coefficient (ADC) measures the magnitude of diffusion, and as such it confirms what is seen on DWI – if the 'ischaemia' demonstrated on DWI is not secondary to an artefact known as T2 shine-through. Thus, ADC and DWI work as positive and negative pictures of each other.

Table 1.1 T1-weighted sequences commonly used in neuro-MRI

Sequence	Acronyms	Common principles
Conventional spin echo	SE, CSE	Uses basic T1 properties
Time-of-flight magnetic resonance angiography	TOF-MRA	Inflow enhancement of blood, with suppression of stationary tissue
Gradient echo	GRE	
Post-gadolinium (Gd)		Gd shortens T1

Adapted from Roberts TPL, Mikulis D. Neuro MR: principles. *J Magn Reson Imaging* 2007; **26**: 823–37.

Table 1.2 T2-weighted sequences commonly used in neuro-MRI

Sequence	Acronyms	Common principles
Conventional spin echo	SE, CSE	Long acquisition times
Fast spin echo (rapid acquisition with relaxation enhancement)	FSE, RARE	Many times faster than CSE, but still retains diagnostic spatial resolution
Fluid-attenuated inversion recovery	FLAIR	A long T1 and inversion recovery prepulse are employed to negate the signal from cerebrospinal fluid (CSF)
Constructive interference in steady-state imaging (fast imaging with steady-state acquisition)	CISS, FIESTA	High-resolution sequence allowing multiplanar reconstruction. Good for structures surrounded by CSF (e.g. cranial nerves)

Adapted from Roberts TPL, Mikulis D. Neuro MR: principles. *J Magn Reson Imaging* 2007; **26**: 823–37.

PROTOCOLS

Table 1.3 summarizes protocols for neuro-MRI.

RECOMMENDED READING

e-MRI: MRI Physics Interactive Tutorial. Available at: www.imaios.com/en/e-Courses/e-MRI/.

Mikulis D, Roberts TPL. Neuro MR: protocols. *J Magn Reson Imaging* 2007; **26**: 838–47.

Roberts TPL, Mikulis D. Neuro MR: principles. *J Magn Reson Imaging* 2007; **26**: 823–37.

Table 1.3 Protocols for neuro-MRI

Protocol	Sequence
Standard or screening brain	Sagittal T1-weighted Axial T2-weighted Axial FLAIR T2*-weighted (maybe) DWI (maybe)
Stroke	Sagittal T1-weighted Axial T2-weighted Axial FLAIR Axial GRE Axial DWI
Multiple sclerosis	Sagittal T1-weighted Axial T2-weighted Axial FLAIR Sagittal T2-weighted
Temporal lobes	Sagittal T1-weighted Axial T2-weighted Coronal T2-weighted Coronal FLAIR
Tumour	Axial T2-weighted Axial and coronal T1-weighted pre- and post-Gd
Cranial nerves	**Face:** Axial and coronal T1-weighted pre-contrast Axial and coronal T1-weighted fat-saturated post-Gd Coronal T2-weighted fat-saturated **Head:** Axial T2*-weighted Axial CISS
Pituitary	**Brain:** Axial T2-weighted **Pituitary:** Sagittal T1-weighted pre-Gd Coronal T1-weighted pre- and post-Gd

Protocol	Sequence
Orbits	**Brain:** Axial T2-weighted **Orbits:** Axial STIR Coronal T1-weighted pre-Gd Axial and Coronal T1-weighted fat-saturated post-Gd
Internal auditory meatus (IAM) screening	Axial T2-weighted Axial CISS
IAM tumour	**Brain:** Axial T2-weighted **IAM:** Axial T1-weighted pre- and post-Gd Coronal T1-weighted post-Gd
Circle of Willis	Axial T2 whole brain 3D-TOF
Magnetic resonance venography (MRV)	Axial T2 whole brain Coronal T1-weighted 3D-TOF MRV
Carotids	Axial T1-weighted fat-saturated MRA
Horner's syndrome	Axial T2-weighted brain Coronal T1-weighted orbits Coronal STIR orbits Sagittal T2-weighted C-spine Axial T1-weighted fat-saturated neck Coronal STIR brachial plexus
Skull base	Axial T1-weighted Coronal T1-weighted Coronal STIR Axial T1-weighted post-Gd Coronal T1-weighted fat-saturated post-Gd

2 NEUROANATOMY

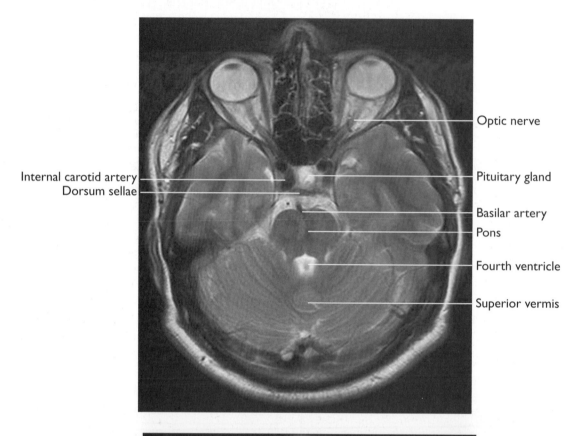

Optic nerve

Internal carotid artery
Dorsum sellae

Pituitary gland

Basilar artery
Pons

Fourth ventricle

Superior vermis

Figure 2.1

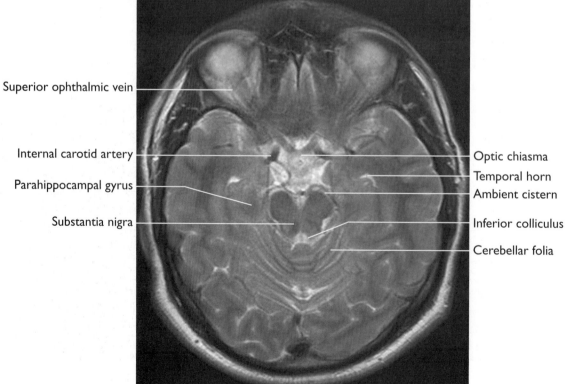

Superior ophthalmic vein

Internal carotid artery

Optic chiasma

Parahippocampal gyrus

Temporal horn
Ambient cistern

Substantia nigra

Inferior colliculus

Cerebellar folia

Figure 2.2

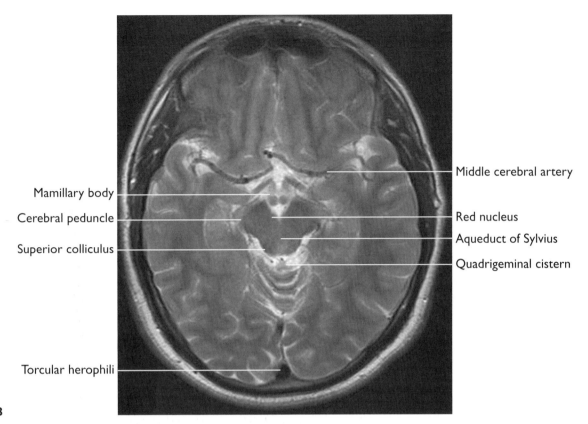

Middle cerebral artery

Mamillary body

Cerebral peduncle

Superior colliculus

Red nucleus

Aqueduct of Sylvius

Quadrigeminal cistern

Torcular herophili

Figure 2.3

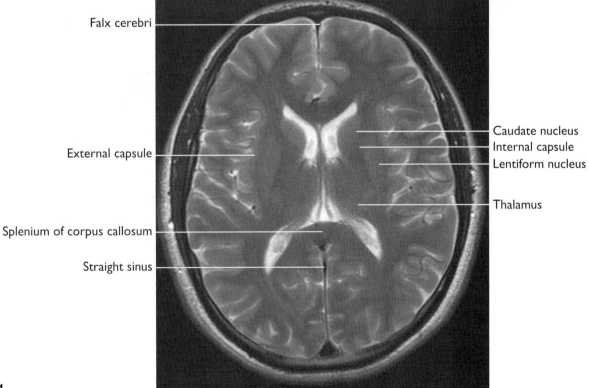

Falx cerebri

Caudate nucleus
Internal capsule
Lentiform nucleus

External capsule

Thalamus

Splenium of corpus callosum

Straight sinus

Figure 2.4

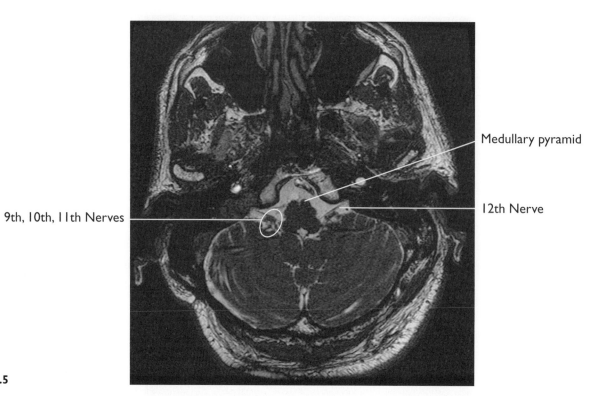

9th, 10th, 11th Nerves

Medullary pyramid

12th Nerve

Figure 2.5

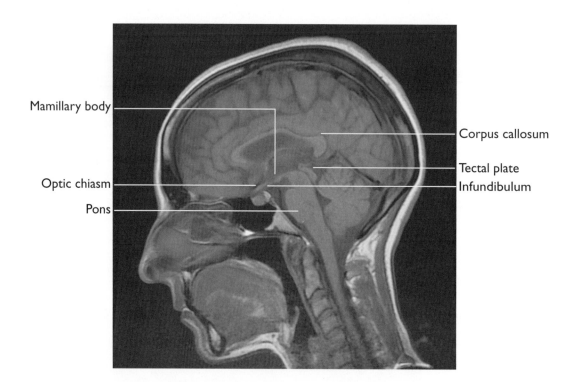

Mamillary body

Optic chiasm

Pons

Corpus callosum

Tectal plate

Infundibulum

Figure 2.6

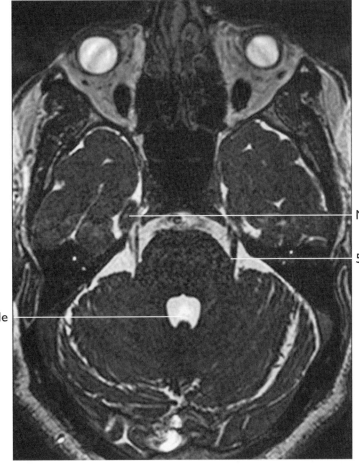

Meckel's Cave

5th Cranial Nerve

4th ventricle

Figure 2.7

3 VASCULAR PATHOLOGIES

EXTRACRANIAL ARTERIAL DISSECTION

Carotid dissection accounts for 10–20% of strokes in adults under 45 years of age. It is caused by a tear in the intima layer of the vessel wall, which allows blood to dissect longitudinally through the media, creating a false lumen. Stroke can occur secondary to narrowing of the true lumen or from embolization of blood clots forming at the site of the tear. The most common cause is rotational neck trauma, but it is also recognized to occur spontaneously in patients with collagen vascular disorders such as Ehlers–Danlos syndrome. The most common location for dissection is the cervical segment of the internal carotid artery (ICA) just distal to the carotid bulb, since this area is most susceptible to stretching during neck extension. An additional at-risk area is the vertebral artery between the C1 vertebra and the skull base. Dissections rarely extend intracranially beyond the point of entry of the ICA into the petrous temporal bone.

Key sequences

- Fat-saturated (FS) T1-weighted axial – to visualize the intramural haematoma
- Magnetic resonance angiography (MRA) (contrast-enhanced or time-of-flight, TOF) – to define the vessel lumen

Imaging findings

There is a narrowed eccentric flow void surrounded by a crescent-shaped hyperintense periarterial rim (an intramural haematoma, representing methaemoglobin).

The haematoma shows temporal evolution of its MR signal.

Tapered luminal narrowing or vascular occlusion is seen on both source images and maximum-intensity projections on MRA. Also look for intimal flap and pseudoaneurysm formation.

Hints and tips

An acute intramural haematoma (in the first 48 hours) can appear hypointense on T2- and T1-weighted images and therefore difficult to delineate from a flow void. Vessel wall thickening and luminal narrowing may be the only indicators of dissection at this stage.

A false-positive diagnosis may originate from misinterpretation of T1 hyperintense fat surrounding the vessel, which can mimic an intramural haematoma. The use of fat-suppression sequences helps avoid this pitfall in most cases.

When TOF-MRA is used, it is important to review the source data carefully in order to distinguish intramural haematoma from flow within the true lumen (flow generally has a more intense signal than haematoma).

Brain imaging, including diffusion-weighted imaging (DWI), should be performed to assess for signs of cerebral infarction secondary to haemodynamic compromise.

Further reading

Flis C, Jager HR, Sidhu PS. Carotid and vertebral artery dissections: clinical aspects, imaging features and endovascular treatment. *Eur J Radiol* 2007; **17**: 820–34.

Case 1: Extracranial arterial dissection

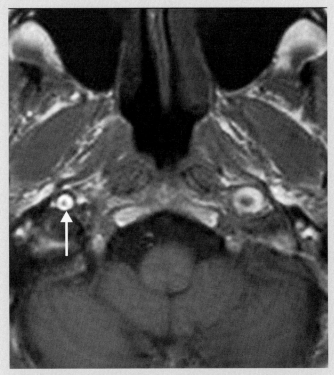

Case 1.1 FS T1-weighted axial image showing bilateral intramural haemorrhage in the carotid vessel wall (arrows). High signal on T1-weighted imaging indicates the presence of methaemoglobin.

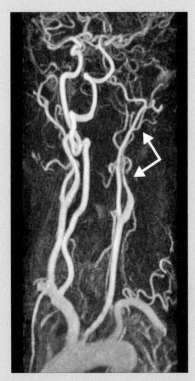

Case 1.2 Note the tapering of the lumen of the left internal carotid artery on contrast-enhanced MRA.

ISCHAEMIC STROKE

The majority of strokes are caused by embolic occlusion of cerebral blood supply, which initiates an ischaemic cascade with cytotoxic oedema and neuronal cell death. Thrombolysis with intravenous tissue plasminogen activator (tPA) is licensed for use in early ischaemic stroke, and careful selection of patients is crucial to improve safety and efficacy. Computed tomography (CT) retains a primary role in the evaluation of patients with acute stroke, but MRI, particularly DWI, is more sensitive and specific than CT for the detection of acute cerebral ischaemia.

Key sequences

- T2-weighted and fluid-attenuated inversion recovery (FLAIR) axial
- T2*-weighted gradient echo – to assess for haemorrhage
- DWI
- MRA (contrast-enhanced or TOF) of intra- and extracranial circulation

Imaging findings

There is a hyperintense signal in white matter on T2-weighted imaging and FLAIR within the first few hours.

Grey–white matter differentiation is lost and there is sulcal effacement and a mass effect.

There is loss of arterial flow void, with major vessel occlusion (intravascular thrombus).

An area of abnormal blooming is seen with acute haemorrhage on T2*-weighted images.

Ischaemic tissue appears high signal on DWI, with corresponding low signal on the apparent diffusion coefficient (ADC) map image.

Hints and tips

Conventional MRI is less sensitive than DWI in the first few hours after a stroke and may result in false-negative findings.

Comparison of DWI with the ADC map image should always be performed, since high DWI signal can reflect high T2 signal in the underlying tissues (T2 shine-through) and not infarction (in which the ADC map image is bright).

Thrombolytic therapy is most beneficial in patients with cytotoxic oedema involving less than one-third of the middle cerebral artery (MCA) territory.

Tissues in which ADC values are reduced almost always undergo irreversible infarction, and decrease in ADC values is only rarely reversible with thrombolysis.

With T2*-weighted sequences, cerebral microhaemorrhages are increasingly detectable in patients with acute stroke. The risk of thrombolysis in this group remains unclear, since current criteria are based on CT evidence of haemorrhage.

Further reading

Srinivasan A, Goyal M, Al Azri F, and Lum C. State-of-the-art imaging of acute stroke. *Radiographics* 2006; **26**: S75–95.

Thurnher M, Castillo M. Imaging in acute stroke. *Eur Radiol* 2005; **15**: 408–15.

Case 2: Ischaemic stroke

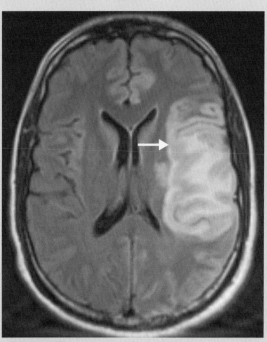

Case 2.1 Axial T2-weighted axial image demonstrating infarction due to branch vessel occlusion in the left middle cerebral artery territory.

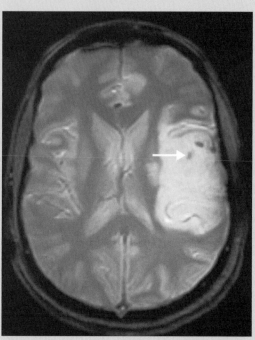

Case 2.2 T2* image showing foci of haemorrhagic transformation.

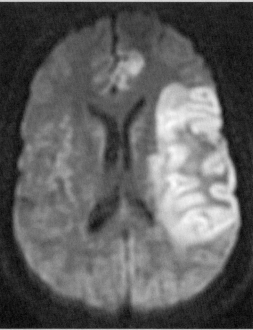

Case 2.3 DWI sequence reveals restricted diffusion in the area of infarct.

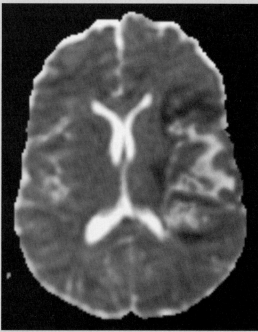

Case 2.4 ADC map confirms acute restriction of diffusion as signal drop-out areas.

CEREBRAL VENOUS SINUS THROMBOSIS

Cerebral venous sinus thrombosis has a varied and often non-specific clinical presentation. The superior sagittal and transverse sinuses are most frequently involved. Predisposing factors include oral contraceptive use and pregnancy in women of childbearing age. Direct spread of infection (e.g. mastoiditis) is a frequent cause in children. No cause is identified in up to 35% of cases. MRI is superior to CT for detecting the subtle parenchymal abnormalities that are often associated.

Key sequences

- T1- and T2-weighted, FLAIR, and T2*-weighted axial/coronal
- TOF, phase contrast or contrast-enhanced venography

Imaging findings

The normal sinus flow void is absent on conventional sequences.

Early thrombus (day 1–5) is isointense on T1-weighted images and hypointense on T2-weighted images.

Thrombus signal evolves over time (hyperintense on T1- and hyperintense on T2-weighted images by day 7).

Focal areas of high T2 signal (venous ischaemia) may be seen in areas not directly drained by the occluded sinus.

Segments of flow void are a sign of thrombus on TOF/phase contrast venography.

Central intraluminal filling defects are a sign of thrombus on contrast venography.

Hints and tips

Anatomical variants can mimic sinus thrombosis, including sinus hypoplasia and atresia (look for the size of the bony ridge on CT or MRI) and can usually be differentiated by reviewing the source images.

'Flow gaps' may result from fat, fibrous bands and arachnoid granulations. Arachnoid granulations appear as well-demarcated areas of low signal on T1-weighted images and high signal on T2-weighted images and display central curvilinear contrast enhancement.

Two-dimensional (2D) TOF techniques are most sensitive to flow perpendicular to the plane of acquisition. Non-perpendicular acquisition can cause nulling of the venous signal and the appearance of 'flow gaps'.

Deep cerebral vein thrombosis is associated with an extremely poor prognosis – thalamic oedema is the imaging hallmark of this condition.

Further reading

Leach JL, Fortuna RB, Jones BV et al. Imaging of cerebral venous thrombosis: current techniques, spectrum of findings, and diagnostic pitfalls. *Radiographics* 2006; **26**: S19–41.

Renowden S. Cerebral venous sinus thrombosis. *Eur Radiol* 2004; **14**: 215–26.

Case 3: Cerebral venous sinus thrombosis

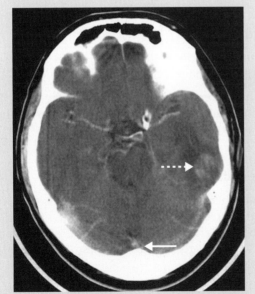

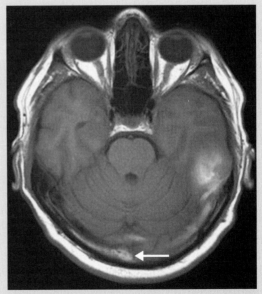

Case 3.1 Contrast-enhanced CT scan of a patient presenting with venous sinus thrombosis. The full arrow points at a filling defect in the inferior sagittal sinus. The dotted arrow demonstrates an area of venous haemorrhagic infarction with surrounding oedema.

Case 3.2 T1-weighted axial image showing high-signal thrombus (arrow) in the inferior sagittal sinus. Also note the associated haemorrhagic cortical venous infarct in the left temporal region.

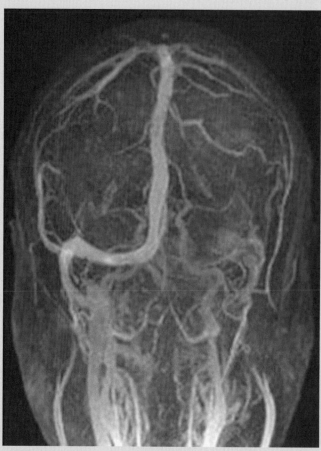

Case 3.3 Magnetic resonance venography on the same patient confirming that the left transverse sinus is occluded.

BERRY ANEURYSM

Berry aneurysms are saccular aneurysms that commonly form on the arteries of the circle of Willis, at the base of the brain. They may rarely be seen in association with adult polycystic kidney disease and coarctation of the aorta, but are not usually associated with any specific predisposing condition. Large aneurysms may cause symptoms as a result of local pressure effects: for example, aneurysm of the posterior communicating artery can cause painful third cranial nerve palsy. More often, aneurysms remain asymptomatic and are identified for the first time following spontaneous rupture and subarachnoid haemorrhage. CT angiography is increasingly utilized as the modality of choice in the acute setting. Aneurysms may be detected incidentally on MRI examinations performed for another indication. MRA or CT angiography may also be used to monitor aneurysm size.

Key sequences

- T1- and T2-weighted and FLAIR axial/coronal/sagittal
- TOF or contrast-enhanced MRA

Imaging findings

A rounded lesion with internal signal void is seen on T2-weighted images, closely associated with a vessel.

Partially thrombosed aneurysms display high T1 signal due to thrombus or an 'onion skin' appearance due to multiple layers of thombus of different ages.

Hints and tips

A giant aneurysm with partial thrombosis may mimic a solid destructive skull base tumour. CT angiography may be especially useful in this setting, since it is less subject to flow-related artefact and bone detail may be assessed.

Further reading

Wardlaw JM, White PM. The detection and management of unruptured intracranial aneurysms. *Brain* 2000; **123**: 205–21.

Case 4: Berry aneurysm

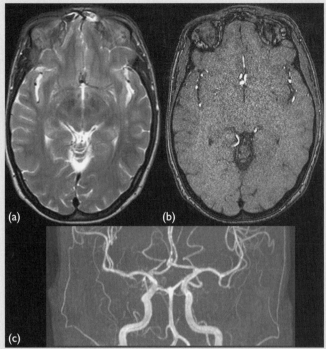

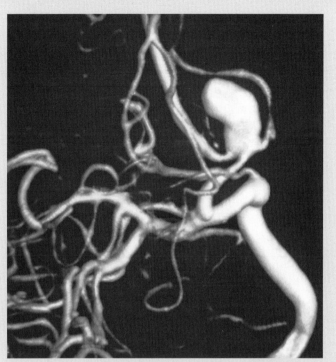

Case 4.1 (a) T2-weighted imaging demonstrates flow voids in the anterior communicating artery territory consistent with small Berry aneurysms. (b, c) MRA confirms these and their location.

Case 4.2 3D reformat of MRA showing a large wide-based aneurysm and its relationship to the parent vessel.

SMALL-VESSEL ISCHAEMIA

This occurs to some degree as a normal part of the aging process, although it may be accelerated in those with cerebrovascular risk factors such as smoking and hypertension. Atherosclerotic brain changes are seen on MRI in up to 50% of patients older than 50 years and are thought to be the result of hypoxic ischaemic injury and resultant microangiopathy. What is considered normal depends upon the age of the patient. Ischaemic white matter lesions present as lacunar infarcts (arteriolar sclerosis of small penetrating end arteries) or more diffuse changes in the deep cerebral white matter. It is important to recognize the typical findings that are very prevalent in old age so as not to mistake them for inflammatory or other pathology.

Key sequence

- T2-weighted and FLAIR sagittal

Imaging findings

There are punctate or confluent foci of high T2 signal in the deep white matter of the centra semiovale.

The Fazekas classification is a useful guide to the significance of these lesions:

- Fazekas I: punctate white matter, high-T2-signal foci (normal in ageing)
- Fazekas II: confluent white matter, high T2 signal (abnormal in age < 75 years)
- Fazekas III: extensive confluent white matter, high T2 signal (always abnormal)

Other features of age-related change are:
- periventricular high-T2-signal 'caps' around the frontal and occipital horns of the lateral ventricles
- mild cerebral atrophy with compensatory ventricular dilatation
- dilated perivascular spaces

Hints and tips

Age-related white matter lesions are very common, and only if the clinical findings strongly suggest an inflammatory, infectious or toxic aetiology should these diagnoses be strongly considered for high-T2 white matter foci.

Unlike multiple sclerosis, age-related white matter lesions do not touch the ventricles, do not touch the cortex and are not found in the corpus callosum. Small-vessel disease sometimes involves the brainstem, but usually in a symmetrical and central fashion, in contrast to multiple sclerosis, which typically has a peripheral distribution.

Further reading

Bot JCJ, Barkhof F, Nijeholt GL et al. Differentiation of multiple sclerosis from other inflammatory disorders and cerebrovascular disease: value of spinal MR imaging. *Radiology* 2002; **223**: 46–56.

Polman CH, Reingold SC, Edan G et al. Diagnostic criteria for multiple sclerosis: 2005 revisions to the 'McDonald Criteria'. *Ann Neurol* 2005; **58**: 840–6.

Case 5: Small-vessel ischaemia

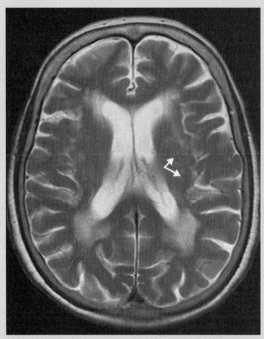

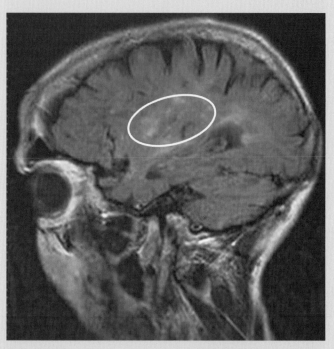

Case 5.1 T2-weighted axial image showing punctate high-signal foci in the deep white matter bilaterally representing Fazekas type I changes of small-vessel ischaemia. Also note the periventricular ischaemic changes.

Case 5.2 T2-weighted sagittal image showing more confluent high-signal foci within the deep white matter, signifying Fazekas type II changes. Also note that these lesions do not touch the ventricles (as seen in multiple sclerosis).

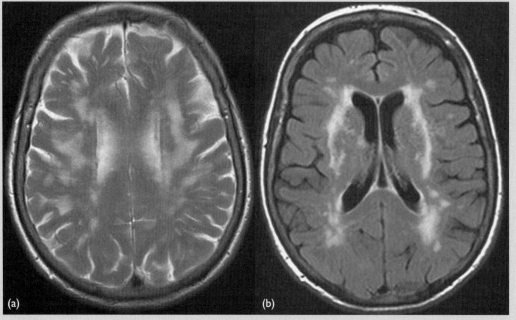

Case 5.3 Extensive confluent Fazekas type III changes demonstrated on T2-weighted (a) and FLAIR (b) axial images.

DEMENTIA

MRI has revolutionized the management of dementia by making possible early diagnosis and classification of its subtypes, thus guiding appropriate treatment. MRI can exclude other conditions that can mimic dementia, such as normal-pressure hydrocephalus.

Key sequences

- T1-weighted high-resolution volumetric, keeping the plane orthogonal to the long axis of the hippocampus to assess atrophic change here
- FLAIR to assess cortical atrophy, hyperintense lesions in the white matter and infarctions
- T2-weighted to assess for small infarctions
- Axial FLAIR and axial whole-brain T2 to assess parenchyma and microangiopathy load

Imaging findings

A clear understanding of the anatomy is essential, since different processes can affect typical anatomic sites.

Medial temporal atrophy and parietal atrophy are associated with Alzheimer's disease.

Frontal lobe atrophy is a feature of frontotemporal lobar degeneration.

White matter lesions and infarcts are consistent with a diagnosis of vascular dementia.

Hints and tips

Various quantitative scales have been described to assess degrees of cortical atrophy, medial temporal atrophy and white matter lesions.

Look for 'strategic infarcts', that is, infarcts in regions that deal with specific cognitive functions.

In patients with Alzheimer's disease, there is a specific route of atrophic progression involving the anteromedial temporal lobe and entorhinal cortex first, then the neocortex and then the sensory cortex. Thus, repeat imaging showing this progression may be helpful.

Further reading

Keyserling H, Mukundan S. The role of conventional MR and CT in the work-up of dementia patients. *Magn Reson Imaging Clin N Am* 2006; **14**: 169–82.

Kantarci K, Jack CR Jr. Neuroimaging in Alzheimer disease: an evidence-based review. *Neuroimaging Clin N Am* 2003; **13**: 197–209.

Case 6: Dementia

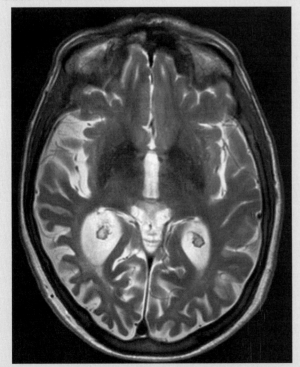

Case 6.1 T2-weighted axial image showing micro-infarcts in the basal ganglia bilaterally, suggesting vascular dementia as the most likely cause in this patient. Also note the early atrophic changes in the cortex of the temporal lobes.

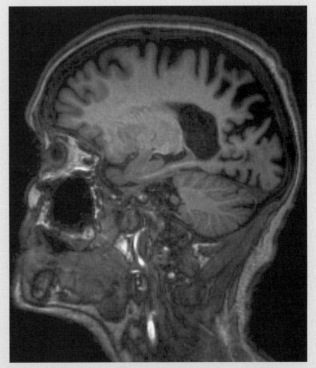

Case 6.2 T1-weighted sagittal image showing atrophic changes of frontotemporal dementia.

4 NEOPLASMS

VESTIBULAR SCHWANNOMA

Vestibular schwannoma is a benign slow-growing tumour that develops from the Schwann sheath of the inferior vestibular nerve in the internal auditory canal. It is the most frequent tumour of the cerebellopontine angle accounting for 70 to 80% of all masses here and typically presents with sensorineural deafness. There is an association with type 2 neurofibromatosis, and bilateral schwannomas are pathognomonic of this condition. As the tumour grows, it smoothly erodes the porus acousticus and then expands as a round or oval component into the cerebellopontine cistern.

Key sequences

- High-resolution T2-weighted fast spin echo (FSE) axial
- T1-weighted post-gadolinium axial

Imaging findings

The intracanalicular portion and the larger cerebellopontine cistern component have an 'ice cream-on-cone' appearance.

Occasionally, a small purely intracanalicular tumour is seen.

Schwannomas are isointense on T1-weighted and high signal on T2-weighted images.

Large lesions (>25 mm) invariably contain cystic components.

There is avid homogeneous enhancement in small lesions on post-gadolinium images. Larger lesions show a heterogeneous enhancement pattern.

Hints and tips

The following important observations aid treatment planning:

- Tumour size is assessed most reproducibly on axial slices by measuring the two largest diameters of the extracanalicular portion of the tumour, parallel and perpendicular to the posterior surface of the petrous temporal bone.
- The distance between the lateral extremity of the intracanalicular portion of the tumour and the fundus is significant because it affects hearing prognosis and may modify the surgical approach.
- Identification of the facial nerve and its position relative to the tumour is best done on post-contrast sequences, which amplify differences of signal intensity between the tumour and the nerve.

Further reading

Bonneville F, Savatovsky J, Chiras J. Imaging of cerebellopontine angle lesions: an update. Part 1: enhancing extra-axial lesions *Eur Radiol* 2007; **17**: 2472–82

Case 7: Vestibular schwannoma

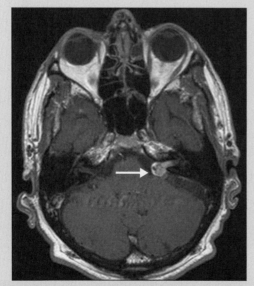

Case 7.1 Post-contrast T1-weighted axial image showing the typical 'ice cream-on-cone' appearance of a left-sided vestibular schwannoma.

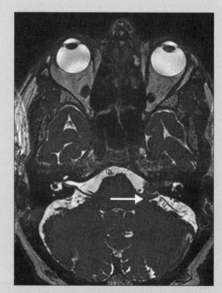

Case 7.2 Left-sided vestibular lesion on an image obtained using a 3D high-resolution volumetric T2-weighted sequence.

PITUITARY ADENOMA

Pituitary tumours are relatively common. Clinical manifestations depend upon hormone production and tumour size. Tumours arising from the anterior lobe of the gland are more common, and include those that secrete prolactin, growth hormone and corticotropin (adrenocorticotropic hormone, ACTH) to cause Cushing's syndrome. Tumours less than 1 cm in size are termed microadenomas, while macroadenomas are larger than 1 cm.

Key sequences

- T1- and T2-weighted axial/coronal/sagittal through the pituitary fossa
- Dynamic contrast-enhancement imaging

Imaging findings

Most adenomas are of low T1 and high T2 signal compared with normal pituitary tissue.

A convex outline and stalk deviation are supportive features of a pituitary microadenoma.

The normal pituitary gland and stalk enhance strongly in the early phase of dynamic imaging compared with microadenomas, which show little enhancement.

Macroadenomas expand out of the pituitary fossa, either superiorly to elevate and compress the optic chiasma or laterally into the adjacent cavernous sinus.

Hints and tips

On unenhanced images, encasement of the internal carotid artery is suggestive of tumour invasion into the cavernous sinus.

On contrast-enhanced images, the normal cavernous sinus displays avid enhancement and better displays the extent of tumour invasion.

The abrupt transition between the air-filled sphenoid bone and the dense cortical bone of the sella floor causes a distortion in the local magnetic field and a subtle increase in signal intensity in the pituitary gland on T1-weighted images. Spin echo imaging is preferred to avoid this artefact.

Further reading

Steiner E, Imhof H, Knosp E et al. Gd-DTPA enhanced high resolution MR imaging of pituitary adenomas. *Radiographics* 1989; **9**: 587–98.

Case 8: Pituitary adenoma

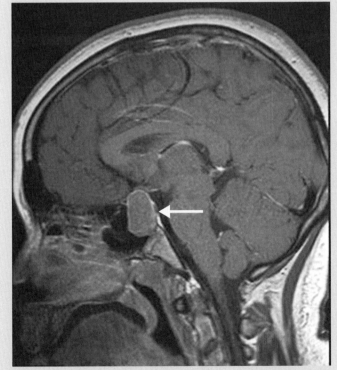

Case 8.1 T1-weighted sagittal image showing an enhancing pituitary adenoma.

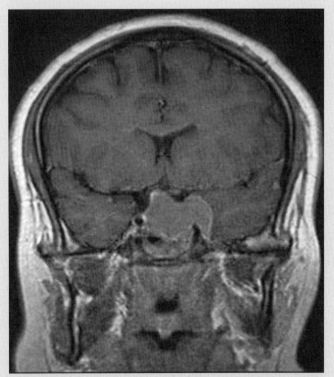

Case 8.2 Coronal imaging is regularly used to assess the exact local spread of pituitary tumours and their effect on surrounding structures. In this case, the tumour is seen to extend into the left cavernous sinus.

HIGH-GRADE GLIOMA (GLIOBLASTOMA MULTIFORME)

Glioblastoma is the most common primary brain tumour, with a peak incidence in the sixth decade. It is a high-grade (WHO grade 4) diffusely infiltrating neoplasm that arises in the deep white matter and is invariably unresectable for cure at time of diagnosis. These lesions have a high metabolic rate and prominent neovascularity, and usually undergo central necrosis, which accounts for their typical enhancement pattern on MRI.

Key sequences

- T1-weighted axial/coronal/sagittal (depending on tumour location)
- T2-weighted axial/coronal/sagittal
- T1-weighted post-contrast

Imaging findings

A large complex mass lesion of mixed signal intensity is seen on T1- and T2-weighted imaging.

There is extensive surrounding oedema and a mass effect.

Central cystic elements reflect tumour necrosis.

There is a thick (>10 mm) enhancing rim with an irregular margin.

The tumour has a tendency to invade white matter tracts and cross the midline via the corpus callosum – 'butterfly glioma'.

Hints and tips

Distinguishing features between glioma and abscess are that an abscess rim is usually thin (2–7 mm) and smooth on its outer and inner aspects and an abscess contains fluid that shows restricted diffusion on appropriate imaging. Clinical signs such as fever are also useful in helping distinguish them.

Additional differential diagnoses include solitary metastasis – sometime differentiation is very difficult without biopsy. Metastases have greater vasogenic oedema for their size, and of course may be multiple.

Further reading

Altman DA, Atkinson DS, Brat DJ et al. Best cases from the AFIP: Glioblastoma multiforme. *Radiographics* 2007; **27**: 883–8.

Case 9: High-grade glioma (glioblastoma multiforme)

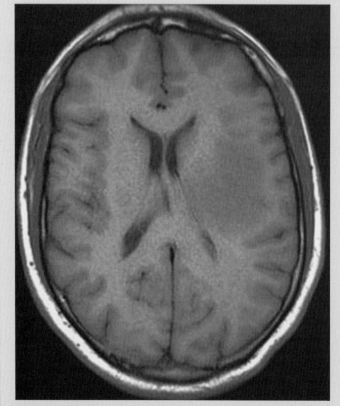

Case 9.1 T1-weighted image demonstrating a low-signal area in the left parietal lobe with effacement of the adjacent sulcal pattern.

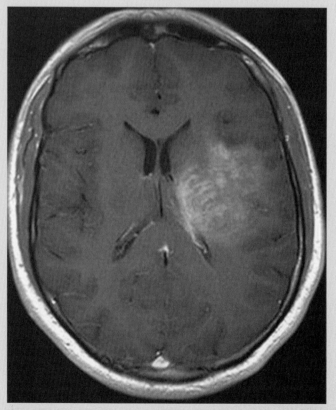

Case 9.2 There is enhancement of the left parietal lesion, delineating a glioma.

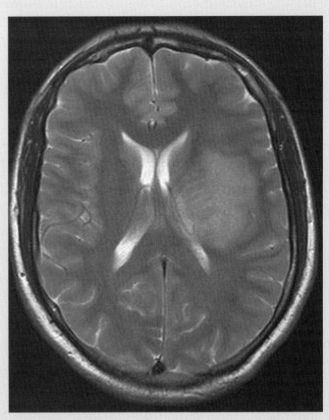

Case 9.3 The lesion demonstrates high signal intensity on a T2-weighted image.

MENINGIOMA

Meningiomas are the most common non-glial primary tumour of the brain. They arise from meningothelial cells of the arachnoid membrane, which is attached to the inner layer of the dura mater. In the majority of cases, their aetiology is unknown, although some occur as a manifestation of genetically inherited conditions such as neurofibromatosis type 2. They are slow-growing, well-localized, WHO grade 1 lesions that are often resectable for cure. They typically manifest clinically in the fourth to sixth decades of life, and are roughly twice as common in females as in males. Most common locations are over the cerebral convexities and parasagittal regions.

Key sequences

- T1-weighted axial/coronal/sagittal (depending on tumour location)
- T2-weighted axial/coronal/sagittal
- T1-weighted with contrast

Imaging findings

There is a localized extra-axial lesion with a broad base of dural attachment.

The lesion is isointense to hypointense on T1-weighted images and isointense to hyperintense on T2-weighted images.

A thin cerebrospinal fluid (CSF) cleft is seen separating the tumour from underlying brain parenchyma.

Twenty percent of meningiomas contain calcifications – areas of signal void on both T1- and T2-weighted images.

Perilesional oedema may be present in the underlying brain parenchyma.

There is avid homogeneous enhancement post-contrast.

Seventy percent display the 'dural tail sign' – a curvilinear region of dural enhancement adjacent to the main body of the tumour

Some meningiomas degenerate and develop cystic change within them. A small proportion also develop perilesional cysts, making the differential diagnosis difficult.

Hints and tips

Dural tail enhancement is thought to be caused by a reactive process rather than by dural infiltration by tumour, as was originally thought. Surgical resection of all enhancing dura mater is therefore not necessary. This enhancement is not specific for meningiomas – it has also been described in schwannomas, lymphoma, sarcoidosis and peripheral gliomas.

The imaging features of meningiomas may be atypical in terms of signal characteristics, tumour location and behaviour. Unusual locations include orbital, intraventricular and paranasal sinus lesions.

Rarely, meningiomas are malignant – metastases to extracranial sites such as the lungs have been described.

Further reading

O'Leary S, Adams WM et al. Atypical imaging appearances of intracranial meningiomas. *Clin Radiol* 2007; **62**: 10–17

Case 10: Meningioma

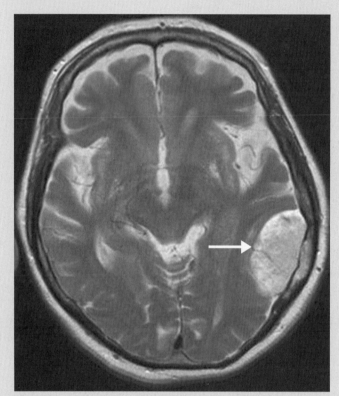

Case 10.1 T2-weighted axial image demonstrating a well-defined extra-axial lesion in the left parietal region.

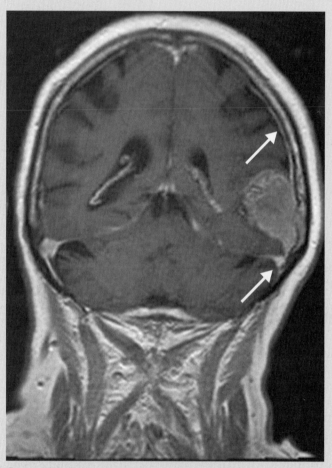

Case 10.2 Post-contrast T1-weighted coronal image showing strong contrast enhancement in the meningioma. Also note the dural tail associated with the tumour (arrows).

BRAIN METASTASES

Metastatic lesions are typically subcortical, occurring in or near the grey–white matter (corticomedullary) junction. This reflects infiltration of intravascular particulate material in this region, at the transition from abundant vessels in the cortical grey matter into the relatively sparse vasculature of the white matter. Tumour angiogenesis causes blood–brain barrier abnormalities, resulting in contrast enhancement and considerable perilesional vasogenic oedema. Because

of their typical location, even small metastases are likely to cause neurological symptoms, including seizures. The most common primary tumours are breast cancer, small cell lung cancer and melanoma. MRI is the most sensitive imaging modality for the detection of brain metastases.

Key sequences

- T2-weighted axial
- T1-weighted axial with contrast

Imaging findings

Small well-demarcated foci of high T2 signal are seen, with distinct 'pushing margins'.

There is extensive (disproportionate) surrounding oedema.

The lesions display homogeneous or rim enhancement.

Hints and tips

Increasing the dose of contrast agent and using delayed imaging protocols may reveal additional metastatic lesions.

Melanoma metastases have distinctive signal characteristics because of the paramagnetic effects of melanin, which shortens both T1 and T2 relaxation times. They are high signal on T1-weighted imaging and low signal on T2-weighted imaging.

Further reading

Smirniotopoulos J, Murphy FM, Rushing EJ et al. From the Archives of the AFIP: Patterns of contrast enhancement in the brain and meninges. *Radiographics* 2007; **27**: 525–51.

Case 11: Brain metastases

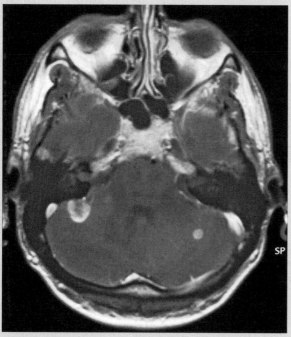

Case 11.1 Post-contrast T1-weighted axial image revealing multiple rim-enhancing lesions in the posterior fossa of the brain, consistent with metastases.

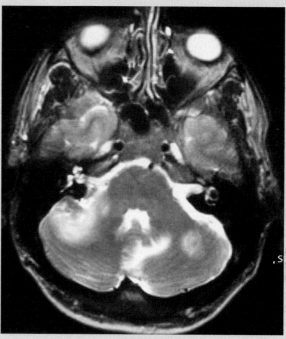

Case 11.2 T2-weighted axial image in the same patient revealing high-signal oedema surrounding these deposits.

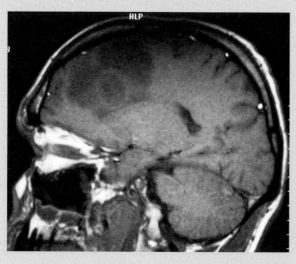

Case 11.3 Another patient with a known primary tumour in the lung. Note the extensive oedema surrounding the solitary brain metastasis in the frontal lobe.

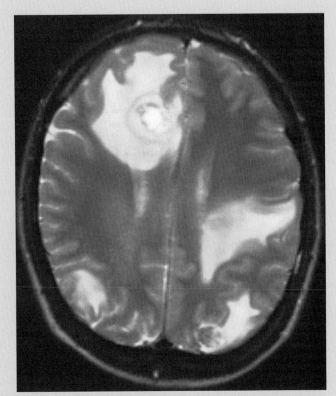

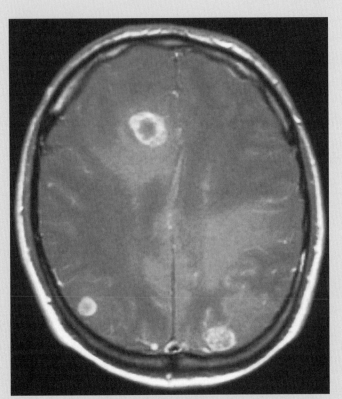

Case 11.4 High-signal cytotoxic oedema around the metastases. The T2-weighted image demonstrates multiple deposits.

Case 11.5 Post-contrast T1-weighted image from the same patient. Metastases show the typical rim-enhancement characteristic.

BRAIN LYMPHOMA

The frequency of primary central nervous system (CNS) lymphoma is on the rise. This is most likely a result of its strong association with long-term immunosuppressive therapy in post-transplant patients and with immunocompromised states such as AIDS. Primary CNS lymphoma occurs almost exclusively in the brain. The spinal cord is a rare site. Any age group can be affected by primary CNS lymphoma. Secondary cerebral involvement on the other hand is not uncommon in patients with non-Hodgkin's lymphoma (in up to 15% of cases at some point during the course of their illness).

Key sequences

- T1-weighted axial/coronal/sagittal
- T2-weighted with contrast

Imaging findings

The distribution of cerebral lymphoma is typical: more than 50% occur in the cerebral white matter in close proximity to and or involving the corpus callosum and the ependymal lining of the ventricles; these often spread across the midline in a butterfly pattern. In approximately 15% of cases, it localizes to the deep cortical grey matter of

the basal ganglia, thalamus and hypothalamus, developing in the posterior fossa of the brain in 11% of cases and being multifocal in 15%.

Lesions are typically hypo- or isointense on T1-weighted images, demonstrating enhancement post-contrast.

Lesions associated with immunocompromised states may appear ring-enhancing.

Plaque-like tumour deposits in the extracerebral spaces are features of secondary CNS lymphoma.

Hints and tips

Secondary cerebral lymphoma more commonly involves the extracerebral spaces and the spinal epidural and subarachnoid spaces. Imaging for suspected lymphoma should therefore cover the whole spine.

Further reading

Hobson DE, Anderson BA, Carr I, West M. Primary lymphoma of the central nervous system: Manitoba experience and literature review. *Can J Neurol Sci* 1986; **13**: 55–61.

Husband JE, Reznek RH, eds. *Imaging in Oncology*, 2nd edn. Taylor & Francis, 2004.

Case 12: Brain lymphoma

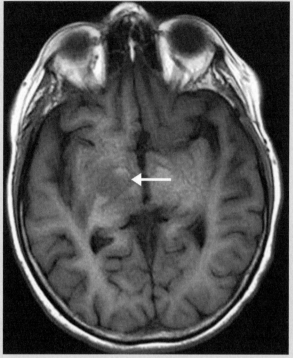

Case 12.1 T1-weighted axial image in a young confused patient demonstrating a subtle area of low signal intensity (arrow).

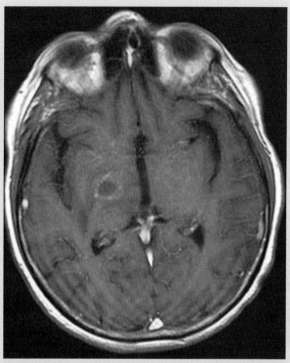

Case 12.2 Post-contrast T1-image confirming the presence of a single rim-enhancing lesion in the same location. This was proven on biopsy to be a primary brain lymphoma.

CRANIOPHARYNGIOMA

Craniopharyngiomas are common supratentorial tumours of childhood that arise from squamous epithelial rests lining the involuted Rathke's pouch. Although tumours of childhood (first and second decades), they are known to show a second peak in the fifth decade of life. They occur with equal frequency in males and females. Patients often present with headaches (due to obstruction of CSF flow), visual disturbances (due to compression of the chiasma) and disorders of the endocrine system.

Key sequences

- T1- and T2-weighted
- T1-weighted with contrast
- Sagittal and coronal sections help determine the relationship of the tumour to the optic chiasm and pituitary gland.

Imaging findings

The typical location for a craniopharyngioma is the suprasellar region. Rarely do these tumours occur at other intracranial sites.

As a rule, craniopharyngiomas demonstrate heterogeneous signal intensity. Various patterns have been observed: cystic being more common than others (hypointense on T1-weighted and hyperintense on T2-weighted images). The presence of protein or blood products in the lesion may produce increased signal intensity on T1-weighted imaging.

Heterogeneous post-contrast enhancement of the lesion is a feature.

Calcification is a common finding in these tumours.

Hints and tips

Rathke's cleft cysts, thrombosed aneurysms and cystic gliomas are the main differential diagnoses to consider at the time of reporting.

Further reading

Karavitaki N, Cudlip S, Adams CBT, Wass JAH. Craniopharyngiomas. *Endocr Rev* 2006; **27**: 371–97.

Case 13: Craniopharyngioma

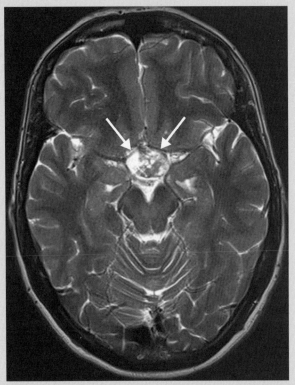

Case 13.1 Craniopharyngiomas (arrows) are heterogeneous tumours on T2-weighted images.

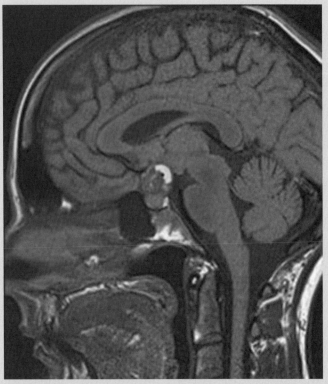

Case 13.2 T1-weighted image sagittal demonstrating a solid mixed-signal suprasellar lesion.

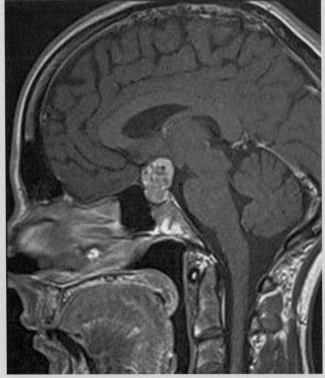

Case 13.3 Craniopharyngiomas enhance after contrast administration.

5 DEVELOPMENTAL CONDITIONS

CAVERNOUS ANGIOMA

This is a vascular malformation consisting of variable-sized intercapillary spaces, sinusoids, and larger cavernous spaces with no normal intervening brain tissue. Cavernous angiomas are prone to internal thrombosis and haemorrhage, and may present clinically with seizures and focal neurological deficits. Angiomas are commonly multiple and have an association with Osler–Weber–Rendu syndrome. A proportion are associated with genetic mutation, and are heritable. They are 'slow-flow' lesions and therefore not routinely identified at cerebral angiography. MRI is the imaging study of choice.

Key sequences

- T2*-weighted axial (the most sensitive sequence for detecting blood breakdown products)

Imaging findings

Cavernous angiomas are usually well-defined lobulated lesions with complex signal intensity caused by internal blood products of various ages.

Haemosiderin may be cleared from the centre of an angioma and deposited peripherally. Haemosiderin causes significant T2 shortening and causes a black 'halo' (or 'bloom') around the lesion.

There is little or no mass effect and no surrounding vasogenic oedema unless complicated by haemorrhage.

Further reading

Vilanova J, Barceló J, Smirniotopoulos J et al. Hemangioma from head to toe: MR imaging with pathologic correlation. *Radiographics* 2004; **24**: 367–85.

Case 14: Cavernous angioma

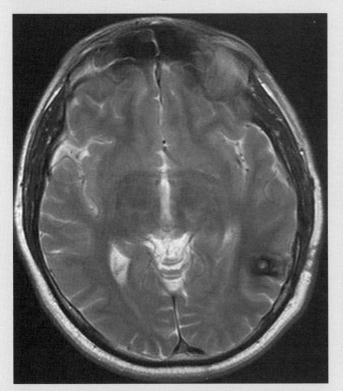

Case 14.1 Cavernomas appear as well-defined lobulated lesions with complex signal intensity due to internal blood products of different ages.

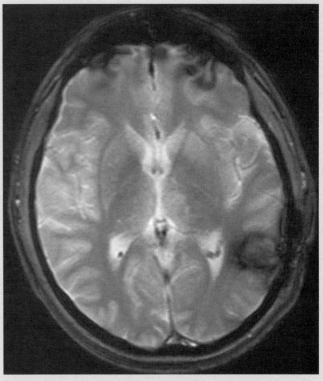

Case 14.2 Haemosiderin causes significant T2 shortening and a 'black halo' or 'bloom' around the lesion on T2*-weighted images.

ARACHNOID CYST

This is a benign developmental intra-arachnoid cerebrospinal fluid (CSF) collection caused by a focal splitting of the arachnoid membrane. The most common location is the floor of the middle cranial fossa, and around 10% are found in the cerebellopontine angle. Arachnoid cysts are usually asymptomatic, but slow expansion and pressure effects can cause headaches and focal neurological signs. Intracystic haemorrhage is a recognized complication, and has been described following minor head trauma. This may present as a neurosurgical emergency requiring decompression and cyst marsupialization.

Key sequences

- T1-weighted axial
- T2-weighted axial
- Fluid-attenuated inversion recovery (FLAIR) axial

Imaging findings

There is an extra-axial mass lesion compressing and displacing adjacent brain parenchyma.

The cyst contents are isointense to CSF on all pulse sequences.

Arachnoid cysts should be distinguished from epidermoid cysts at the cerebellopontine angle – epidermoid cysts appear bright on FLAIR, whereas arachnoid cysts are dark.

Major vessels may be seen to 'float' within the cyst.

A slowly enlarging mass may be associated with adjacent lobar hypoplasia and there may therefore be a disproportionately minor mass effect for the size of the lesion.

Further reading

De K, Berry K, Denniston S. Haemorrhage into an arachnoid cyst: a serious complication of minor head trauma. *Emerg Med J* 2002; **19**: 365–6.

Case 15: Arachnoid cyst

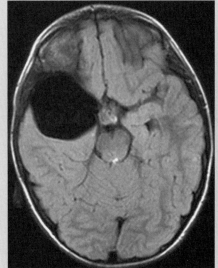

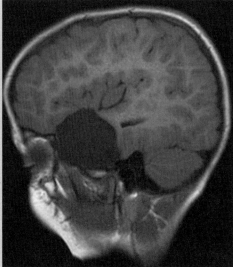

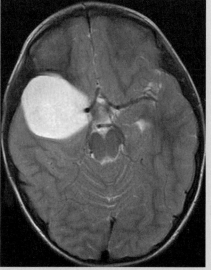

Case 15.1 Arachnoid cysts are isointense to CSF on all pulse sequences. This is a T1-weighted image.

Case 15.2 Sagittal image showing an arachnoid cyst.

Case 15.3 T2-weighted image showing an arachnoid cyst.

COLLOID CYST

Colloid cysts typically arise in the anterior aspect of the third ventricle in close proximity to the foramen of Monro. The peak incidence is in the 3rd to 4th decade, with an equal sex preponderance. Symptoms are due to the intermittent hydrocephalus that occurs owing to the ball-valve effect of the tumour with the foramen of Munro. Sudden death is a well-reported phenomenon.

Key sequences

- T1-weighted
- T1-weighted with contrast
- Sagittal imaging is crucial.

Imaging findings

The typical mass is hyperintense on T1- and hypointense on T2-weighted images. Colloid cysts can, however, display varying signal intensities on different pulse sequences.

Other more unusual forms include lesions displaying hyperintense outer rims and hypointense cores on T2-weighted images.

Hints and tips

Flow artefacts from the CSF in the region of the foramen of Munro can simulate the appearances of a colloid cyst and should be viewed with caution.

Colloid cysts may rarely occur in the lateral and fourth ventricles or even in an extraventricular location.

Further reading

Maeder PP, Holtas SL, Basibuyuk LN et al. Colloid cysts of the third ventricle: correlation of MR and CT findings with histology and chemical analysis. *Am J Neuroradiol* 1990; **11**: 575–81.

Case 16: Colloid cyst

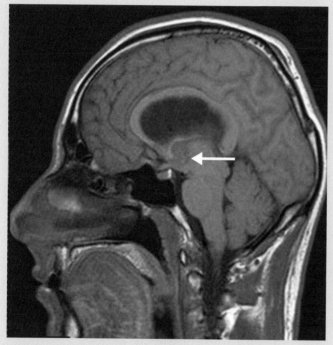

Case 16.1 T1-weighted sagittal image reveals a hyperintense lesion in the region of the third ventricle.

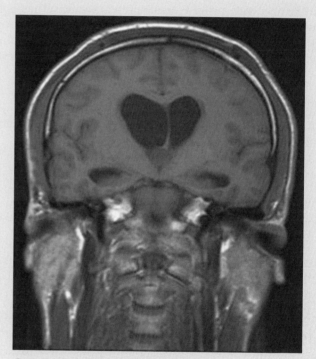

Case 16.2 Coronal image of the same.

6 VASCULITIS/DEMYELINATION

MULTIPLE SCLEROSIS

Multiple sclerosis is an idiopathic inflammatory disease of the central nervous system characterized by patches of inflammation and subsequent demyelination throughout the brain and/or spinal cord. It usually follows a relapsing, remitting clinical course with repeated episodes of neurological dysfunction. Most patients present in early to middle age, with a slight female preponderance. The diagnosis of multiple sclerosis includes some demonstration, by clinical or radiological means, that lesions are separated in both space and time. MRI is the most sensitive imaging test.

Key sequences

- T2-weighted and fluid-attenuated inversion recovery (FLAIR) sagittal
- T1-weighted post-contrast axial

Imaging findings

Plaques are typically ovoid lesions between 5 and 15 mm in size.

They are low signal on T1-weighted images (if established) and high signal on T2-weighted, proton density (PD)-weighted and FLAIR sequences.

Orientation perpendicular to the margins of the lateral ventricles is characteristic (Dawson's fingers).

Other common locations are juxtacortical, U-fiber, temporal lobe and brainstem.

In the active phase, plaques may display mild surrounding oedema and a mass effect.

Plaques usually enhance during the active phase, which lasts for 2–6 weeks. The enhancement pattern may be homogeneous or ring-like.

Hints and tips

Other causes of periventricular high-T2-signal lesions include small-vessel ischaemia, Virchow–Robin spaces (dark on FLAIR), vasculitis, sarcoidosis, Lyme disease and acute disseminated encephalomyelitis (ADEM).

McDonald MRI criteria for multiple sclerosis

See Table 6.1

Table 6.1

Number of clinical attacks	Lesions	Additional requirement for diagnosis
2 or more	2 or more	None
2 or more	1	Dissemination in space on MRI/ 2 or more lesions on MRI + active CSF
1	2 or more	Dissemination in Time on MRI/ Another clinical episode
1	1	Dissemination in space/ 2 or more lesions on MRI + active CSF/ Dissemination in time (MRI or clinical)
0	1 or more	Disease progression for 1 year and 2 of: 9 T2 lesions 4 T2 lesions + positive VEP Spinal cord lesions Active CSF

Further reading

Pretorius PM, Quaghebeur G. The role of MRI in the diagnosis of MS. *Clin Radiol* 2003; **58**: 434–48.

Simon JH. Update on multiple sclerosis. *Magn Reson Imaging Clin N Am* 2006; **14**: 203–24.

Case 17: Multiple sclerosis

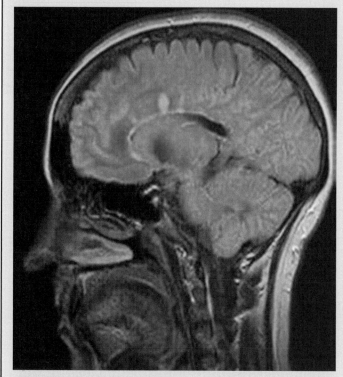

Case 17.1 FLAIR sagittal image demonstrating high-signal ovoid plaque lesions oriented perpendicular to the margins of the lateral ventricles.

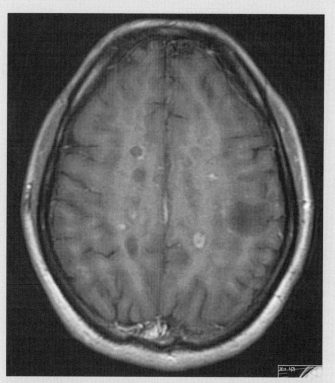

Case 17.2 These ovoid lesions (Dawson's fingers) enhance with contrast in the active phase.

ACUTE DISSEMINATED ENCEPHALOMYELITIS (ADEM)

ADEM is a postviral (postvaccination or parainfectious) immune-mediated phenomenon that pathologically follows a process of demyelination. It presents in a non-specific way but has a rapid clinical progression, and therefore making an early diagnosis is crucial. Up to 30% of patients with ADEM will go on to develop full-blown multiple sclerosis.

Key sequences

- T2-weighted
- FLAIR
- T1-weighted with contrast

Imaging findings

There are widespread, bilateral but asymmetric lesions, typically located in the subcortical areas of the brain, and hyperintense on T2-weighted images.

Lesions may become confluent and affect surrounding structures such as the basal ganglia.

Lesions may enhance after contrast administration, particularly at the periphery.

In very severe cases, haemorrhagic transformation of the lesions may be noted.

Hints and tips

Contrast enhancement of lesions is a marker of acute activity.

The lesions often spare the periventricular white matter.

Imaging findings improve with clinical recovery; however, some lesions may persist in adormant state.

It may be impossible to distinguish multiple sclerosis from ADEM on the basis of a single MRI study.

Further reading

Filippi M, DeStefano N, Dousset V, McGowan JC, eds. *MR Imaging in White Matter Diseases of the Brain and Spinal Cord.* New York: Springer-Verlag, 2005.

Case 18: Acute disseminated encephalomyelitis (ADEM)

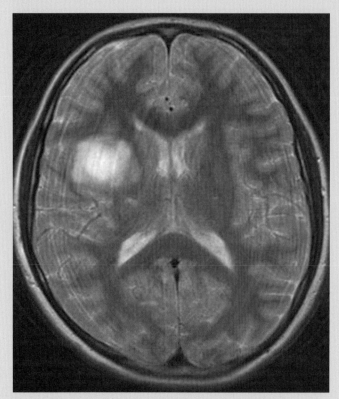

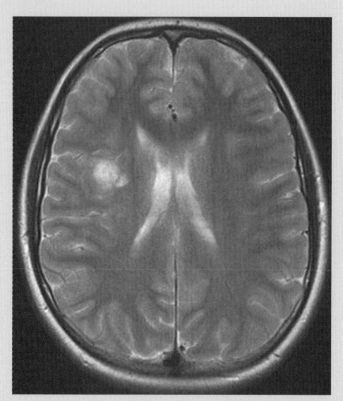

Case 18.1 T2-weighted FLAIR image of a young patient presenting with rapidly progressive ascending weakness showing a hyperintense lesion in the deep white matter of the right parietal lobe. Lesions of ADEM can be asymmetric or bilateral.

Case 18.2 In the same patient, there is regression of high-signal change after a course of steroids.

REVERSIBLE LEUKOENCEPHALOPATHY SYNDROME

This syndrome describes acute neurological changes in the setting of sudden or prolonged arterial hypertension that overcomes the autoregulatory capacity of the cerebral vasculature. It is also recognized to occur as a complication of immunosuppressive drug therapy. The relative paucity of sympathetic innervation in the posterior circulation is thought to account for the preponderance of posterior cerebral changes. Clinical manifestations include headache, nausea, vomiting, seizures, visual changes and coma. Prompt control of blood pressure or the causative drug often results in complete neurological recovery with resolution of the neuroimaging abnormalities. Left untreated, there is a risk of progressive neurological deterioration leading to infarction.

Key sequences

- T1- and T2-weighted and FLAIR axial/sagittal/coronal
- Diffusion-weighted imaging (DWI)

Imaging findings

There is subcortical white matter oedema (low T1, high T2 and FLAIR signal), predominantly in the posterior temporal, parietal, and occipital lobes.

In severe cases, changes can also be seen to involve the basal ganglia, cerebellar hemispheres and brainstem.

Hints and tips

The affected areas are of low signal (normal or increased diffusion) on DWI, indicating vasogenic oedema rather than ischaemia.

Further reading

Vázquez E, Lucaya J, Castellote A et al. Neuroimaging in pediatric leukemia and lymphoma: differential diagnosis. *Radiographics* 2002; **22**: 1411–28.

Case 19: Reversible leukoencephalopathy syndrome

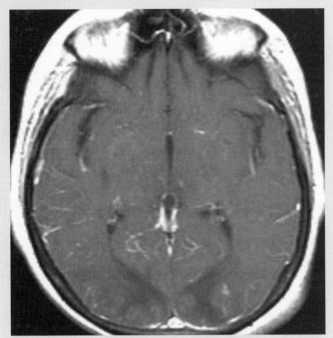

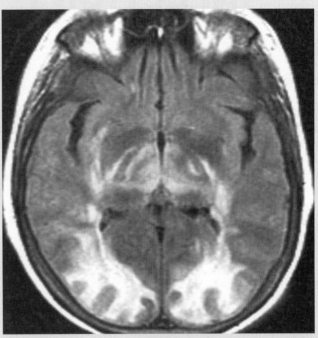

Case 19.1 T1-weighted image showing patchy non-enhancing low-signal change in the posterior fossa. Image courtesy of Dr Alice Smith, Attending Neuroradiologist, Washington DC, USA.

Case 19.2 Bilateral symmetric high-signal changes on FLAIR imaging confirm posterior leukoencephalopathic change. These completely resolved on follow-up MRI. Image courtesy of Dr Alice Smith, Attending Neuroradiologist, Washington DC, USA.

7 INFECTIONS

CEREBRAL ABSCESS

Pyogenic infections of the central nervous system (CNS) usually arise from septic emboli transmitted haematogenously. Less frequently, transdural spread may occur from adjacent sinus infections. After an initial cerebritis, a normal immune response induces angiogenic neovascularity and collagen deposition to form a capsule of granulation tissue around the infected area. A brain abscess is potentially fatal and requires urgent neurosurgical review.

Key sequences

- T1- and T2-weighted and fluid-attenuated inversion recovery (FLAIR) axial/sagittal/coronal
- T1-weighted post-contrast axial/sagittal/coronal
- Diffusion-weighted imaging (DWI)

Imaging findings

Typically, an abcess appears as a parenchymal mass lesion with extensive surrounding oedema and mass effect.

Classically, it displays a uniformly thin rim of enhancement with smooth inner and outer walls. The rim is typically hypointense on T2-weighted images.

Hints and tips

The differential diagnosis of a ring-enhancing intracranial mass lesion is wide and includes primary brain tumours (e.g. glioblastoma), metastases, resolving haematoma, infarction and radiation necrosis.

DWI is a useful adjunct to help narrow the differential diagnosis. This shows an abscess as having markedly high DWI signal with corresponding low signal on the apparent diffusion coefficient (ADC) map image.

Only acute ischaemic stroke classically has the same DWI and ADC signal characteristics as an abscess, but ring enhancement in acute stroke is unusual.

Further reading

Stadnik TW, Demaerel P, Luypaert RR et al. Imaging Tutorial: Differential diagnosis of bright lesions on diffusion-weighted MR images. *Radiographics* 2003; **23**: e7.

Case 20: Cerebral abscess

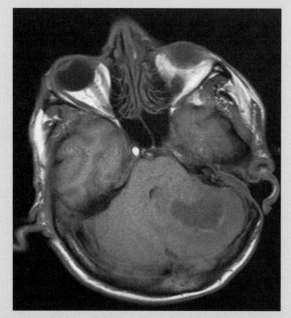

Case 20.1 T1-weighted axial image showing an intracranial abscess as a low-signal area in the left cerebellar hemisphere.

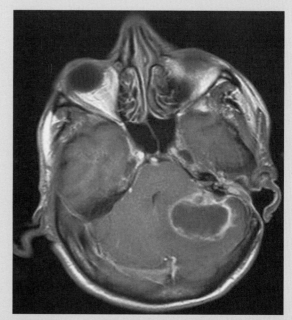

Case 20.2 On contrast administration, there is rim enhancement of the lesion.

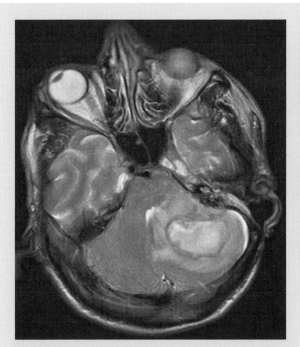

Case 20.3 T2-weighted image revealing extensive local oedema associated with this lesion.

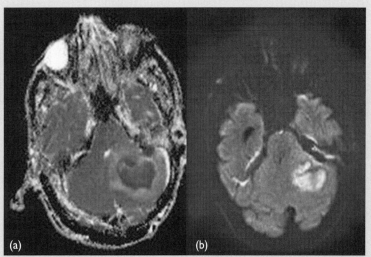

Case 20.4 (a) There is restricted diffusion on DWI. (b) The corresponding ADC mapping.

HERPES ENCEPHALITIS

Herpesvirus is thought to spread intracranially via the olfactory pathways following reactivation of dormant virus in cranial nerve ganglia. It produces superficial grey matter disease, and pathological specimens show petechial haemorrhages and inflammation in affected areas. Clinical symptoms and signs are non-specific and a high index of suspicion is required since, without prompt treatment, mortality rates approach 50%. MRI is the most sensitive imaging modality, but findings may not be apparent in the early stages of infection.

Key sequences

- T2- and T2*-weighted and FLAIR axial
- T1-weighted post-contrast
- DWI

Imaging findings

There is high T2 and FLAIR signal, which most often begins in the medial temporal and frontal lobes. The lentiform nucleus is characteristically spared.

Progression to bilateral disease and parietal lobe involvement is typical.

Contrast enhancement in a cortical gyral pattern, particularly around the sylvian fissure, is characteristic.

There is marked hyperintensity on DWI and reduced ADC values.

Hints and tips

The cortical gyral enhancement pattern in herpes encephalitis often lags behind the onset of signs and symptoms and may be suppressed by steroid medication. The absence of enhancement does not exclude encephalitis.

The differential diagnosis between acute ischemic stroke and herpes encephalitis can be problematic. Clinical presentation (acute onset in ischaemic stroke, more progressive in herpes encephalitis) and biological tests (polymerase chain reaction for herpes simplex virus) are especially useful to distinguish these conditions.

Further reading

Stadnik TW, Demaerel P, Luypaert RR et al. Imaging Tutorial: Differential diagnosis of bright lesions on diffusion-weighted MR images. *Radiographics* 2003; **23**: e7.

Case 21: Herpes encephalitis

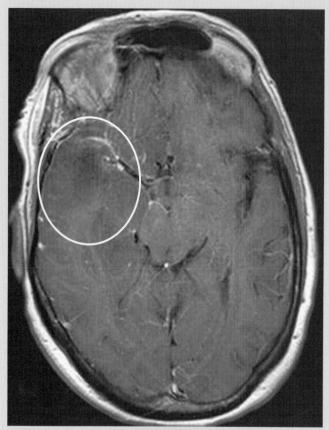

Case 21.1 Post-contrast T1-weighted image showing a low-signal area in the right temporal lobe. This is associated with subtle leptomeningeal enhancement.

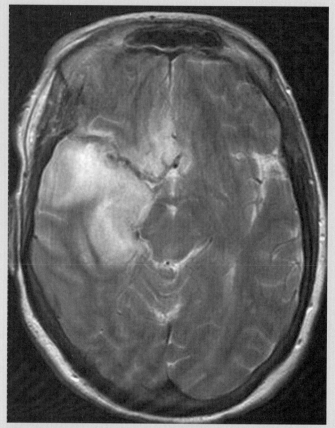

Case 21.2 T2-weighted axial image confirming extensive high-signal change in the same territory.

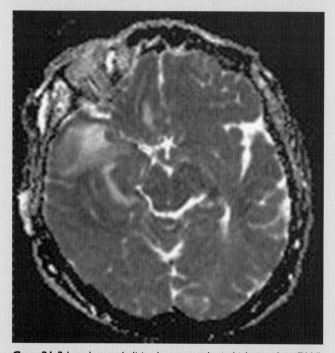

Case 21.3 Local encephalitic change results in high signal on DWI.

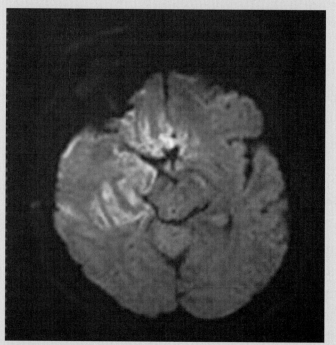

Case 21.4 The corresponding ADC maps shows low signal in the encephalitic focus.

MENINGITIS

CNS infection is a commonly encountered diagnosis. Pathogens infiltrate the pia and arachnoid mater linings of the brain either through blood or lymph or through structures without a blood–brain barrier, such as the choroid plexus and circumventricular structures. Direct extension from orbits, sinuses and mastoids, although less common, is a life-threatening complication of otherwise straightforward inflammatory processes. The early pathophysiological events are hyperaemia of the linings of the brain, followed by the formation of thick exudates that settle in the dependent aspects of the brain.

Key sequences

- FLAIR
- T1-weighted with contrast

Imaging findings

Of note, imaging may be unremarkable in the early days and if treatment for clinically suspected meningitis was begun early. Imaging may be carried out, not to make the diagnosis, but to look for complications of infection, and to follow treatment.

There is marked contrast enhancement of the leptomeninges and narrowed basal cisterns

There is enlargement of subarachnoid spaces with enhancing inflammatory exudates. The involved cerebrospinal fluid (CSF) spaces may not suppress fully on FLAIR sequence.

Subdural collections may be present, as may hydrocephalus (usually communicating in nature) and ventriculitis (enhancement of the ependymal ventricular lining).

Secondary parenchymal infarction may ensue, secondary to focal vasculitis.

Other complications may be noted: abscess, generalized cerebral swelling and herniation syndromes.

Hints and tips

A 'normal' appearing MRI study should be reported with caution if the clinical presentation suggests meningitis, since it could lead to misdiagnosis.

Ependymal and meningeal enhancement per se can be a non-specific sign and is encountered in other conditions such as tumours, chemotherapy, shunt placement and post lumbar puncture.

Further reading

Grossman RI, Yousem DM. *Neuroradiology: The Requisites*, 2nd edn. St Louis, MO: Mosby, 2003.

Case 22: Meningitis

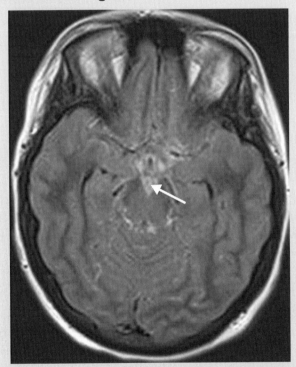

Case 22.1 FLAIR axial image showing lack of suppression of CSF signal in the interpeduncular cistern, indicating replacement of CSF by infectious/inflammatory exudate (arrow).

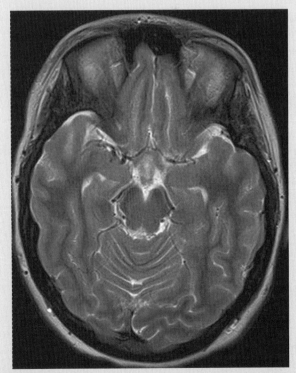

Case 22.2 T2-weighted image from the same patient demonstrating high-signal changes in the corresponding areas.

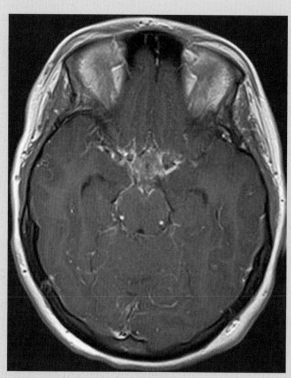

Case 22.3 Post-contrast T1-weighted image showing abnormal enhancement of the suprasellar cistern.

HIV ENCEPHALOPATHY

HIV encephalitis and HIV leukoencephalopathy are two distinct histopathological patterns of brain involvement in HIV infection or the AIDS dementia complex. These can be distinguished clinically and radiologically. Patients typically present with disturbances in cognition, behavioural changes and non-specific motor disturbances. Early MRI may help to distinguish vague early presentations of HIV from often wrongly diagnosed and treated 'psychiatric illnesses'.

Key sequences

- T2-weighted axial
- Post-contrast T1-weighted

Imaging findings

The presence of diffuse or patchy high-signal abnormalities in the periventricular and deep white matter regions of the brain is the hallmark of HIV-related brain involvement. The frontal lobe is the most common site for such changes.

High signal is noted on T1- and T2-weighted images.

Progression of these changes can be seen in patients who commence antiretroviral therapy, even though they may show clinical improvement.

Hints and tips

HIV encephalopathy does not result in a mass effect or enhancement. If these findings are present, another diagnosis must be considered.

Progressive multifocal leukoencephalopathy lesions may show post-contrast enhancement.

There is a wide differential diagnosis for brain lesions in patients with AIDS dementia complex. One must not forget the possibility of opportunistic pathogens such as fungi and viruses.

Further reading

Smith AB, Smirniotopoulos JG, Rushing EJ. Central nervous system infections associated with human immunodeficiency virus infection: radiologic–pathologic correlation. *Radiographics* 2008; **28**: 2033–58.

Thurnher MM, Schindler EG, Thurnher SA et al. Highly active antiretroviral therapy for patients with AIDS dementia complex: effect on MR imaging findings and clinical course. *AJNR Am J Neuroradiol* 2000; **21**: 670–8.

Case 23: HIV encephalopathy

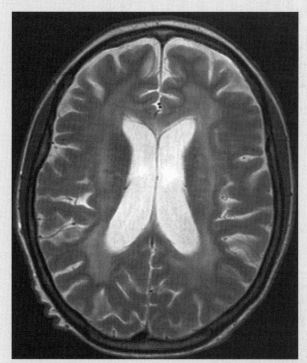

Case 23.1 T2-weighted axial image revealing ventricular and sulcal prominence, features of atrophy, as well as confluent periventricular high-signal changes in the deep white matter of the brain. Image courtesy of Dr N McConachie, Consultant Neuroradiologist, Queen's Medical Centre, Nottingham, UK.

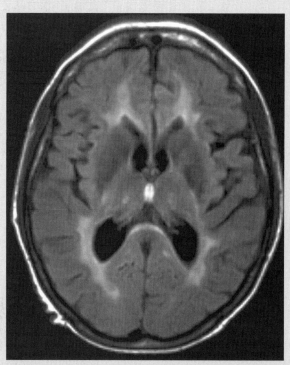

Case 23.2 T1-weighted axial image showing high-signal periventricular changes. Image courtesy of Dr N McConachie, Consultant Neuroradiologist, Queen's Medical Centre, Nottingham, UK.

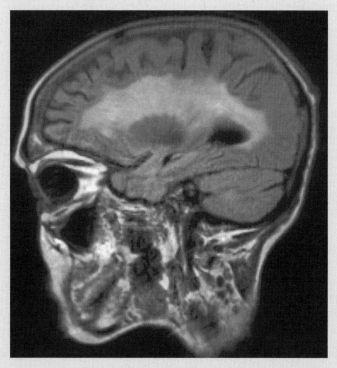

Case 23.3 Sagittal section from the same patient demonstrating the extent of high-signal change and its typical association with the ventricles. Image courtesy of Dr N McConachie, Consultant Neuroradiologist, Queen's Medical Centre, Nottingham, UK.

8 CONGENITAL CONDITIONS

CHIARI I MALFORMATION

The hallmark of the Chiari I malformation is herniation of the cerebellar tonsils below the level of the foramen magnum. Slight tonsillar ectopia is common, but descent greater than 5 mm is considered significant. Symptoms associated with this anomaly are related to spinal cord and/or cerebellar compromise and alteration of cerebrospinal fluid dynamics, and usually become manifest in early adulthood. However, cough headache may be the only symptom. Despite caudal elongation of the tonsils, the fourth ventricle remains in its normal position. Associated anomalies include Klippel–Feil syndrome (block vertebrae).

Key sequences

- T1- and T2-weighted sagittal and axial through the craniocervical junction
- T1- and T2-weighted sagittal covering the whole spine

Imaging findings

There is descent of the cerebellar tonsils >5 mm beneath the foramen magnum.

Hydrocephalus occurs in a quarter of cases.

Syringomyelia may be concomitantly present in up to 60% of patients

Hints and tips

Chiari II malformation is characterized by cerebellar hypoplasia, caudal displacement and narrowing of the fourth ventricle and a variety of other central nervous system (CNS) abnormalities. Over 90% of cases have hydrocephalus and presentation is in early childhood.

Further reading

Poe LB, Coleman LL, Mahmud F. Congenital central nervous system anomalies. *Radiographics* 1989; **9**: 801–26.

Case 24: Chiari I malformation

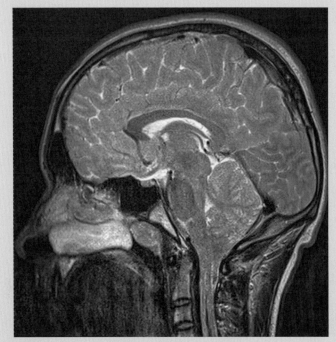

Case 24.1 Sagittal sections are best for confirming descent of the cerebellar tonsils beneath the foramen magnum.

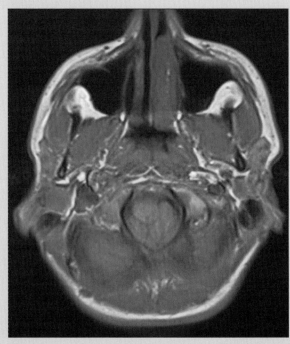

Case 24.2 An axial image at the cervicocranial junction is evaluated to confirm the presence and extent of tonsillar descent.

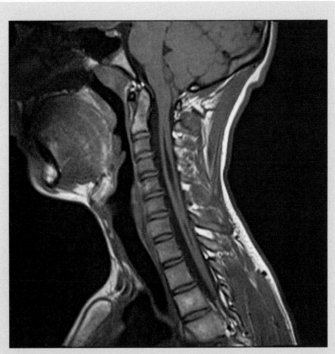

Case 24.3 Up to 60% of patients with Chiari I malformation have an associated syrinx.

TUBEROUS SCLEROSIS

Tuberous sclerosis is an autosomal dominant neurocutaneous syndrome characterized by the development of a range of hamartomatous lesions in different organ systems. The diagnosis is usually established on the basis of criteria applied to physical or radiological findings. Intracranial lesions are seen in up to 100% of affected individuals and comprise four main abnormalities: cortical tubers, subependymal nodules, subependymal giant cell astrocytomas and white matter abnormalities.

Key sequences

- T1- and T2-weighted

Imaging findings

Cortical tubers: These are cortically based nodules with low T1 and high T2 signal. They most commonly involve the frontal lobes, but can occur anywhere. Imaging appearances may vary on MRI, and occasionally lesions may be more conspicuous on computed tomography (especially if they are calcified).

Subependymal nodules and giant cell astrocystoma: These show high T1 and isohigh T2 signal. Giant cell astrocytoma classically arises in the foramen of Munro and causes obstructive hydrocephalus.

White matter abnormalities: These are low-T1- and high-T2-signal areas associated with cortical tubers. Radial white matter bands are distinct lesions that appear as thin or curvilinear regions of high T2 signal and usually involve the frontal lobes.

Hamartomas may also be seen

Hints and tips

Less common CNS manifestations include cerebral and cerebellar atrophy, infarction, aneurysms, dysgenesis of the corpus callosum, and microcephaly.

Further reading

Umeoka S, Koyama T, Miki Y et al. Pictorial review of tuberous sclerosis in various organs. *Radiographics* 2008; **28**: e32.

Case 25: Tuberous sclerosis

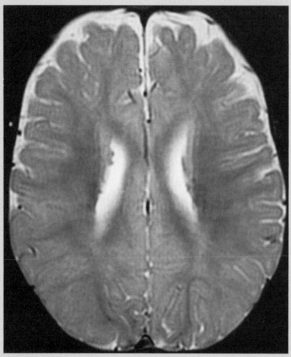

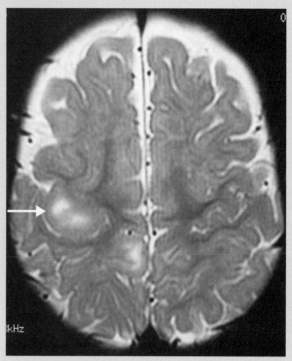

Case 25.1 T2-weighted axial image showing subependymal hamartomas (arrowheads). These are present in nearly 95% of patients with tuberous sclerosis. They are most commonly located near the caudate nucleus. They are often calcified, which explains the low signal on T2-weighted images.

Case 25.2 Different patterns of white matter lesions are seen in tuberous sclerosis. This image shows confluent tumefactive changes. Also note the associated radial bands.

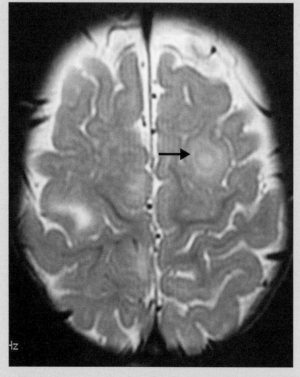

Case 25.3 Cortical tubers are the most characteristic lesion seen in tuberous sclerosis. They may show age-related changes and, as in this case, can often distort the local gyral pattern.

STURGE–WEBER SYNDROME (LEPTOMENINGEAL ANGIOMATOSIS)

Sturge–Weber syndrome is one of the neurocutaneous syndromes, a phakomatosis that is characterized by facial port wine stain and is associated with seizures, buphthalmos, glaucoma and hemiplegia. This is a sporadic condition seen with equal frequency in males and females. The intracranial pathology includes vascular angioma. Vascular congestion within the angioma predisposes to local hypoxia of the cortex and secondary dystrophic calcification. While computed tomography is good in the detection of calcification, MRI is better at demonstrating the true extent of the disease.

Key sequences

- T2-weighted
- T1-weightedwith contrast
- MR angiography may be combined to give better definition

Imaging findings

There is enhancement of the pia mater.

The cortex enhances with secondary ischaemia.

In some cases, there are prominent medullary and subependymal veins.

Hints and tips

Look for associated ocular abnormalities: glaucoma with buphthalmos and choroidal angiomas.

The calcification in Sturge–Weber syndrome is not contained within the angioma per se, but in the underlying cortex. This may be seen better on T2-weighted images.

Further reading

Adams ME, Aylett SE, Squier W, Chong W. A spectrum of unusual neuroimaging findings in patients with suspected Sturge–Weber syndrome. *AJNR Am J Neuroradiol* 2009; **30**: 276–81.

Case 26: Sturge–Weber syndrome (leptomeningeal angiomatosis)

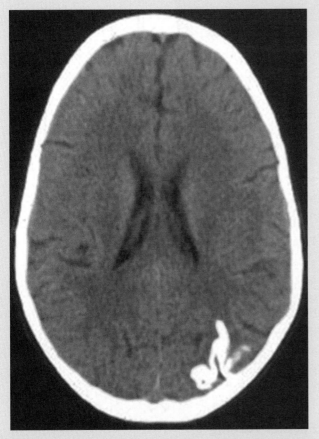

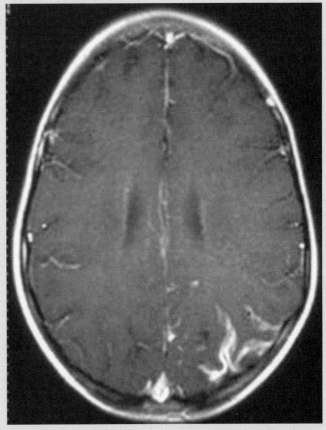

Case 26.1 Non-contrast computed tomography best demonstrates the gyriform calcification typically seen in the occipital and posterior parietal lobes on the same side of a facial angioma.

Case 26.2 Post-contrast T1-weighted image revealing contrast enhancement of a pial leptomeningeal angioma.

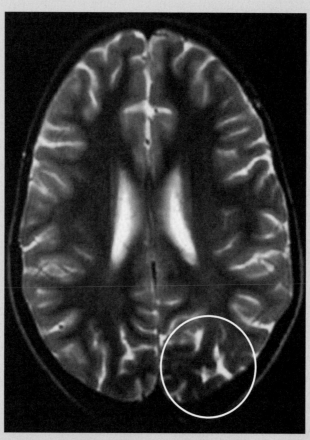

Case 26.3 The circled area demonstrates subtle high signal intensity in the affected region.

NEUROFIBROMATOSIS TYPE 1 (NF1)

NF1 is one of the neurocutaneous phakomatoses. In fact, it is the most common variety of these. The implicated chromosome is number 17 and inheritance is autosomal dominant. Brain lesions typically seen are optic nerve gliomas, non-optic gliomas (e.g. astrocytoma), plexiform neurofibromas, hamartomas, sutural defects, hypoplastic sinuses, occlusive arterial disease and arteriovenous malformations.

Key sequences

- T1- and T2-weighted
- Post-contrast T1-weighted

Imaging findings

Optic nerve gliomas typically appear hypo/isointense on T1-weighted and hyperintense on T2-weighted images. Contrast enhancement characteristics are highly variable.

Non-optic gliomas commonly occur in the brainstem.

Plexiform neurofibromas are the most characteristic findings. Within the brain, these are typically seen on the trigeminal nerve as tortuous worm-like lesions along the axis of the nerve. Skeletal abnormalities are often seen in conjunction with plexiform neurofibromas. (look for sphenoid wing dysplasia). Plexiform neurofibromas demonstrate avid contrast enhancement.

High-signal basal ganglia changes are commonly associated findings.

Hints and tips

Having described the above, the only findings that one may encounter on MRI could be 'unexplained bright objects' typically in the posterior fossa, temporal lobe and basal ganglia. By themselves, these have poor diagnostic value, and clinical correlation is often necessary.

These patients have an increased risk of developing neoplasms, including leukaemia. These should be carefully looked for on any form of imaging.

Further reading

Korf BR. Malignancy in neurofibromatosis type 1. *Oncologist* 2000; **5**: 477–85.

Osborne AG. *Diagnostic Neuroradiology*. St Louis, MO: Mosby, 1994.

Case 27: Neurofibromatosis type 1

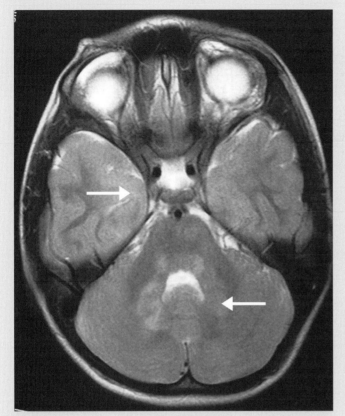

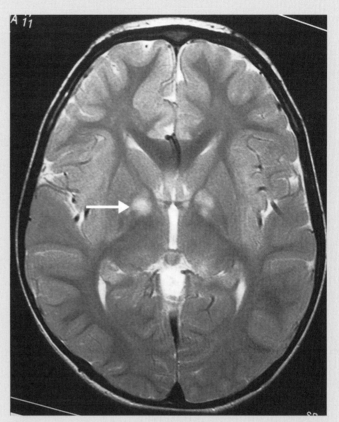

Case 27.1 T2-weighted image initially reported as showing 'unexplained bright objects (arrows)' on a patient clinically diagnosed with neurofibromatosis type 1 (NF1).

Case 27.2 High-signal changes within the basal ganglia are a feature of NF1.

NEUROFIBROMATOSIS TYPE 2 (NF2)

NF2 is transmitted in an autosomal dominant fashion, the culprit chromosome being number 22.

Key sequences

- Post-contrast T1-weighted
- T2-weighted

Imaging findings

The diagnostic criteria for NF2 are as follows:
- a first-degree relative with the condition *plus*
- either a single acoustic neuroma or any two of the following: schwannoma, neurofibroma, meningioma, glioma or juvenile posterior subcapsular lens opacity

The presence of bilateral acoustic schwannomas is diagnostic.

Schwannomas appear as isointense or low-signal masses on T1-weighted images and isointense to high-signal masses on T2-weighted images. They demonstrate avid but heterogeneous contrast enhancement.

Hints and tips

Always cover the spine when imaging for possible neurofibromatosis, since spinal lesions, including intradural tumours, are common associations.

Further reading

Osborne AG. *Diagnostic Neuroradiology*. St Louis, MO: Mosby, 1994.

Case 28 Neurofibromatosis type 2

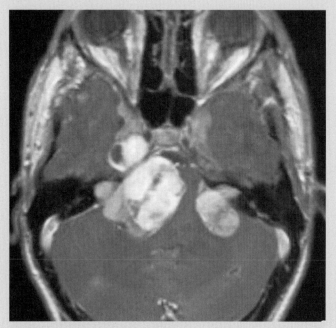

Case 28.1 Post-contrast T1-weighted axial image showing bilateral acoustic schwannomas as enhancing cerebellopontine tumours.

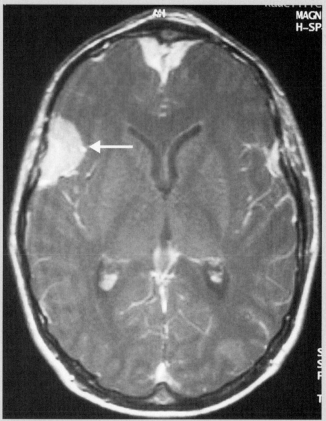

Case 28.2 Meningiomas are common associations in neurofibromatosis type 2 patients.

9 INTRACEREBRAL HAEMORRHAGE

INTRODUCTION

Intracerebral haemorrhage (ICH) is a serious event that accounts for approximately 5–15% of strokes and that is associated with a poor clinical outcome with high mortality rates.

It is typically classified into primary (spontaneous) ICH associated with hypertension or amyloid angiopathy, and secondary ICH associated with various causes such as coagulation disorders, vascular malformations, trauma, ischaemia, vasculitis, cerebral venous sinus thrombosis and neoplasms.

Key sequences

- T2*-weighted-GRE axial as a screening sequence.
- T1- and T2-weighted sequences to determine haemorrhage age.

Imaging findings

Haemorrhage signal is primarily affected by the magnetic properties of blood and its breakdown products. Five stages are usually distinguished:

1. Findings in the hyperacute phase (< 12–24h) might be discreet, since the initial haemorrhage is a liquid consisting of red blood cells with nearly fully oxygenated haemoglobin with diamagnetic properties. T1 as well as T2 are long.

2. Later in the acute phase (1–3 days), the clotting blood with an increasing haematocrit and paramagnetic intracellular deoxyhaemoglobin lead to a magnetic non-uniformity with T2 shortening while T1 is still long. A surrounding oedema may also be visible from this phase on.

3. In the following early subacute phase (3–7 days), paramagnetic intracellular methaemoglobin leads to dipole–dipole interactions with T1 shortening while the persistent magnetic non-uniformity causes T2 shortening.

4. The late subacute phase (7–14 days) is characterised by cell lysis with a high water content and a loss of magnetic compartmentation with free methaemoglobin. Consequently, T2 is long and T1 short. Furthermore, a hypointense rim due to macrophages laden with haemosiderin may be visible both in T1- and T2-weighted images.

5. Finally, the chronic phase is characterised by the aforementioned haemosiderin halo and a rather isointense haemorrhage core.

Hints and tips

T2*-GRE sequences feature similar signal changes as T2-weighted images but are more sensitive to susceptibility effects and require much shorter acquisition times. Therefore, they are very useful in the context of emergency diagnosis of hyperacute ICH as well as chronic haemorrhages and microbleedings.

Every acute ICH is an emergency that necessitates a control examination in order to exclude rehaemorrhage.

Further reading

Kidwell CS, Wintermark M. Imaging of intracranial haemorrhage. *Lancet Neurol* 2008; **7**(3):256–67.

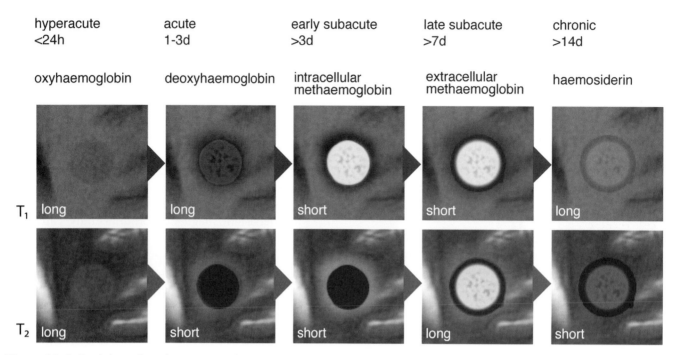

	hyperacute <24h	acute 1-3d	early subacute >3d	late subacute >7d	chronic >14d
	oxyhaemoglobin	deoxyhaemoglobin	intracellular methaemoglobin	extracellular methaemoglobin	haemosiderin
T₁	long	long	short	short	long
T₂	long	short	short	long	short

Figure 9.1: Stylised chronological appearance of intraparenchymal haemorrhage in MRI.

Case 29: 63 year old with two episodes of visual field loss within four weeks.

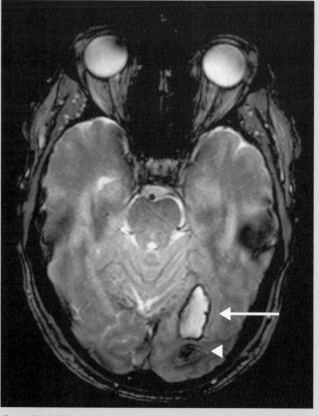

Case 29.1 Axial T1w image showing two haematomas of different age in the left occipital lobe (arrow: late subacute; arrowhead: early subacute).

Case 29.2 T2*-GRE image showing two haematomas of different age in the left occipital lobe (arrow: late subacute; arrowhead: early subacute).

UNIT III
Body MRI

Nikhil Bhuskute

Hepatobiliary sections edited by
Ashley Guthrie

1 ANATOMY

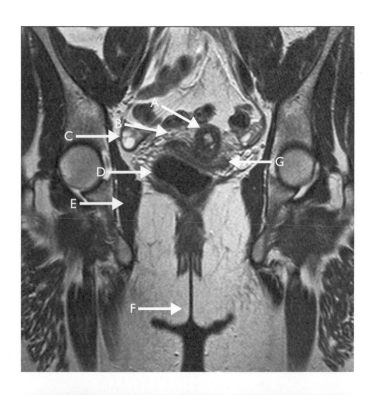

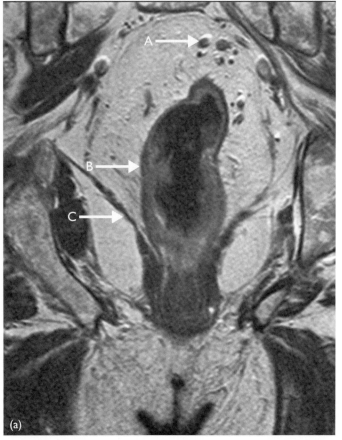

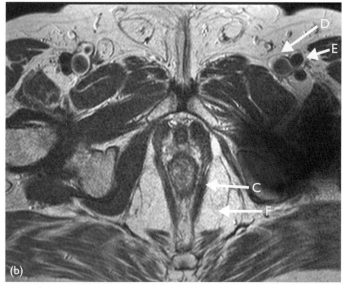

Figure 1.1 A, cervix with endocervical canal (note the dark stromal ring); B, broad ligament; C, right ovary with physiological follicles; D, bladder wall; E, pelvic sidewall; F, vulva; G, uterus (note the thickness of the endometrial lining).

Figure 1.2 A, lymph nodes in mesorectal envelope; B, rectum (note the malignant rectal wall thickening); C, levator ani; D, femoral vein (look for deep vein thrombosis in oncology assessments, since the patient may need a preoperative inferior vena cava filter); E, femoral artery; F, ischiorectal fossa.

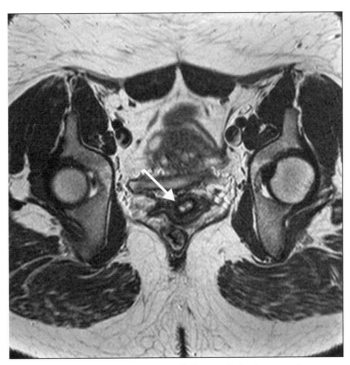

Figure 1.3 The dark stroma ring of the cervix is the most important landmark for cervical cancer staging.

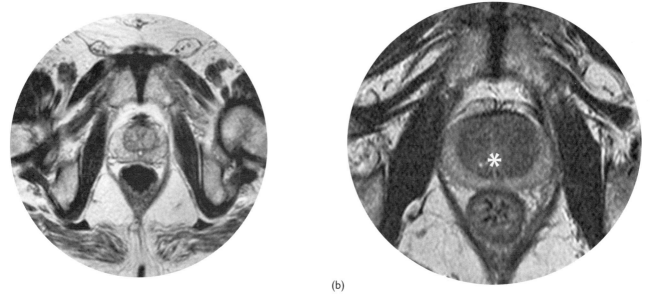

(a)

(b)

Figure 1.4 (a) The prostate demonstrates central and peripheral zones. Malignancy generally involves the peripheral zones, while benign prostatic enlargement typically involves the central zone as shown in (b) (asterisk).

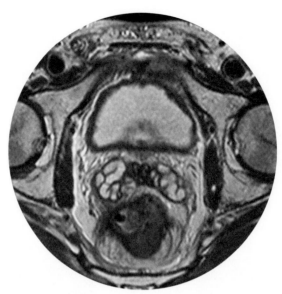

Figure 1.5 Hyperintense seminal vesicles sitting between bladder and rectum. Tumour invasion (low signal on T2-weighted images) and haemorrhage (high signal on T1-weighted images) are common findings.

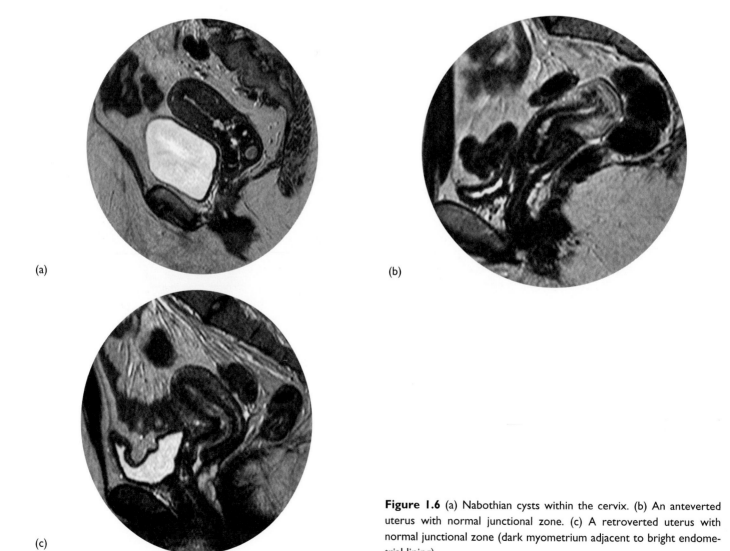

(a)

(b)

(c)

Figure 1.6 (a) Nabothian cysts within the cervix. (b) An anteverted uterus with normal junctional zone. (c) A retroverted uterus with normal junctional zone (dark myometrium adjacent to bright endometrial lining).

2 ABDOMINAL

FOCAL NODULAR HYPERPLASIA (FNH)

FHN is a common solid benign liver tumour, second only in frequency to haemangioma. FNH can be considered as a proliferation of hepatocytes with an abnormal pattern of other, normal, liver tissue. Hence, FNH contains normally functioning hepatocytes and Kupffer cells. On gross pathology, the hallmark feature of FNH is a central stellate scar with radiating fibrous septae dividing the tumour into lobules. The central scar contains an arterial malformation with spiderlike branches supplying the component nodules and also has an abnormal bile duct remnant. This central scar may also be seen on MRI.

Key sequences

- Fast imaging with steady-state precession (FISP) for general overview and further sequence planning
- T1-weighted gradient echo (GRE)* in-phase and out-of-phase axial
- Half Fourier acquired single-shot turbo spin echo (HASTE)/single-shot fast spin echo (SS-FSE)† axial, coronal and sagittal
- T1-weighted gadolinium (Gd)-enhanced and 3D GRE fat-saturated (FS) unenhanced, arterial and venous phases, oblique coronal (along the plane of the main portal vein bifurcation)
- Reticuloendothelial system (Kupffer cell) agents, i.e. superparamagnetic iron oxides (SPIOs) such as Endorem (Guerbet) and Resovist (Schering), can be used with T2*-weighted sequences, pre and 10 minutes post SPIO administration. (Note that Resovist is being withdrawn, while Endorem is still available but requires a longer delay.)
- Other hepatocyte-specific agents (gadobenate, gadoxetic acid and mangafodipir trisodium) can be used. All of these are paramagnetic and hence cause T1 shortening (hyperintensity).

Imaging findings

On T1-weighted images, FNH is isointense to hypointense, while on T2-weighted images, the lesion is slightly hyperintense to isointense.

The central stellate scar is hypointense on T1-weighted images while in most cases it is hyperintense on T2-weighted images. Dynamic Gd-enhanced images show early intense enhancement that becomes isointense during the portal venous phase and isointense on delayed images. The central scar may show late and prolonged enhancement.

On administration of SPIO, there is uptake by Kupffer cells, and hence the lesion is hypointense on T2*-weighted sequences.

On administration of hepatocyte-specific agents, there is uptake in the normally functioning hepatocytes within the FNH. The biliary remnants within FNH, however, do not communicate with the remaining biliary tree, and as a result the these agents are retained in the FNH longer than in normal liver parenchyma, leading to persistent hyperintensity on T1-weighted images.

Hints and tips

Persistent enhancement on delayed imaging after hepatocyte-specific agents is pathognomonic. The use of SPIO may improve characterization in difficult cases

In FNH, the central scar tends to be hyperintense on T2-weighted images, while in fibrolamellar hepatocellular carcinoma (HCC), which is the closest mimic, the central scar is hypointense on all sequences.

A significant proportion of FNH are atypical and may overlap with features of adenomas. In such cases, the use of tissue-specific agents to aid diagnosis is critically important.

Further reading

Robinson PJA, Ward J. *MRI of the Liver: A Practical Guide.* London: Informa Healthcare, 2006.

---

*GRE sequences use a gradient to generate a radiofrequency echo with a flip angle of less than 90°. These sequences allow faster imaging, but are prone to susceptibility artefacts.

†Spin echo (SE) sequences use a 90° excitation pulse followed by a 180° refocusing pulse. In HASTE (Siemens) and SS-FSE (GE Medical systems and Phillips), only half of **k**-space is filled to generate the image, thereby reducing total acquisition time. Images can therefore be sometimes blurred.

Case 1: Focal nodular hyperplasia (FNH)

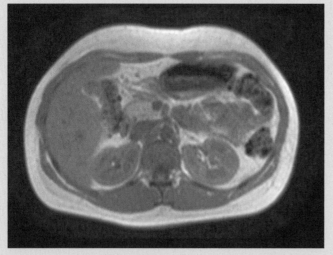
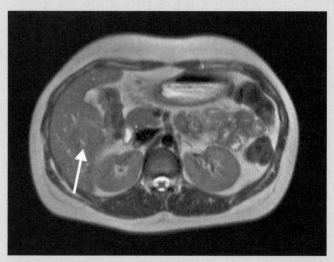

Case 1.1 (a, b) T1- and T2-weighted axial images showing a well-defined mass, with a hyperintense central scar on the T2-weighted image (arrow), as typically seen in FNH.

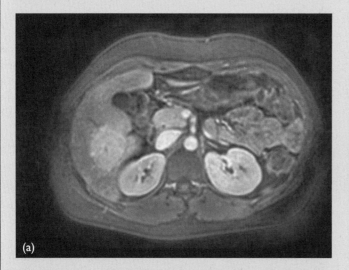
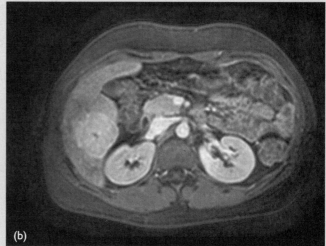

(a)

(b)

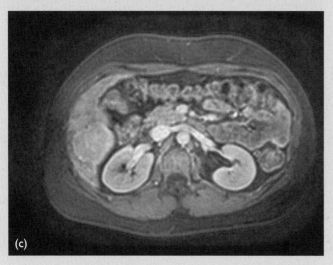

(c)

Case 1.2 (a–c) Dynamic Gd-enhanced images showing intense homogeneous enhancement of the FNH, with late and prolonged enhancement of the central scar.

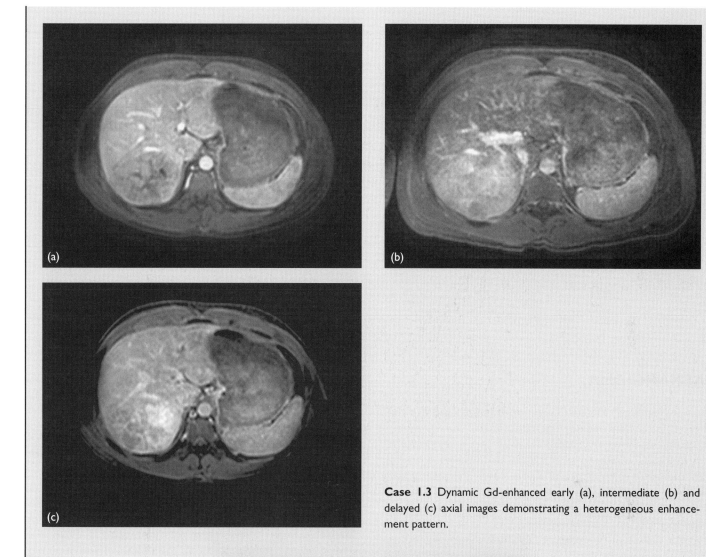

Case 1.3 Dynamic Gd-enhanced early (a), intermediate (b) and delayed (c) axial images demonstrating a heterogeneous enhancement pattern.

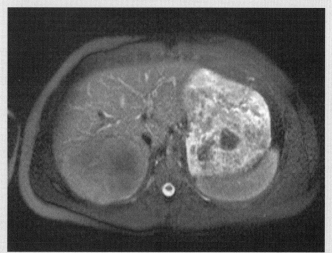

Case 1.4 T2-weighted image showing a fibrolamellar hepatocellular carcinoma (HCC) with a hypointense central scar (compare with the FNH).

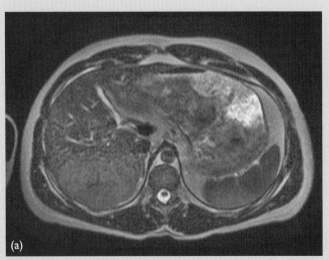
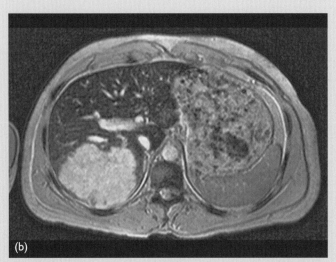

Case 1.5 (a, b) T2*-weighted images before and 10 minutes after administration of SPIO showing the signal dropout from the normal liver. The fibrolamellar HCC is seen as a hyperintense lesion owing to its failure to take up SPIO.

HAEMANGIOMA

Haemangioma is the most common benign liver tumour other than cysts. Most haemangiomas are congenital in origin; however, some familial forms are known. Cavernous haemangiomas originate from the endothelial cells and are composed of multiple, large vascular channels lined by a single layer of endothelial cells. These are often multifocal and are often found in patients with FNH. In the majority of cases, haemangiomas are asymptomatic; however, they can be symptomatic when complicated by rupture, acute thrombosis or consumptive coagulopathy (i.e. Kasabach–Merritt syndrome).

Key sequences

- The sequences used to diagnose haemangiomas and differentiate them from other focal liver lesions are similar to those used for FNH.

Imaging findings

On T1-weighted images, haemangiomas are hypointense, and may be smooth or lobulated, homogeneous or sometimes septated.

On T2-weighted images, haemangiomas are hyperintense similar to cerebrospinal fluid (CSF). Occasionally, in the cases of a heavily hyalinized haemangioma, which may represent an end stage of haemangioma involution, the T2 signal is not as hyperintense as CSF and the appearance may be similar to that of a metastasis. Some large haemangioma may demonstrate a fluid–fluid level owing to sedimentation of blood products.

On dynamic imaging, the characteristic feature of haemangiomas is a discontinuous peripheral nodular enhancement with progressive, centripetal fill-in.

Hints and tips

Haemangiomas derive their vascular supply from the hepatic artery; hence, post-Gd, the enhancement matches the extent in other arteries, and intrahepatic vessels should be used for comparison.

Haemangiomas that show early, homogeneous contrast enhancement on dynamic MRI closely mimic other hypervascular liver tumours but retain contrast and so remain conspicuous, while other hypervascular tumours rapidly become isointense or wash out.

Atypical haemangiomas are less bright on T2-weighted images and enhancement may be heterogeneous.

In cirrhotic livers, haemangiomas are rare and tend to have atypical features; hence, a nodular enhancement pattern should be suspicious for malignancy and further liver-specific contrast agents may be needed.

Further reading

Robinson PJA, Ward J. *MRI of the Liver: A Practical Guide.* London: Informa Healthcare, 2006.

Case 2: Haemangioma

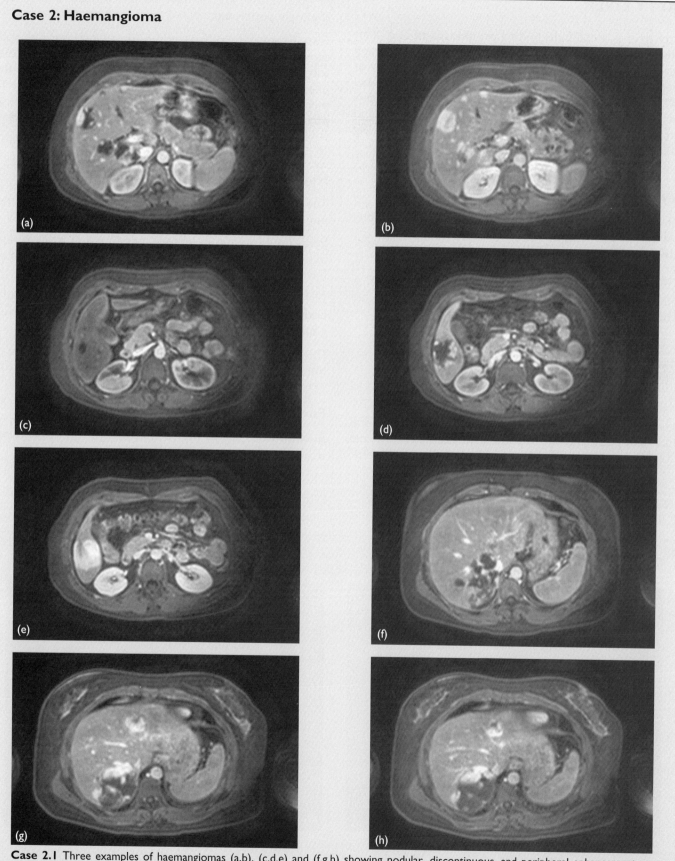

Case 2.1 Three examples of haemangiomas (a,b), (c,d,e) and (f,g,h) showing nodular, discontinuous, and peripheral enhancement on dynamic post contrast imaging.

FATTY LIVER

Fatty liver is a common finding on ultrasound and computed tomography. Not infrequently, fatty infiltration focally or fatty sparing mimics inflammatory, vascular or neoplastic conditions. In such cases, MRI is an essential tool in differentiating other causes from fatty liver. MRI is useful in diagnosing focal or diffuse fatty infiltration and can be used to quantify, but is not reliable in identifying steatohepatitis (e.g. non-alcoholic steatohepatitis)

Key sequences

- Fast spin echo (FSE) for general overview and further sequence planning
- T1- and T2-weighted GRE axial and coronal
- T1-weighted GRE in-phase and out-of-phase axial. At this point, if the lesion is completely characterized as fatty liver or focal fatty sparing, further sequences are not required.

Imaging findings

A higher than normal intensity of liver on T1- images or T2-weighted images is suggestive of fat content.

When fat and water coexist in a voxel owing to chemical shift on in-phase and out-of-phase sequences, there is signal dropout from fat on out-of-phase imaging. Spectrographic or quantitative studies have been described, but are not routinely performed.

Fatty liver can be diffuse or multifocal, perivascular, subcapsular, or due to focal fat sparing. A perivascular distribution of fat with a tramline-like configuration in the imaging plane, a ring-like appearance perpendicular to the imaging plane that completely disappears on out-of-phase imaging and the absence of a mass effect on adjacent vessels provides a confident diagnosis.

Hints and tips

The spleen is used as an internal reference for signal intensity.

Focal fatty infiltration or focal fatty sparing is often seen in segment 4, in the gallbladder fossa, adjacent to the falciform ligament and in non-portal-vein inflow areas.

Watch out for fat-containing tumours (e.g. HCC and adenoma) – these show heterogeneous enhancement and exert a mass effect on adjacent structures.

Do not forget biochemical markers such as raised transaminases.

Further reading

Robinson PJA, Ward J. *MRI of the Liver: A Practical Guide.* London: Informa Healthcare, 2006.

Case 3: Fatty liver

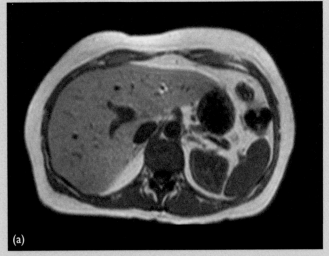 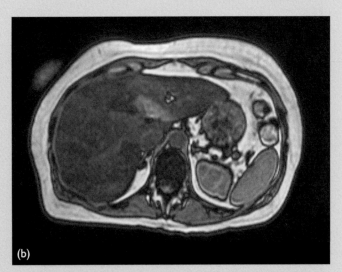

Case 3.1 (a, b) In-phase and out-of-phase axial images demonstrating signal dropout from fatty areas within the liver. Note that there is no dropout of subcutaneous fat signal, because fat and water have to coexist in a voxel for a chemical shift to take place, which is not the case where pure fat exists (e.g in subcutaneous and mesenteric fat).

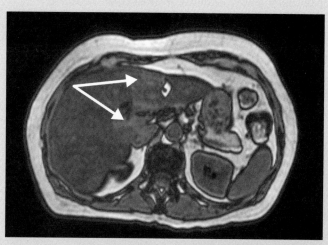

Case 3.2 Out-of-phase image showing signal dropout from most of the fatty liver but focal areas of fatty sparing (arrows) with no signal loss adjacent to the falciform ligament and caudate lobe.

CIRRHOSIS AND NODULES WITHIN

Cirrhosis is the end result of insult to the liver by various causes, the most common being toxins such as alcohol, infections such as viral hepatitis and biliary disorders such as primary sclerosing cholangitis (PSC). The condition is characterized by dysfunctioning hepatocytes with formation of fibrous tissue, followed by regenerative nodules. It is now recognized that, like the adenoma-to-cancer pathway in the colon, nodules pass through the sequence from regenerative to dysplastic to HCC. Dysplastic nodules can show low- or high-grade dysplasia. Regenerative nodules and some low-grade dysplastic nodules derive their blood supply from the portal venous flow, while high-grade dysplastic nodules and HCC increasingly derive their supply from the hepatic artery, with important imaging implications. Cellular function within HCC is altered, which is reflected in the uptake of liver-specific contrast agents.

Key sequences

- These are similar to those used for FNC.

Imaging findings

Unlike the homogeneous intermediate signal of normal liver on both T1- and T2-weighted images, cirrhotic liver shows heterogeneous signal due to accumulation of fat, iron, fibrous tissue, glycogen and bile. The typical cirrhotic liver demonstrates atrophy of segment 4, caudate lobe enlargement (due to inferior vena cava-based blood supply), capsular retraction (due to volume loss of the right lobe) and fibrosis. Occasionally, focal hypertrophy may be seen in PSC.

Dysplastic nodules are classically hyperintense on T1-weighted images and hypointense on T2-weighted images relative to the regenerating background nodular liver. Iso-intensity on T1-weighted images can also be seen. On images obtained using liver-specific contrast agents such as SPIO, these nodules show hypointense signal as the functioning Kupffer cells take up the iron particles. These nodules show vascularity similar to that of remaining liver

High-grade dysplasia and malignant nodules show variable signal on T1-weighted images and are typically hyperintense on T2-weighted images. These nodules do not take up iron particles, and remain hyperintense on images obtained using SPIO. On dynamic Gd-enhanced imaging, they show arterial phase enhancement. When smaller than 2 cm, these are more difficult to identify, but generally nodules larger than 2 cm with heterogeneous signal should be treated with suspicion for HCC. Only 50% of HCCs are visible on unenhanced images.

Fibrosis in the liver is hypointense on T1-weighted and hyperintense on T2-weighted images. It is best seen on SPIO-enhanced images as reticular morphology, but may become confluent, particularly in segment 4. Fibrosis also shows delayed enhancement. These features differentiate it from infiltrative HCC. Vascular invasion is helpful towards diagnosing the latter.

Hints and tips

Look for other supportive evidence of cirrhosis in the form of varices, portal cavernous transformation, splenomegaly, siderotic nodules in the spleen (Gandy–Gamna bodies) and ascites.

Look for specific causes for cirrhosis, such as hypointense liver on T2-weighted images in haemochromatosis and biliary beading in PSC.

Dysplastic nodules should not be T2-bright; if bright nodules are present then suspect high-grade dysplasia or neoplasia. Small arterialized nodules should be noted and carefully followed up.

Further reading

Robinson PJA, Ward J. *MRI of the Liver: A Practical Guide.* London: Informa Healthcare, 2006.
Guthrie JA. Cirrhosis and focal liver lesions: MRI findings. *Imaging* 2004; **16**: 351–63.

Case 4: Cirrhosis and nodules within

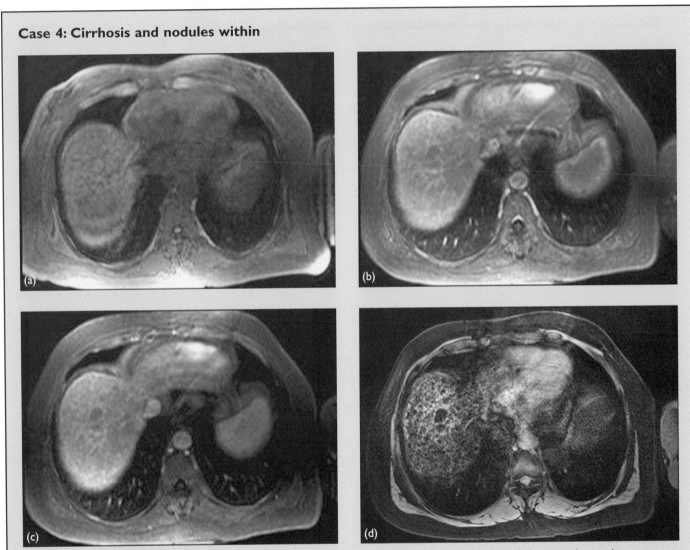

Case 4.1 This benign dysplastic nodule (regenerative) is hyperintense on the T1-weighted image (a) and does not show enhancement on early and 4 minutes post-Gd images (b, c). On the SPIO- plus Gd-enhanced image (d), the nodule is hypointense, since it has accumulated SPIO owing to the presence of normal Kupffer cells

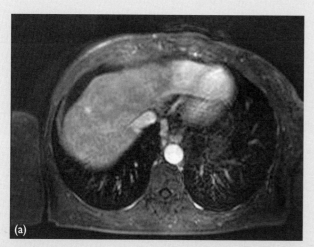
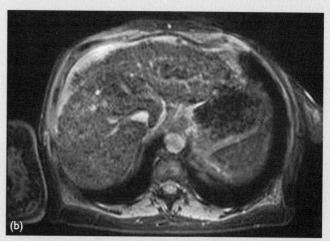

Case 4.2 (a) Early Gd-enhanced image of a hypervascular nodule. (b) Ten minutes after SPIO administration, the nodule is hyperintense – as a high-grade dysplastic nodule, it lacks functioning Kupffer cells.

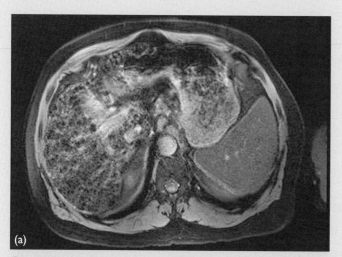
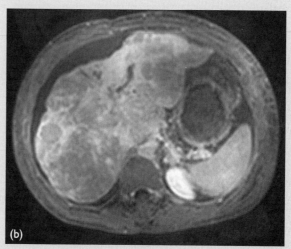

Case 4.3 (a, b) Two different examples showing the hyperintense reticulation within the liver on images 10 minutes after administration SPIO plus Gd. This is fibrosis. The image (b) shows multiple enhancing nodules with early enhancement of the parenchymal strands – this is an example of hepar lobatum carcinomatosum, a rare infiltrating metastasis, in this case from breast carcinoma.

HEPATOCELLULAR CARCINOMA (HCC)

HCC is the most common primary liver malignancy in adults. Cirrhosis, hepatitis B or C, and hepatotoxins are known to predispose to the development of this malignancy. It is the second most common primary liver malignancy in children after hepatoblastoma. On pathology, there is development of non-triadal arteries within the portal triads. Normally, the distal arterial supply does not extend beyond the lobular level; hence, these non-triadal arteries become the dominant supply of the HCC. This explains the contrast enhancement of the tumour on arterial phase.

Key sequences

• These are similar to those used for FNH.

Imaging findings

HCC has variable appearances on MRI. Imaging features depend upon the content of the tumour (i.e. fat, blood and pigments), the host response to the tumour and the status of the native liver.

The majority of HCCs are hypointense on T1-weighted images and hyperintense or mixed intensity on T2-weighted images and show Gd enhancement, the pattern of which is variable.

On SPIO-enhanced images, HCC appears hyperintense owing to failure to accumulate iron within the tumour cell.

A small proportion of HCCs can be hyperintense on T1-weighted images owing to the presence of fat, copper or glycoprotein.

The majority of HCCs show a capsule, which can be seen as a hyperintense 'ring sign' on T2-weighted images.

Hints and tips

HCC can be difficult to distinguish from its differential diagnoses of haemangioma, adenoma, FNH, cholangiocarcinoma and an area of fibrosis.

Look for local lymph nodes, peritoneal disease, invasion of portal, splenic or hepatic veins, bile duct invasion, and arteriovenous shunting.

Look for any arterial or venous anomalies in order to forewarn the surgeons.

Remember that HCC can be multifocal.

Pay attention to dysplastic nodules in a cirrhotic liver. These may be siderotic or non-siderotic. A small focus of evolving HCC within a dysplastic nodule has signal intensity characteristics exactly opposite to those of the nodule. This is a 'nodule-in-nodule' sign.

Further reading

Robinson PJA, Ward J. *MRI of the Liver: A Practical Guide.* London: Informa Healthcare, 2006.
Guthrie JA. Cirrhosis and focal liver lesions: MRI findings. *Imaging* 2004; **16**: 351–63.

Case 5: Hepatocellular carcinoma

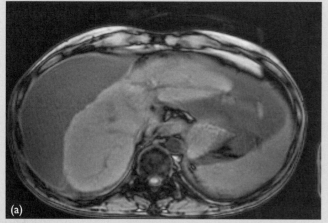
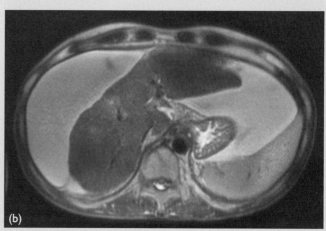

Case 5.1 (a) T1-weighted axial image of a cirrhotic liver with an area of hypointensity, which appears bright on the T2-weighted image (b). Also note the presence of a large ascites (asterisk).

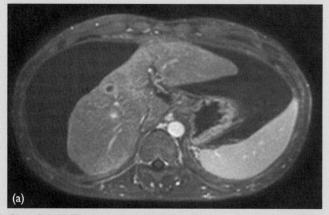
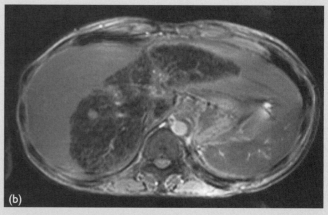

Case 5.2 (a) The same liver as in Case 5.1 on a Gd-enhanced T1-weighted image with the 'ring sign'. (b) HCC cells fail to accumulate SPIO, and hence appear hyperintense on a background of dark liver that has taken up SPIO.

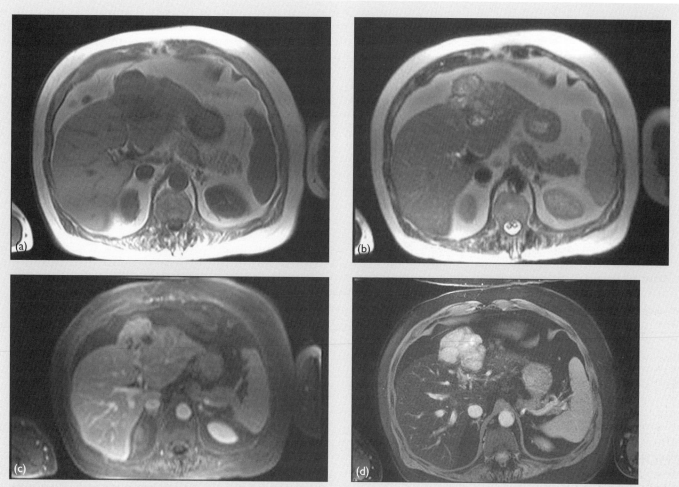

Case 5.3 Another example of a large HCC in a non-cirrhotic liver. The tumour is hypointense on the T1-weighted image (a) and hyperintense on the T2-weighted image (b). It shows heterogeneous enhancement on the post-Gd image (c) and is hyperintense 10 minutes after administration of SPIO and Gd (d).

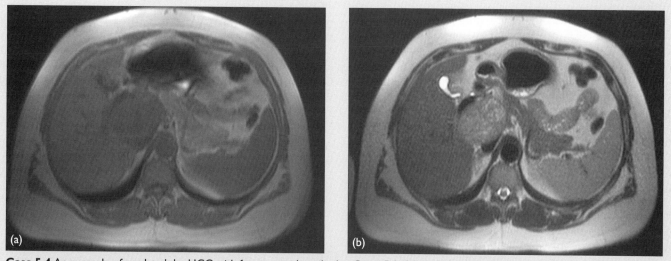

Case 5.4 An example of caudate lobe HCC with features as described in Cases 5.1–5.3: (a) T1-weighted; (b) T2-weighted; (c) Gd-enhanced; (d) 10 minutes after administration of SPIO and Gd. Note here the involvement of the right portal vein.

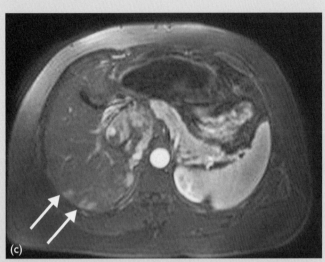 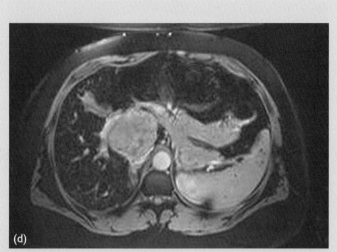

Case 5.4 On the Gd-enhanced image (c), note the wedge-shaped areas (arrows) in the subcapsular region that show normal SPIO uptake. This is transient intrahepatic intensity difference (THID). Tumour often blocks the peripheral portal vein branches, resulting in an increased wedge-shaped enhancement on post-Gd T1-weighted arterial phase imaging.

CHOLANGIOCARCINOMA

Cholangiocarcinoma accounts for one-third of primary liver tumours. There is a strong association with PSC. The tumour can be intrahepatic situated centrally or peripherally or extrahepatic. The majority in the Western population are of hilar type.

Key sequences

- FSE for general overview and further sequence planning
- T1-weighted GRE in-phase and out-of-phase axial
- T1- and T2-weighted GRE axial, coronal and oblique coronal (in the plane of the portal vein bifurcation)
- T1-weighted Gd-enhanced and FS unenhanced, arterial and venous phases, oblique coronal (along the plane of the main portal vein) and delayed axial and coronal
- MRCP sequences (see below)

Imaging findings

On T1-weighted images, the tumour is iso- or hypointense.

On T2-weighted images, the tumour is of mixed intensity, with the central more fibrotic part remaining hypointense and the viable peripheral portion hyperintense.

Not uncommonly, there is no discrete mass, and the only suspicion is of a dominant stricture within the biliary tree. These can be difficult to distinguish from the strictures of PSC. In such cases, dynamic Gd-enhanced sequences can be of help. A mass or stricture that shows persistent enhancement in delayed images is strongly suspicious of cholangiocarcinoma.

Small tumours within the lower common bile duct are best seen on T1-weighted FS images as a hypointense mass against the high signal of the pancreatic head.

Hints and tips

HCC and metastasis uncommonly cause obstruction of the intrahepatic duct.

Hilar tumours are usually infiltrative, the peripheral intrahepatic type are generally mass-forming and the least common intraluminal type are of papillary nature.

In the hilar type, look for venous involvement or biliary stricture.

Distal (lower common bile duct) tumours present similar to pancreatic adenocarcinoma without pancreatic duct dilatation.

Look for hilar nodes and peritoneal deposits.

Further reading

Robinson PJA, Ward J. *MRI of the Liver: A Practical Guide.* London: Informa Healthcare, 2006.

Case 6: Cholangiocarcinoma

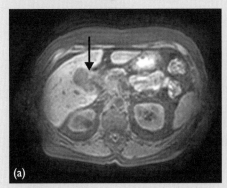 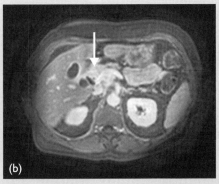 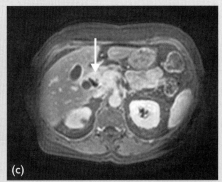

Case 6.1 (a–c) Pre, early and delayed dynamic enhanced images showing progressive and persistent delayed enhancement of the hilar cholangiocarcinoma (arrow).

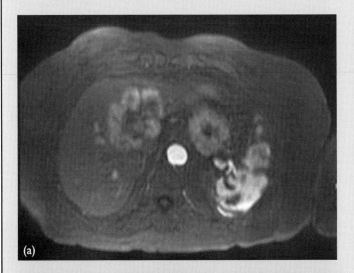 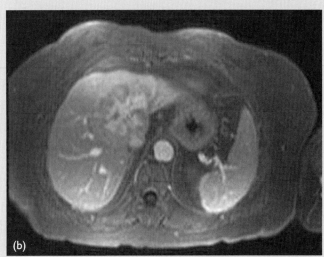

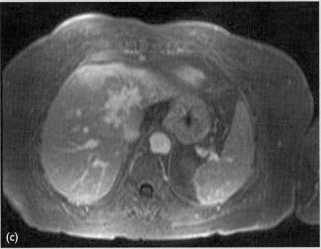

Case 6.2 (a–c) Early, mid and delayed dynamic volumetric interpolated breath-hold examination (VIBE) images showing intrahepatic cholangiocarcinoma. There is persistent enhancement on the 10-minute delayed image (c) – typical of cholangiocarcinoma.

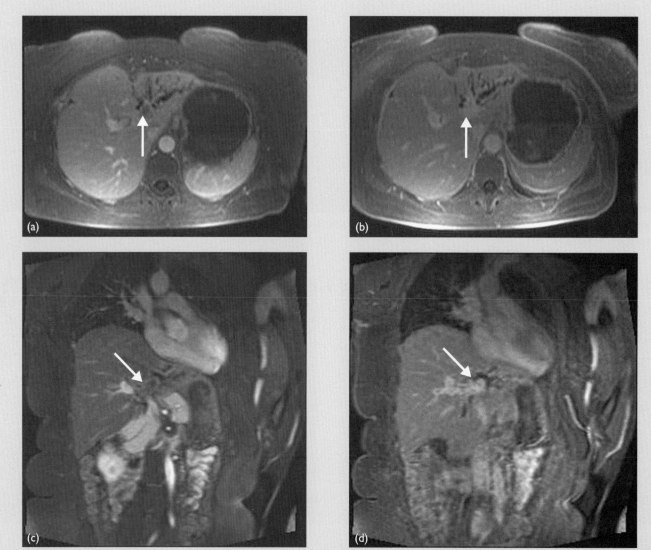

Case 6.3 (a–d) Early and delayed dynamic post-contrast images showing persistent enhancement in an infiltrative central cholangiocarcinoma (arrow).

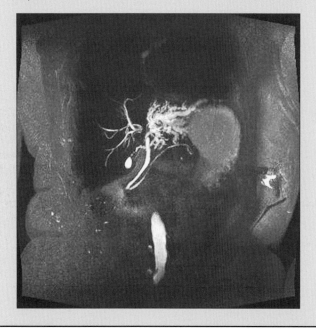

Case 6.4 MRCP image showing left lobe duct stricture with dilatation of the left-lobe intrahepatic ducts.

LIVER METASTASES

The liver, owing to its large blood supply, is the second most common site for metastatic disease after the lymph nodes, and can receive metastases from virtually any cancer. Morphologically, these can be mass lesions or of infiltrative type. Metastases can be hypo- or hypervascular compared with the liver parenchyma. Hypovascular metastases are best identified in the portovenous phase of a contrast study, while, because hypervascular metastases may still be visible in the portovenous phase, they are best identified in the arterial phase of the study.

Key sequences

- These are similar to those used for FNH.

Imaging findings

Most liver tumours, benign or malignant, are generally hypointense on T1-weighted and hyperintense on T2-weighted images; exceptions to this general rule are melanoma metastases (due to melanin) or mucinous or haemorrhagic metastases, which are hyperintense on T1-weighted images.

Heavily T2-weighted images in particular help to differentiate small metastases from haemangiomas and benign cysts, since these are both more hyperintense than malignant lesions. With larger lesions, heterogeneous signal, central hyperintense areas of necrosis, and irregular and indistinct margins all favour a metastatic lesion.

Dynamic Gd-enhanced sequences improve identification and also help characterization. Metastases demonstrate heterogeneous enhancement, with no enhancement in necrotic areas. Hypervascular lesions are most prominent in the arterial phase of dynamic imaging and show a rapid washout of contrast, becoming isointense in the portal phase.

Mucinous metastases are bright on T2-weighted images, but usually only rim-enhance.

The use of SPIO further aids the detection of metastasis. Because of the lack of Kupffer cells in metastases, they do not take up the SPIO. As a result, the normal liver, which has taken up SPIO, has a signal drop due to magnetic susceptibility and the metastases stand out as hyperintense lesions in a dark liver.

Hints and tips

The use of MRI to detect liver metastases is usually reserved for cases likely to benefit from surgical resection of the metastases. Dynamic Gd-enhanced imaging is useful.

Metastasis often blocks the peripheral portal vein branches, resulting in a wedge-shaped area of increased enhancement on post-Gd T1-weighted arterial phase imaging. This transient intrahepatic intensity difference (THID), although also seen in some benign causes, should prompt a search for a small lesion at the apex of the wedge.

Rarely, primaries such as breast carcinoma and lymphoma, pre- or post-treatment, can give a cirrhotic appearance to the liver, with or without venous obstruction. This is diffuse carcinomatosis along with intense fibrous reaction and is called hepar lobatum carcinomatosum (see Case 4.3b).

Further reading

Robinson PJA, Ward J. *MRI of the Liver: A Practical Guide.* London: Informa Healthcare, 2006.

Case 7: Liver metastasis

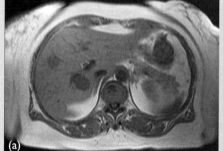 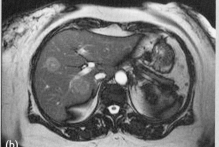 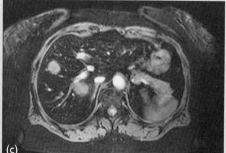

Case 7.1 Two lesions of different sizes, which are hypointense on the T1-weighted image (a) and slightly hyperintense on the T2-weighted image (b). Both of these lesions are hyperintense on the 10 minutes post SPIO plus Gd image (c), suggesting the absence of functioning Kupffer cells. This is typical of metastases.

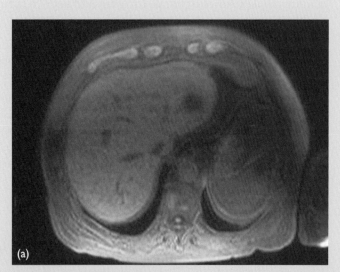
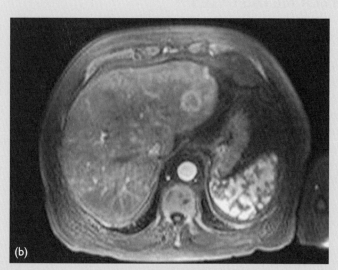

Case 7.2 (a, b) FS T1-weighted images before and after Gd administration demonstrating rim enhancement of the segment 2 lesion.

MAGNETIC RESONANCE CHOLANGIOPANCREATOGRAPHY (MRCP)

MRCP is widely used in the evaluation of biliary tree obstruction. The diagnostic information achieved with MRCP is comparable to that from diagnostic endoscopic retrograde cholangiopancreatography (ERCP) and has practically replaced the latter. Indications for MRCP include obstructive jaundice, post-biliary-surgery complications, follow-up of PSC and post-liver-transplant biliary fibrosis.

Key sequences

- T2-weighted true FISP axial and coronal
- T2-weighted turbo SE thin collimation in the axial plane and a 3D reconstruction maximum intensity projection (MIP) image from this data
- A thick slab of T2-weighted HASTE/SS-FSE
- Occasionally, T1-weighted sequences may be required if there is suspicion of biliary casts, particularly post-surgery.

Imaging findings

Biliary calculi are readily identified as dark filling defects within the high-signal fluid due to the very high signal-to-background ratio of bile. Calculi up to 2 mm in diameter can be confidently diagnosed with MRCP.

A dominant stricture within an obstructed biliary tree should be carefully evaluated for a cause; here clinical history may prove useful. In follow-up of PSC, a new dominant stricture should raise the possibility of cholangiocarcinoma, while a dominant stricture in a post-biliary-surgery case offers a differential between iatrogenic cause, vascular insufficiency (e.g. in liver transplant) or extrinsic causes such as collections or lymph nodes.

In the case of common bile duct dilatation, a narrowing smoothly tapering to an obstruction usually suggests a benign cause, while a shouldering raises suspicion of a neoplastic process.

A dilated double duct (pancreatic duct and common bile duct) should raise suspicion of an ampullary or pancreatic head neoplasm.

Hints and tips

Always evaluate source images carefully, because the sensitivity for detection of small filling defects decreases with an increase in section thickness owing to volume averaging of high-signal bile surrounding the stone.

Pulsations from the hepatic artery, an en face cystic duct, non-dependent gas and susceptibility artefacts from metallic surgical clips can give the appearance of a pseudostricture or filling defects on MIP images, again emphasizing the importance of investigating the source images.

An impacted stone in the ampulla can be difficult to visualize owing to lack of surrounding high-density fluid and may be misinterpreted as a stricture.

Contraction of the sphincter may cause abrupt cut-off of the duct. Repeating 2D sequences after the 3D reconstruction may help to differentiate.

Further reading

Robinson PJA, Ward J. *MRI of the Liver: A Practical Guide.* London: Informa Healthcare, 2006.
Irie H, Honda H, Kuroiwa T et al. Pitfalls in MR cholangio-pancreatographic interpretation. *Radiographics* 2001; **21**: 23–37.

Case 8: Magnetic resonance cholangiopancreatography

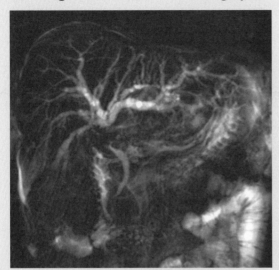

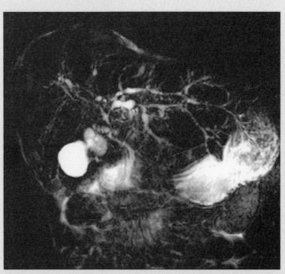

Case 8.1 Intra-hepatic duct dilatation due to complete obstruction of the proximal common bile duct, in this case secondary to external nodal compression.

Case 8.2 Spider's web-like appearance of the intrahepatic biliary ducts with 'beading' typical of primary sclerosing cholangitis.

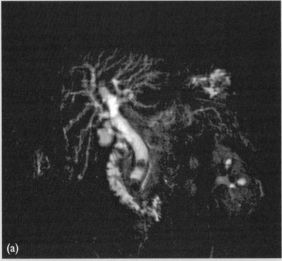

(a)

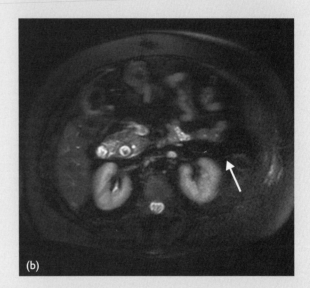

(b)

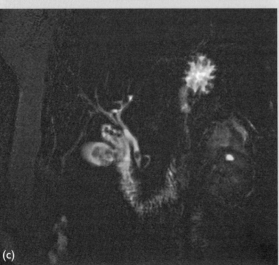

(c)

Case 8.3 (a–c) Hypointense calculus in the distal hyperintense common bile duct causing dilatation of the biliary tree.

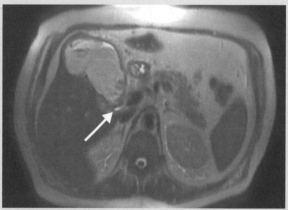

Case 8.4 Compression of the common hepatic duct by a distended gallbladder due to an impacted stone at its neck.

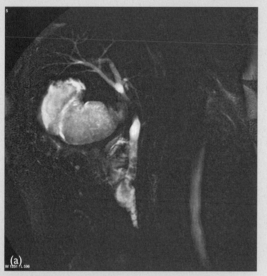

(a)

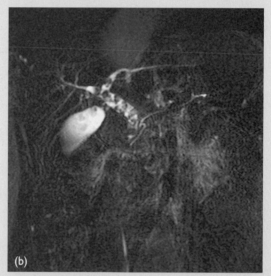

(b)

Case 8.5 (a, b) Examples of multiple calculi within the common bile duct, with pathological thickening of the gallbladder.

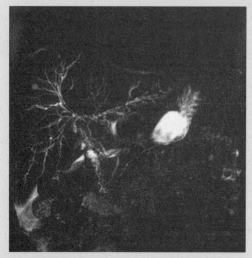

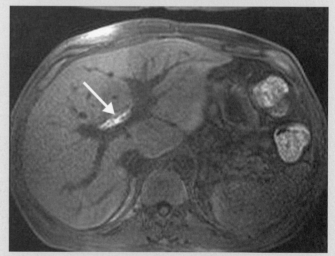

Case 8.6 MRCP image showing a non-dilated intrahepatic biliary tree with multifocal areas of stenoses. This image is of a transplanted liver with worsening liver function tests. In this transplant scenario with biliary stricture, a vascular insult such as hepatic artery stenosis or thrombosis is the most common cause.

Case 8.7 Another example of post-liver-transplant MRI performed for abnormal liver function. Note the hyperintense material on this T1-weighted image (arrow) within the right and left bile ducts – this represents a biliary cast causing obstruction to biliary flow.

RECTAL CANCER

In the past, the outcome of rectal cancer has been poor compared with that of colon cancer because of the higher local recurrence rate. However, in recent years, with the introduction of neoadjuvant treatment options and an improved surgical approach (namely, total mesorectal excision), outcome has improved and is now comparable to that of colon cancer. In order to achieve this, high-quality imaging has had an important role. An essential concept in rectal cancer is the circumferential resection margin (CRM) – this simply means how far the tumour is from the mesorectal fascia. If the CRM is involved or threatened then neoadjuvant therapy is considered, since the presence of tumour in the resection margin is a major prognostic feature for predicting local recurrence. The role of MRI is to stratify therapy by locally staging these tumours and assess preoperatively the likelihood of achieving a clear CRM. MRI also plays important role in assessing local response to neoadjuvant treatments that aim at downgrading tumours to achieve adequate local excision.

Key sequences

- T2-weighted SE sagittal through the pelvis (from sidewall to sidewall) with a large field of view (FOV) and a slice thickness of 5 mm
- T2-weighted SE axial through the pelvis with a large FOV and a slice thickness of 5 mm
- T2-weighted SE oblique axial perpendicular to the rectal mass with a small FOV and a slice thickness of 3 mm to cover tumour and presacral space.
- For low tumours, T2-weighted SE coronal
- For assessment of recurrence, T1-weighted GRE axial through the rectal mass with T1-weighted Gd-enhanced FS in the same plane

Imaging findings

Tumours can be polypoid, annular, bulky or ulcerated. They are of intermediate signal on T2-weighted images, typically slightly higher than that of muscle. Rectal cancers can display a desmoplastic reaction in adjacent mesorectal fat. This is usually spiculated, with a narrow base compared with the broader-based tumour invasion.

Look for the size and position of the rectal mass in the upper, middle or lower third of the rectum and its distance from the anal verge. The relationship of the tumour to peritoneal reflection in the upper two-thirds of the rectum should be closely examined. The peritoneum does not count as CRM, since it is often adherent to the anterior wall of the superior rectum. Treatment options may differ, depending upon these variables.

Look for the low-signal rim in the rectal wall – this is muscularis propria. Invasion of tumour through this upgrades the T stage to T3, and these cases will need neoadjuvant treatment prior to surgery. Describe the site and extent of invasion into the bright mesorectal fat envelope and measure the distance from the outermost tumour margin to the mesorectal fascia (CRM).

Look for lymph nodes within the pelvis and mesorectal fat and if these are close to the enclosing fascia. Nodes often follow the vessels superior to the tumour. Lymph node size is of limited significance; irregular contour and signal intensity are important for tumour involvement.

Post-treatment fibrosis is low signal compared with intermediate signal of recurrence or residual disease, which also enhances post-contrast.

Hints and tips

Identify the tubular tumour extensions along the line of vessels, staged as V1.

High signal within the tumour is suggestive of a mucinous tumour. These tumours generally respond less favourably to neoadjuvant therapy.

For lower-rectal tumours, describe the relationship with the levator ani.

Do not forget to look at any caecal dilatation, synchronous tumours, fistulation or perforation of tumour.

Further reading

Hulse PA, ed. *Handbook of MRI Staging of Pelvic Cancer*. London: Informa Healthcare, 2003.
Husband JE, ed. *Imaging in Oncology*. London: Informa Healthcare, 2004.
Iafrate F, Laghi A, Paolantonio P et al. Preoperative staging of rectal cancer with MR imaging: correlation with surgical and histopathologic findings. *Radiographics* 2006; 26: 701–14.

Case 9: Rectal cancer

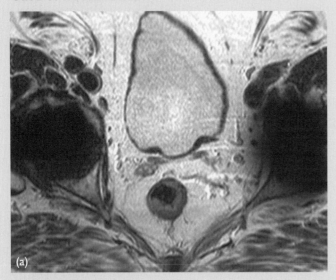

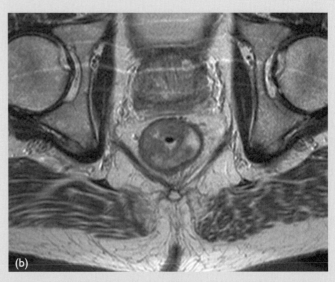

Case 9.1 (a, b) Two different examples of intermediate-intensity rectal tumours on T2-weighted images. Note that the tumours do not breach the hypointense muscularis layer. In (b), there are areas of hyperintensity (arrow) within the tumour, which indicates a likely mucinous type. In both images, note that there is no corruption of the mesorectal fat envelope.

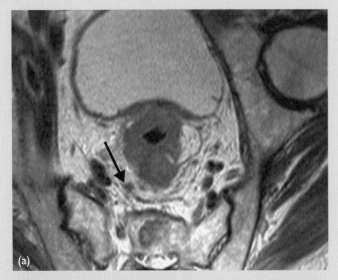

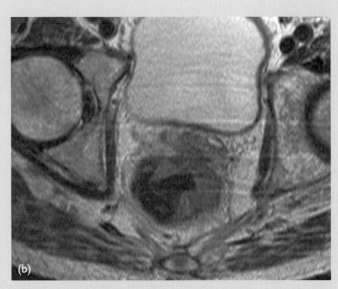

Case 9.2 (a, b) Two different examples of stage III disease on T2-weighted images, with the intermediate-intensity tumours breaching the hypointense muscle layer and extending into the mesorectal fat. In (a), there is a tumour deposit (arrow) on the CRM at the 7 o'clock position. In (b), the tumour invades the seminal vesicles anteriorly; these vesicles normally return a bright T2 signal, but in this case are almost completely engulfed by the tumour.

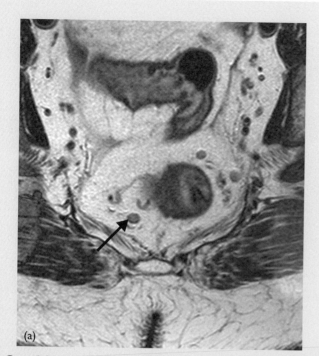
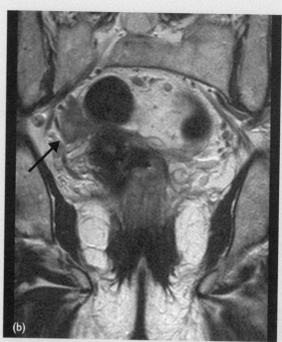

Case 9.3 (a, b) Axial and coronal images demonstrating lymph nodes (arrows) with increased tumour intensity against a background of bright fat.

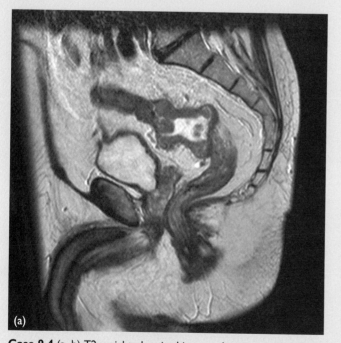
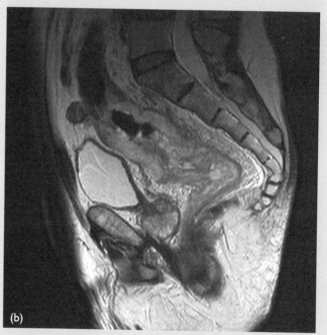

Case 9.4 (a, b) T2-weighted sagittal images showing two examples of rectal tumours extending above the peritoneal reflection.

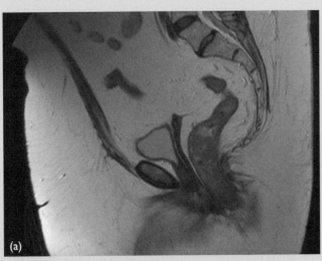

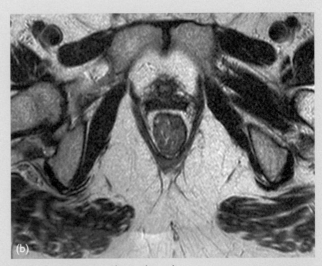

Case 9.5 (a, b) T2-weighted axial and sagittal images showing extension of rectal tumour into the anal canal.

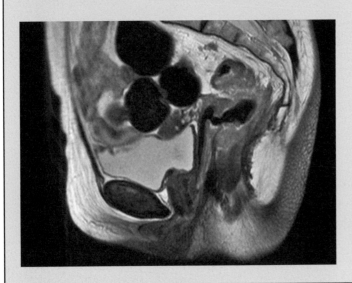

Case 9.6 An example of T4 disease causing fistulation of rectal tumour into the vagina anteriorly.

ANORECTAL (PERIANAL) FISTULA

The role of MRI is to accurately demonstrate the anatomy of the perianal region. In addition, it shows the relationship of fistula to the levator ani and the ischioanal and ischiorectal fossae. In the simple intersphincteric variety, the ischioanal and ischiorectal fossae are not involved. In the trans-sphincteric or suprasphincteric varieties, the ischioanal or ischiorectal fossa is involved by a fistulous track or by an abscess (the latter indicating complex disease). Surgery for these types threatens continence or may require colostomy to allow healing. In translevator fistulae, there is communication above the pelvic diaphragm, and hence a pelvic source of sepsis should be suspected.

Key sequences

- T2-weighted SE sagittal through the pelvis (from sidewall to sidewall) with a large FOV and a slice thickness of 5 mm
- T2-weighted SE axial through the pelvis with a large FOV and a slice thickness of 5 mm
- T2-weighted FS and short-tau inversion recovery (STIR) coronal and oblique axial perpendicular to the area under investigation with a small FOV and a slice thickness of 3 mm
- T1-weighted GRE axial and coronal through the area under investigation (T1-weighted Gd-enhanced FS imaging in the same plane may be needed)
- MR fistulography with T2-weighted images after saline instillation into the fistula tract

Imaging findings

T1-weighted images provide good anatomic details of the sphincters and ischiorectal fat.

T2-weighted and STIR sequences are best for evaluating hyperintense abscesses and fistulous tracts, both primary and secondary, across the hypointense sphincter, muscles and fat (only on STIR)

On contrast-enhanced imaging, the walls of the fistulous tract and abscess wall enhance.

The St James's University Hospital MRI classification of perianal **fistula**s is recommended to classify the anatomy of the fistula, on which the surgical decision making process is based.

Hints and tips

Look for a dumbbell-shaped (on coronal imaging) and circumferential horseshoe-shaped (on axial imaging) fistulous tract.

Look out for causes of non-idiopathic fistulae such as Crohn's disease, tuberculosis, trauma during childbirth, pelvic infection, pelvic malignancy and radiation therapy

Further reading

Morris J, Spencer JA, Ambrose NS. MR imaging classification of perianal fistulas and its implications for patient management. *Radiographics* 2000; **20**: 623–35; discussion 635–7.

Spencer JA, Ward J, Ambrose NS. Dynamic contrast-enhanced MR imaging of perianal fistulae. *Clin Radiol* 1998; **53**: 96–104.

Case 10: Anorectal (perianal) fistula

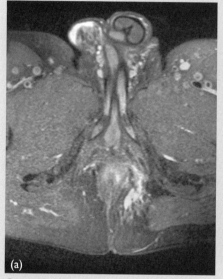
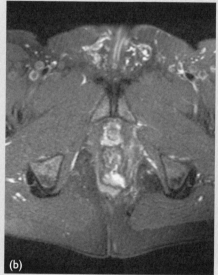
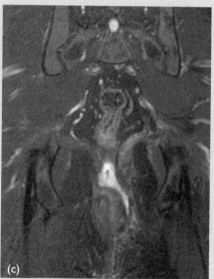

Case 10.1 (a-c) Various examples of intra and inter-sphincteric extention of the peri-anal fistula.

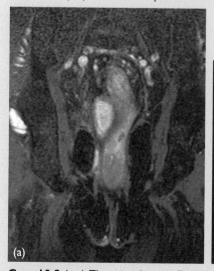
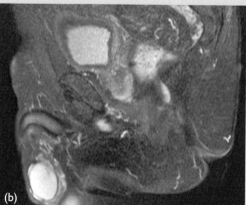
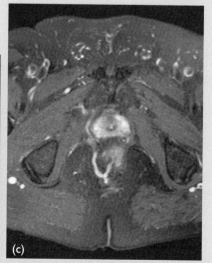

Case 10.2 (a-c) There is a large collection above the levator ani, which is feeding the fistula. Identification and treatment Aof this source of collection is essential for successful treatment.

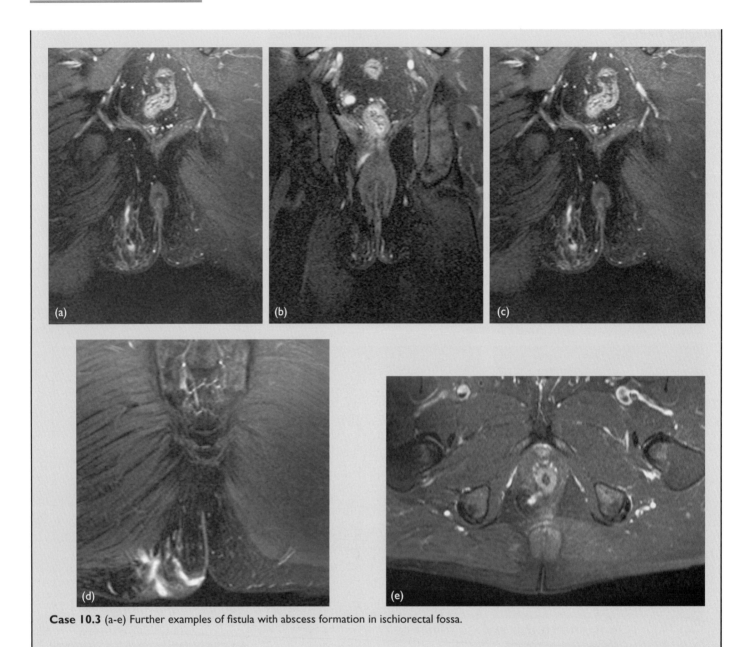

Case 10.3 (a-e) Further examples of fistula with abscess formation in ischiorectal fossa.

ADRENAL ADENOMA

Adrenal adenomas are the most common adrenal lesions. They are benign tumours of the adrenal gland, arising from its cortex, and are not known to exceed 5 cm in size. They are called 'functioning' when they produce hormones (leading to Conn's and Cushing syndromes, among others). Adrenal adenomas may be associated with multiple endocrine neoplasia type 1 (MEN1), Beckwith–Wiedemann syndrome and Carney complex. The closest differential diagnoses are adrenal metastases (chiefly from non-small cell lung, renal and hepatocellular carcinoma),

adrenocortical carcinoma and phaeochromocytomas (these arise from the medulla).

Key sequences

- T2-weighted rapid acquisition with relaxation enhancement (RARE) axial and coronal
- T1-weighted chemical shift in- and out-of-phase coronal and axial
- Volumetric interpolated breath-hold examination (VIBE),* performed before and after administration of Gd, only if further evaluation is needed

---

*VIBE is a 3D GRE sequence. It is used to provide dynamic contrast-enhanced thin-section images with fat saturation and a high signal-to-noise ratio.

Imaging findings

Adrenal adenomas are hypointense on T1-weighted images and of variable intensity on T2-weighted images. T1- and T2-weighted signal characteristics of benign adrenal adenomas and adrenal metastases overlap significantly.

In-phase and out-of phase imaging must be used to diagnose adenomas with 80–100% sensitivity and 90–100% specificity. Out-of-phase or opposed-phase chemical shift images of lipid-rich adrenal adenomas show decreases in signal intensity – a 20% reduction in signal intensity on an out-of-phase image is diagnostic of an adenoma. As a corollary, MRI cannot be used to definitely characterize lipid-poor adenomas (which, luckily, are very rare entities). In the latter case, one should proceed to administer contrast.

If contrast is administered, adenomas show mild enhancement and rapid washout.

Hints and tips

Signal loss on out-of-phase imaging can be assessed visually by inspecting the spleen or skeletal muscle as a reference standard. Liver is not reliable, because fatty infiltration in the liver is common and will cause the liver to lose signal intensity anyway on out-of-phase images.

Adenomas with organizing haematomas may present a diagnostic dilemma, since they mimic haemangiomas.

Do not get caught out by a collision tumour: a metastatic deposit sitting next to an adenoma.

Remember that the echo time used for out-of-phase imaging should be shorter than that used for in-phase imaging, so that loss of signal intensity reflects the presence of lipid and not T2 decay!

Further reading

Elsayes KM, Mukundan G, Narra VR et al. Adrenal masses: MR imaging features with pathologic correlation. *Radiographics* 2004; **24**(Suppl 1): S73–86.

Case 11: Adrenal adenoma

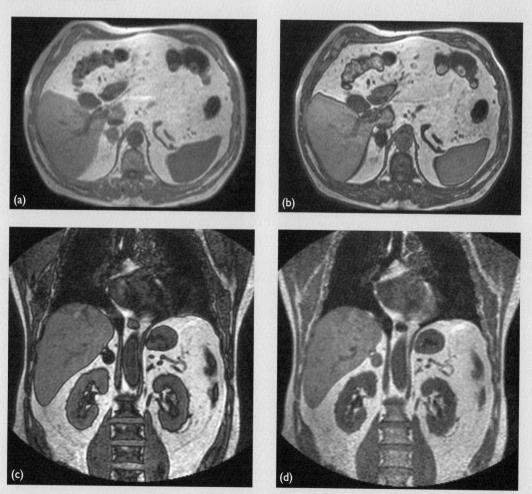

Case 11.1 (a, c) In-phase axial and coronal images showing an intermediate-intensity right adrenal lesion. (b, d) The lesion loses signal completely on out-of-phase imaging, suggesting the presence of fat, a feature of benign adenomas.

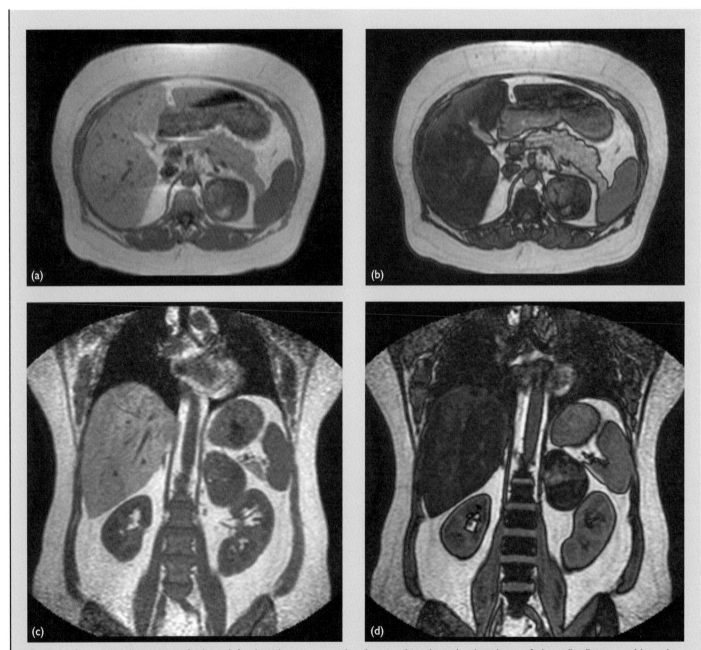

Case 11.2 Another illustration of a large left adrenal mass on axial and coronal in-phase (a, c) and out-of-phase (b, d) images. Note that although the lesion is large, there is signal dropout, suggesting that this is a benign adenoma.

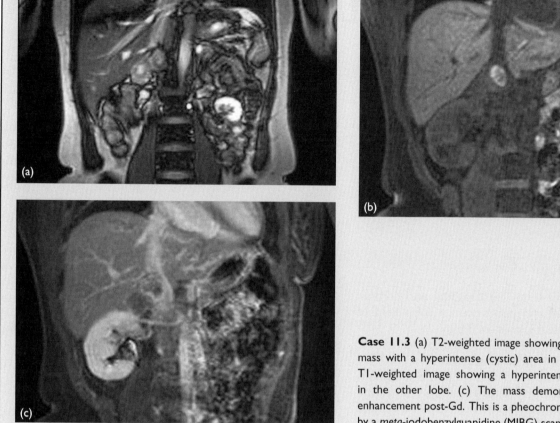

Case 11.3 (a) T2-weighted image showing a bilobed right adrenal mass with a hyperintense (cystic) area in one of its lobes. (b) FS T1-weighted image showing a hyperintense area (haemorrhage) in the other lobe. (c) The mass demonstrates heterogeneous enhancement post-Gd. This is a pheochromocytoma, as confirmed by a *meta*-iodobenzylguanidine (MIBG) scan.

3 UROLOGY AND GYNAECOLOGY

OVARIAN DERMOID

Ovarian dermoid is a neoplasm of germ cell origin, arising from elements of all three germ layers. There are three types of ovarian dermoid: mature cystic teratomas (dermoid cysts), immature teratomas and monodermal teratomas (i.e. those arising from single cell line, such as struma ovarii, carcinoid tumours and neural tumours)

Key sequences

The approach is as for any other indeterminate adnexal mass:
- T2-weighted fast spin echo (FSE) sagittal and coronal through the abdomen and pelvis with a large field of view (FOV) and a slice thickness of 5 mm
- T1-weighted spin echo (SE) axial through the pelvis with a small FOV and a slice thickness of 3 mm
- T1-weighted fat-saturated (FS) axial through the pelvis with a small FOV and a slice thickness of less than 3 mm, with a gadolinium (Gd) enhancement sequence if needed in cases of atypical appearance
- T2-weighted SE axial through the pelvis with a small FOV and a slice thickness of 3 mm. If neither ovary is identified well, add T2-weighted axial sections perpendicular to the long axis of the uterus.

Imaging findings

Appearances are variable, depending upon the proportion of the three germ cell elements.

Fat is the predominant component in most mature dermoid tumours. The sebaceous and haemorrhagic contents are hyperintense on T1-weighted images and similar to retroperitoneal fat. The fatty component can be distinguished from haemorrhage, since the former shows signal loss on FS images. Dense calcific foci such as tooth or material such as hair are hypointense on T1- and T2-weighted images.

The cystic areas are hyperintense on T2-weighted images. The appearances on T1- and T2-weighted sequences mimic those seen in haemorrhagic endometrioma, but the FS images help differentiate mature dermoid from other pathologies.

Up to a third of teratomas in the first and second decades are malignant and a small proportion of older women with teratomas develop squamous cancer in skin elements. Malignant change should be suspected if there is focal thickening or irregularity and especially if the outer margin is irregular or indistinct. When there is a soft tissue component within the cystic component that exceeds 5 cm or if the rate of growth is high, malignant transformation should be suspected.

Hints and tips

In the monodermal struma ovarii variety, some of the cystic spaces may demonstrate low signal on both T1- and T2-weighted images due to the thick gelatinous colloid. No fat is evident in these lesions.

The carcinoid variety of monodermal teratomas usually occur in the postmenopausal age group and are generally solid rather than cystic. Compared with other solid ovarian tumours, these have higher signal on T2-weighted images due to the presence of mucin within them .

Further reading

Outwater EK, Siegelman ES, Hunt JL. Ovarian teratomas: tumor types and imaging characteristics. *Radiographics* 2001; **21**: 475–90.

Case 12: Ovarian dermoid

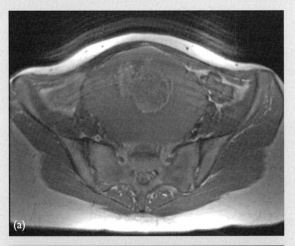

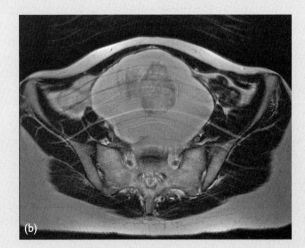

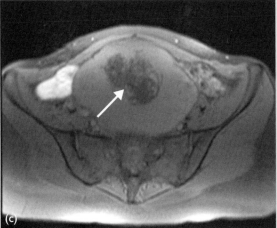

Case 12.1 Large solid-cystic ovarian mass with T1-bright solid central element (a) within T2-bright fluid (b). Note the signal dropout from the central solid component (arrow) on the FS T1-weighted image (c).

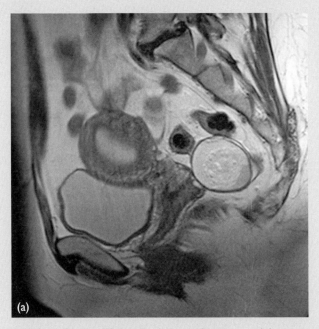

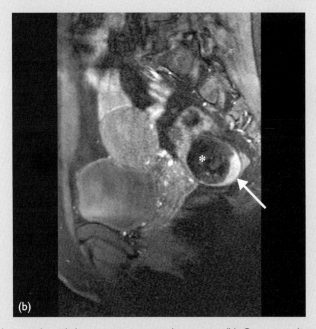

Case 12.2 (a) Sagittal T2-weighted image showing a solid mass in the pouch with heterogeneous signal intensity. (b) Corresponding FS T1-weighted image showing signal dropout from the larger anterior fat component (asterisk), with the hyperintense bright area representing blood products (arrow), probably from haemorrhage due to a recent torsion episode.

FIBROMA

Ovarian fibroma is the most common sex cord stromal tumour. It is most commonly seen in young women and is also known to be associated with Gorlin's syndrome. These tumours present a diagnostic dilemma when identified on other imaging modalities, since they are closely mimicked by both benign and malignant causes such as pedunculated fibroid and malignant ovarian tumours.

Key sequences

The approach is as for any other indeterminate adnexal mass:

- T2-weighted FSE sagittal and coronal sections through the abdomen and pelvis, with a large FOV and a slice thickness of 5 mm
- T1-weighted SE axial through the pelvis with a small FOV and a slice thickness of 3 mm
- T1-weighted FS axial through the pelvis with a small FOV and a slice thickness less than 3 mm, with Gd enhancement if necessary
- T2-weighted SE axial through the pelvis with small FOV and a slice thickness of 3 mm. If neither ovary is identified well, add T2-weighted axial sections perpendicular to the long axis of the uterus.

Imaging findings

Fibroma is seen as a well-demarcated hypointense mass within the adnexa on both T1- and T2-weighted images. This is due to the dense collagen content of the tumour.

Occasionally, hyperintense areas may be seen on T2-weighted images. There are areas of degeneration or oedema.

On contrast-enhanced images, there is no or delayed enhancement of these masses.

Hints and tips

Look for ascites or pleural effusion in cases of Meigs' syndrome.

Fibroma, like any other ovarian tumour, is prone to torsion and hence can show areas of haemorrhage.

Further reading

Imaoka I, Wada A, Kaji Y et al. Developing an MR imaging strategy for diagnosis of ovarian masses. *Radiographics* 2006; **26**: 1431–48.

Case 13 Fibroma

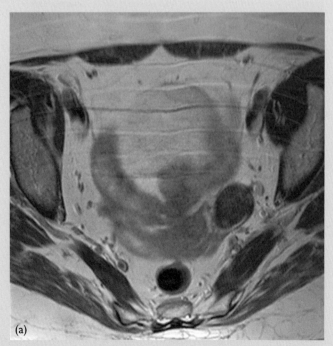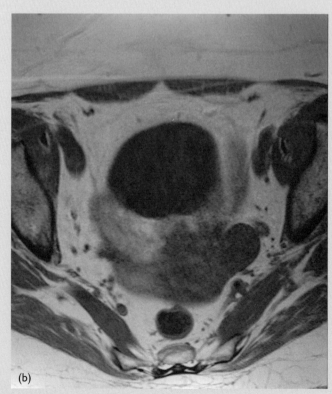

(a) (b)

Case 13.1 (a, b) T2- and T1-weighted axial images showing a hypointense left ovarian fibroma (asterisk).

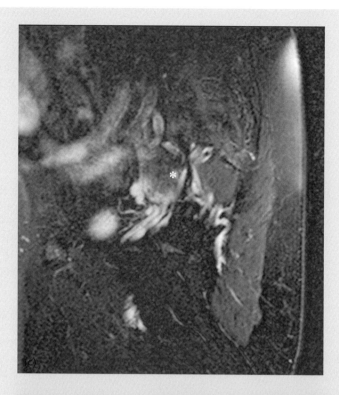

Case 13.1 *continued* (c) On this FS post-Gd T1-weighted sagittal image, there is no enhancement of the fibroma (asterisk), in contrast to the enhancing remaining normal ovarian tissue.

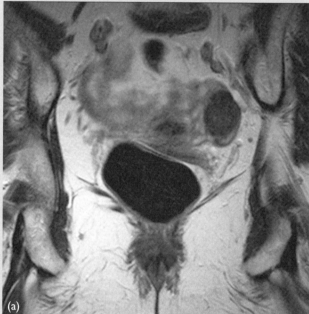

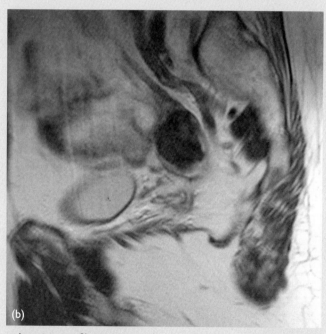

Case 13.2 (a, b) T1-weighted coronal and sagittal images demonstrating a hypointense fibroma arising from the left ovary. The ovarian pedicle supplying to the fibroma on (b) confirms the ovarian origin.

OVARIAN CANCER

Ovarian cancer is the second most common gynaecological malignancy but the leading cause of death from such tumours. More than two-thirds occur above the age of 50 years. Primary ovarian cancers are classified according to the cell line of origin: 85% are epithelial and the remaining are germ cell or sex cord stromal tumours. Computed tomography is used to stage tumours confidently shown by ultrasound scan, while the role of MRI is to characterize ultrasound-indeterminate adnexal masses, particularly in young women with normal or slightly raised CA-125. Ovarian tumours can be cystic, solid or mixed.

Key sequences

- T2-weighted FSE sagittal and coronal through the abdomen and pelvis with a large FOV and a slice thickness of 5 mm
- T1- and T2-weighted SE axial through the pelvis with a small FOV and a slice thickness of 3 mm
- FS T1-weighted axial through the pelvis with a small FOV and a slice thickness less than 3 mm and T1-weighted GRE with Gd enhancement
- T2-weighted SE sagittal from one pelvic sidewall to the other

Imaging findings

Normal postmenopausal ovaries are of small volume and hypointense on T1- and T2-weighted images, since the ovarian stroma is replaced by fibrous tissue.

Solid tumours are hypointense on T1- and T2-weighted images and enhance post-contrast. The strongest signs of malignancy on contrast-enhanced T1-weighted images are the presence of enhancing solid components, 'vegetations' or the presence of necrosis in solid enhancing areas.

The cystic components of malignant ovarian tumours have variable signal, but are usually low to intermediate signal on T1-weighted images and high signal on T2-weighted images. On contrast-enhanced T1-weighted images, mural thickening, septations larger than 3 mm, mural nodularity and papillary projections suggest malignancy. Lesions with multiple fine septa and none of the above are regarded as benign and treated by excision alone.

Large cystic tumours without frank malignant features should be considered borderline and treated by surgical excision and staging.

Large-FOV images are useful to look for ascites, liver surface and parenchymal lesions, and lymphadenopathy. FS Gd-enhanced images are best to look for peritoneal deposits.

Hints and tips

Sex cord tumours, of which the granulosa cell type is the most common, are seen in both the juvenile and adult postmenopausal age groups. These are of mixed intensity with haemorrhage. They may exhibit endocrine activity (oestrogen) and produce endometrial hyperplasia or cancer (e.g. postmenopausal bleeding), and sometimes the diagnosis is made in this way.

Germ cell tumours are rare. They are seen in younger women, as unilateral, predominantly solid masses with varying degrees of necrosis and haemorrhage. Nodal metastases are more frequent than peritoneal disease.

Further reading

Hulse PA, ed. *Handbook of MRI Staging of Pelvic Cancer*. London: Informa Healthcare, 2003.

Husband JE, ed. *Imaging in Oncology*. London: Informa Healthcare, 2004.

Case 14: Ovarian cancer

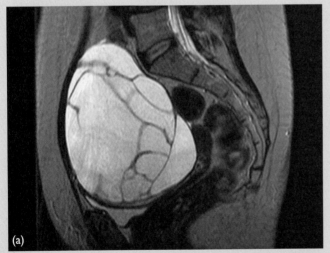
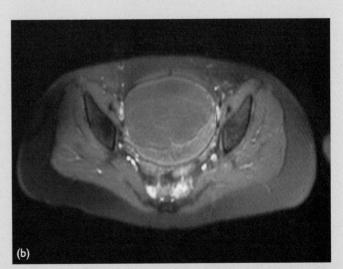

Case 14.1 (a–c) T2-weighted sagittal, FS T1-weighted axial and FS post-Gd T1-weighted axial images showing a large cystic ovarian mass with fine sepations, less than 2 mm in thickness, which show no enhancement post-Gd. These are features of a borderline ovarian cancer, for which only surgery is curative.

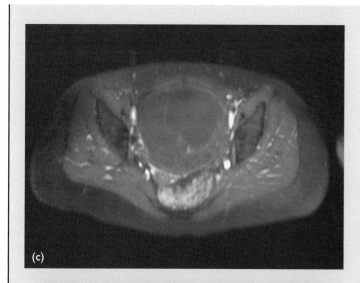

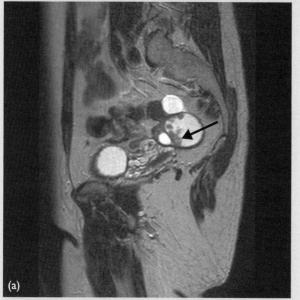

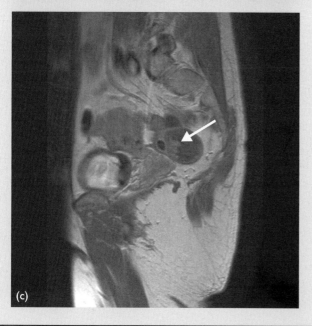

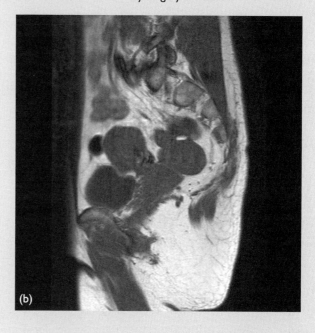

Case 14.1 *continued* (a–c) T2-weighted sagittal, FS T1-weighted axial and FS post-Gd T1-weighted axial images showing a large cystic ovarian mass with fine sepations, less than 2 mm in thickness, which show no enhancement post-Gd. These are features of a borderline ovarian cancer, for which only surgery is curative.

Case 14.2 (a, b) T2- and T1-weighted sagittal images showing a predominantly cystic ovarian mass with solid mural elements (arrow). (c) Post-Gd T1-weighted image showing intense enhancement of this solid mural tissue suggestive of malignancy.

ENDOMETRIOMA

Endometriosis is defined as the presence of endometrial glandular tissue outside the uterus. An MRI examination is required when this entity is encountered as an indeterminate mass on other imaging modalities, usually pelvic ultrasound. MRI works as a problem-solving tool.

Key sequences

- T2-weighted FSE sagittal and coronal through the abdomen and pelvis with a large FOV and a slice thickness of 5 mm
- T1-weighted SE axial through the pelvis with a small FOV and a slice thickness of 3 mm
- FS T1-weighted axial through the pelvis with a small FOV and a slice thickness less than 3 mm, with Gd enhancement if necessary
- T2-weighted SE axial through the pelvis with a small FOV and a slice thickness of 3 mm. If neither ovary is identified well, add T2-weighted axial sections perpendicular to the long axis of the uterus.
- T2-weighted SE sagittal from one pelvic sidewall to the other

Imaging findings

The appearance of endometriomas on MRI is variable and depends on the concentration in the fluid of iron and protein from the products of blood degradation. Most endometriomas have highly concentrated blood products, and MRI demonstrates these as cystic masses with pronounced hyperintensity on T1-weighted images and hypointensity on T2-weighted images. The hypointensity on the T2-weighted images occurs in a gradient from higher to lower signal called shading. This pattern of shading is almost always seen in endometriomas.

Multiple high-signal lesions, usually in the ovaries, on T1-weighted images are also highly suggestive of endometriosis.

Peritoneal implants are initially small serosal lesions and usually escape detection. Larger, fibrotic implants of endometriosis are seen as spiculated nodules of very low signal on T2-weighted images. These commonly occur in the cul-de-sac; less commonly, they appear on the bladder dome, rectum or umbilicus or in pelvic surgical scars. Dilated fallopian tubes are occasionally seen on MRI in patients with endometriosis; these are high signal on T1-weighted images, indicative of bloody fluid.

Further reading

Ghattamaneni S, Weston MJ, Spencer JA. Imaging in endometriosis. *Imaging* 2007; **19**: 345–68.

Case 15: Endometrioma

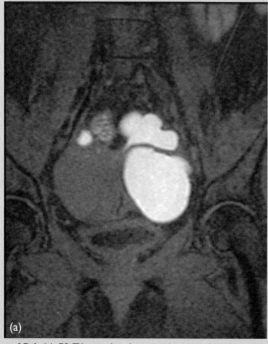
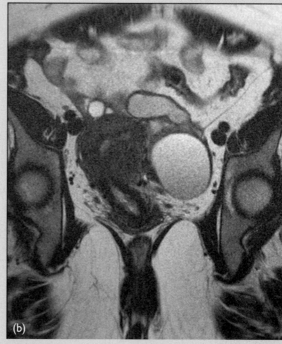

Case 15.1 (a) FS T1-weighted coronal image showing a bright cystic left adnexal mass suggestive of a haemorrhagic component. Note the 'shading' within this cyst on coronal (b) and sagittal.

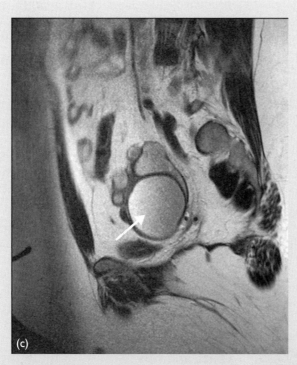

Case 15.1 (c) T2-weighted images (arrow).

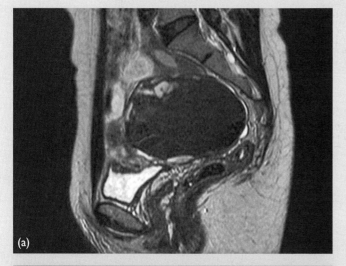

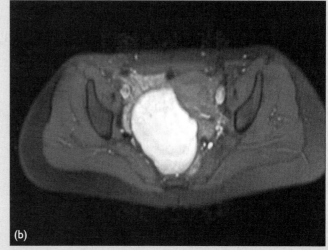

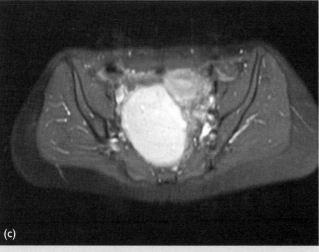

Case 15.2 (a) Sagittal T2-weighted image showing a large hypointense mass. (b, c) The mass is hyperintense on T1-weighted images and shows no enhancement. This represents the fibrotic type of endometrioma.

FALLOPIAN TUBE DISEASE

MRI is used in cases of fallopian pathology when ultrasound fails to make a confident diagnosis of an indeterminate adnexal mass. The common tubal conditions include hydrosalpinx, pyosalpinx, endometriosis and, rarely, malignancy. A systematic approach looking at shape, boundaries and contents is helpful in confidently determining the origin of a complex mass and characterizing it as a specific disease process.

Key sequences

- T2-weighted FSE sagittal through the abdomen and pelvis with a large FOV and a slice thickness of 5 mm
- T1-weighted SE and FS T1-weighted axial through the pelvis with a small FOV and a slice thickness of 3 mm, with a post-Gd T1-weighted sequence if necessary
- T2-weighted SE axial and sagittal through the pelvis with a small FOV and a slice thickness of 3 mm. Problem-solving T2-weighted images in a plane along the length of a suspected tubal mass may be helpful to show its morphology.

Imaging findings

Fallopian pathology manifests as a tortuous or folded fluid-filled tubular structure. Convolutions of the tube can lead to 'beaking' similar to bowel volvulus or a prominent 'waist'. The wall may show thin incomplete mucosal folds or thin fibrinous sepatations. Other features of tubal mass may include low-signal, non-enhancing mural nodules on T2-weighted images.

A thick wall that is hypointense on T1-weighted images and hyperintense on T2-weighted images and enhances on post-Gd T1-weighted images is suggestive of acute salpingitis. In such cases, hyperaemia of the ovarian pedicle and broad ligament can also be seen.

Contents characteristic of the tubal mass help in diagnosis of the cause. The simple fluid of hydrosalpinx is hyperintense on T2-weighted images and low signal on T1-weighted images. On T2-weighted images, pus often shows signal loss and shading due to cellular and proteinaceous component of the fluid. It seldom shows a fluid–fluid level, since the contents do not sediment but may contract into irregular shapes. With endometriosis, there is hyperintensity on T1-weighted images due to the blood components.

Primary fallopian tube malignancy is rare. On T2-weighted images, intermediate-signal solid components within the tubular mass that enhance on post-Gd T1-weighted images should alert for malignancy, which often causes and presents as hydrosalpinx. Also look for peritoneal thickening if tumour spill has occurred.

Hints and tips

The first step in the approach is to clearly identify the ovaries separate from or with the adnexal tubular mass stretched around them. On T2-weighted images, bright physiological cysts are helpful in localizing the ovaries. Then look for shape, wall and contents.

Further reading

Ghattamaneni S, Bhuskute NB, Weston MJ, Spencer JA. Discriminant MRI features of fallopian tube masses. *Clin Radiol* 2009; **64**: 815–31.

Case 16: Fallopian tube disease

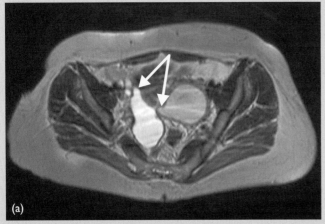 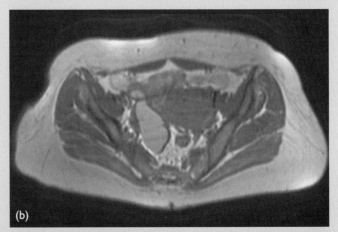

Case 16.1 (a, b) Bilateral tubal dilatation on T2-weighted and T1-weighted axial images. Look for the 'beak sign' (white arrows). The tube on the right is T2- and T1-bright, suggesting a blood/mucinous component, while on the left the tube contents are T1-dark and amorphously bright, suggesting 'pus'.

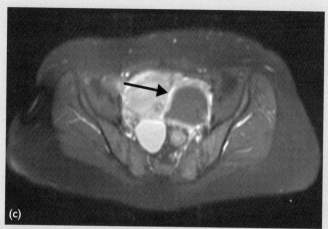

Case 16.1 (c) post-Gd T1-weighted image showing intense enhancement of the right left tubal wall on (black arrow).

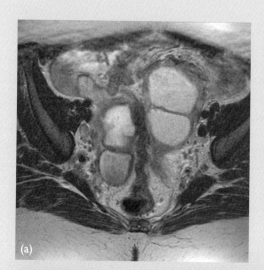

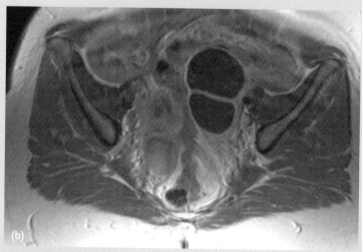

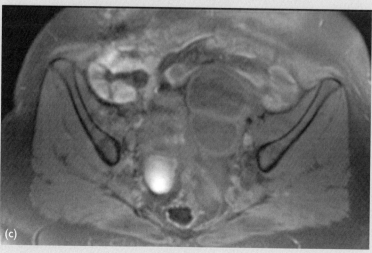

Case 16.2 (a–c) T2-weighted, T1-weighted and FS post-Gd T1-weighted axial images showing bilateral tubo-ovarian masses with similar T2 signal characteristics with thick walls and containing fluid of differing densities, which suggests the presence of blood or complex protein, resulting in shading. Note the wall enhancement on the FS post-Gd T1-weighted image (c), with high signal in the right tube suggestive of subacute blood. These features are all collectively suggestive of infection.

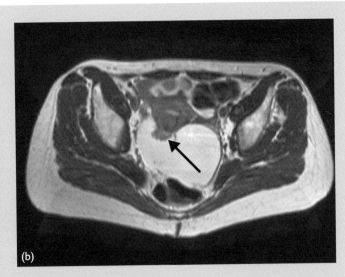

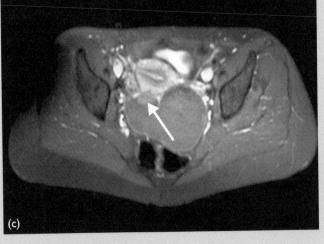

Case 16.3 (a) T2-weighted coronal image showing a thick mucosal fold within the convoluted cyst, suggesting a fallopian origin. Note the solid mural component (arrow) on the T2-weighted axial image (b), which shows enhancement on the post-Gd T1-weighted axial image (c).

UTERINE FIBROID

Uterine fibroids are the most common benign gynaecological tumours. They are oestrogen-dependent and therefore atrophy after the menopause. The use of tamoxifen may continue or rekindle their activity. The role of MRI is to differentiate uterine from ovarian indeterminate adnexal masses to establish a firm diagnosis of fibroids. MRI also helps to provide information regarding the location, type and size of these tumours. It also helps to plan and monitor treatment options such as myomectomy and endovascular embolization.

Key sequences

The role of MRI in fibroids is when they present as an indeterminate mass on pelvic ultrasound or when there is an unexpected increase in fibroid size on ultrasound follow-up scan. MRI is also used in planning and monitoring the response to uterine artery embolization for fibroid uterus.

Consider using the sequences described for an indeterminate adnexal mass.

Imaging findings

Fibroids can be submucosal, interstitial or subserosalin in location, and can be sessile or pedunculated in appearance. They may occur separate from the uterus within the round or broad ligaments.

On T1- and T2-weighted images, uterine fibroids are seen as well-demarcated low- to intermediate-signal masses arising within or from the myometrium of the uterus. A large fibroid presenting as an adnexal mass can be identified from its stalk, which extends to the myometrium. The stalk may show bridging vessels from the uterus, a sign of exophytic fibroid.

Occasionally, on T2-weighted images, large fibroids may demonstrate a peripheral hyperintense ring indicating oedema or patchy hyperintense areas within suggesting degeneration, haemorrhage, highly cellular fibroids or sarcomatous transformation. On contrast enhancement, fibroids usually show slightly delayed enhancement compared with the normal myometrium. Sarcomatous fibroids are difficult to diagnose, with no pathognomic features, although a rapid increase in size compared with prior imaging and intense and early enhancement might raise suspicion.

Post-embolization appearances of favourable response include a reduction in size and perfusion of fibroids. Signal intensity changes consistent with haemorrhagic infarction, namely hyperintense areas on T1-weighted images, are also seen.

Hints and tips

Fibroids (leiomyomas) are also seen at sites away from the uterus, such as intravenous locations, loose detached 'parasitic' fibroid intraperitoneally, urinary bladder, intrapulmonary, vulva, urethra, ovary and retroperitoneum.

Intravascular extension of uterine fibroids has been described. These extensions may be directly into the pelvic veins, progressing upwards into the vena cava. Fast flow-weighted sequences (e.g. fast imaging with steady-state precession: FISP) may show the extent.

Further reading

Kitamura Y, Ascher SM, Cooper C et al. Imaging manifestations of complications associated with uterine artery embolization. *Radiographics* 2005; **25**(Suppl 1): S119–32.

Case 17: Uterine fibroid

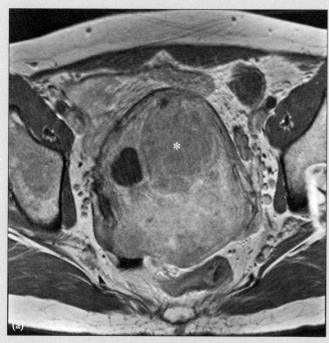 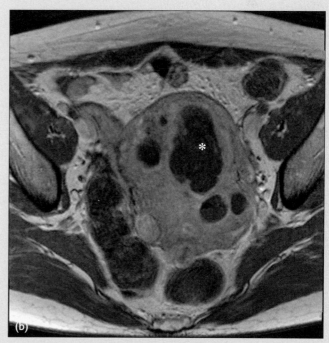

Case 17.1 (a, b) Pre- and 3 months post-embolization T1-weighted Gd-enhanced axial images showing reduced perfusion of a large fibroid (asterisk).

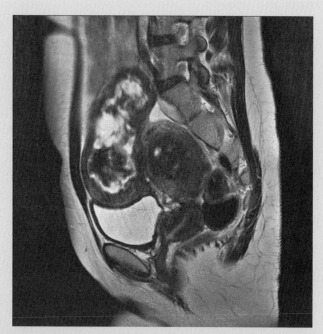

Case 17.2 T2-weighted axial image illustrating high-signal areas within a low-signal large fibroid, suggesting myxoid degeneration.

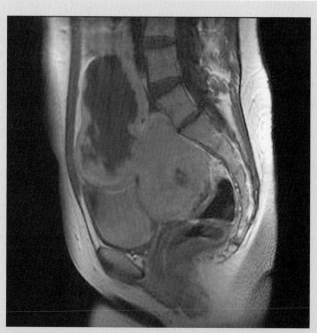

Case 17.3 Post-Gd T1-weighted image of the same case post-embolization illustrating large areas of the fibroid with no perfusion, indicating a good response.

ADENOMYOSIS

Adenomyosis is a common non-neoplastic disorder among women in the menstruating age group. It is characterized pathologically by benign invasion of ectopic endometrium into the myometrium with adjacent smooth muscle hyperplasia. With increasing use of tamoxifen in oestrogen-sensitive breast cancer, the incidence of adenomyosis among postmenopausal women is on the rise. As the junctional zone thickness can increase in days 1–2 of the menstrual phase (a physiological response), MRI should be avoided during this period.

Key sequences

- T2-weighted FSE sagittal and coronal through the abdomen and pelvis with a large FOV and a slice thickness of 5 mm
- T1-weighted SE sagittal and FS T1-weighted axial through the pelvis with a small FOV and a slice thickness of 3 mm
- T2-weighted SE axial through the pelvis with a small FOV and a slice thickness of 3 mm. If neither ovary is identified well, add T2-weighted axial sections perpendicular to the long axis of the uterus.
- T2-weighted SE sagittal from one pelvic sidewall to the other.

Imaging findings

On T2-weighted images, the hypointense junctional zone (JZ) is thickened, representing myometrial hyperplasia.

A JZ thickness greater than 12 mm is highly predictive of adenomyosis, while a thickness less than 8 mm almost rules it out.

T2-hyperintense areas within the JZ represent ectopic endometrium and glandular tissue within the myometrium.

T1-hyperintense areas may be seen within the ectopic endometrial tissue in the JZ. These represent focal haemorrhage and are particularly well seen if scanned during the menstrual phase.

Hints and tips

Adenomyosis can be symmetrical, asymmetrical or focal. The intensity of adenomyosis on T1- and T2-weighted images varies depending upon the time of scanning during the menstrual cycle.

Ill-defined areas of T2 signal within the myometrium may represent focal adenomyomas (cf. well-defined rounded or ovoid areas suggesting fibroids). Close mimics of adenomyosis are focal myometrial thickening and diffuse myometrial hyperplasia. The thickness criteria usually help to distinguish these.

Myometrium contraction can also mimic adenomyosis. While sequential imaging helps in differentiation of this temporary focal thickening of myometrium, it can be difficult to distinguish on a single study.

The presence of adenomyosis can make staging of endometrial cancer difficult.

Case 18: Adenomyosis

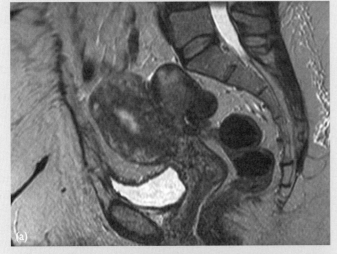

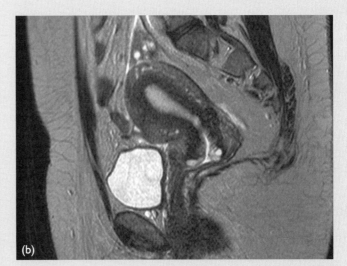

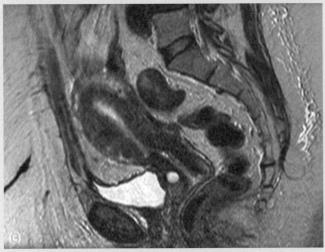

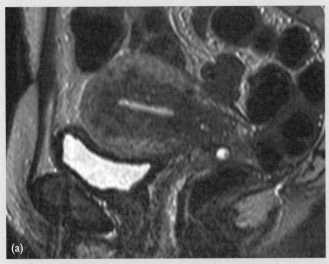

Case 18.1 (a–c) T2-weighted images in different cases showing high signal within the myometrium, while the hypointense junctional zone (arrow) is thickened.

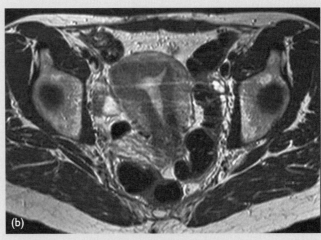

Case 18.2 (a, b) Two more examples of a thickened junctional zone in the sagittal and coronal oblique planes.

ENDOMETRIAL CANCER

Endometrial cancer is a common gynaecological malignancy and its incidence in UK has increased gradually over the last three decades. MRI is used in local staging. The FIGO classification system is used for staging. The depth of myometrial invasion and invasion of cervix stroma are the two most important prognostic factors. The role of MRI is to accurately differentiate outer-half myometrial invasion (FIGO stage IC) and cervical invasion (FIGO stage II) in deciding if lymph node dissection is indicated. Lymph node dissection is associated with complications, but, on the other hand, understaging may lead to a poorer outcome.

Key sequences

- For overview, FISP axial of the abdomen and pelvis and T1-weighted coronal with a large FOV of the retroperitoneum
- T2-weighted SE oblique axial (perpendicular to the long axis of the uterus) with a small FOV and a slice thickness of 3 mm
- T1-weighted SE and FS T1-weighted sagittal and oblique axial through the uterus with a small FOV and a slice thickness less than 3 mm
- Dynamic FS Gd-enhanced T1-weighted sagittal and oblique axial between 60 and 150 s through the uterus with a small FOV and a slice thickness less than 3 mm. (Contrast-enhanced study is not always required and is not routinely performed at our centre.)

Imaging findings

T2-weighted sequences depict the uterine zonal anatomy. Sandwiched between a high-signal endometrium and intermediate-signal myometrium is a low-signal junctional zone (JZ). The demarcation between the uterine body and cervix is defined by a waist in the uterine contour and the entrance of the uterine blood vessels at the level of the internal os. Also, the cervical epithelium is visible as a fourth layer defining the start of the endocervix.

On T2-weighted images, tumour can be seen as a mass or thickening of the endometrium of intermediate signal against the high signal of normal endometrium or endometrial cavity fluid and the low signal of the JZ of the myometrium. If the JZ is intact, there is usually no deep myometrium invasion (i.e. tumour is stage IB or lower). If it is disrupted (JZD), the tumour is usually stage IC or higher.

T1-weighted images help in identifying lymph node involvement.

On dynamic imaging, the uterus enhances avidly while the tumour is relatively less enhancing. There is an intense subendometrial enhancement (SEE), which defines the margins of the tumour. This helps not only to delineate tumour extent but also to differentiate tumours from endometrial debris.

Hints and tips

Coexisting benign disease, such as fibroids or adenomyosis, can result in morphological and signal changes in the myometrium that mimic tumour infiltration.

The abnormality of the JZ in adenomyosis and the absence of this in postmenopausal women makes dynamic contrast-enhanced imaging helpful for problem solving.

With deeper invasion, look for a hypointense infiltrate or mass as parametrial tumour and ovarian deposits (stage III).

Further reading

Hulse PA, ed. *Handbook of MRI Staging of Pelvic Cancer*. London: Informa Healthcare, 2003.

Husband JE, ed. *Imaging in Oncology*. London: Informa Healthcare, 2004.

Case 19: Endometrial cancer

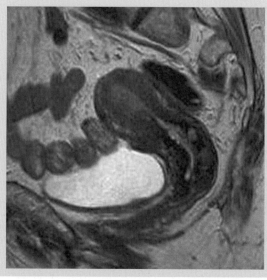

Case 19.1 T2-weighted sagittal image showing a distended bright endometrial cavity with intemediate-density tumour protruding into the cavity.

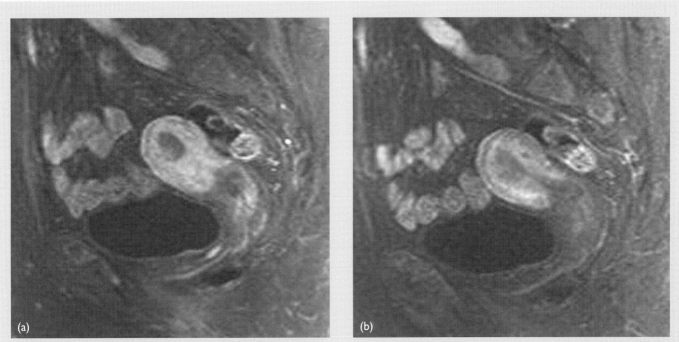

Case 19.2 (a, b) Dynamic FS images in early and delayed phases showing relatively poor enhancement of the endometrial tumour. On the delayed-phase image (b), less than 50% of myometrial invasion is seen, making this a stage Ib tumour.

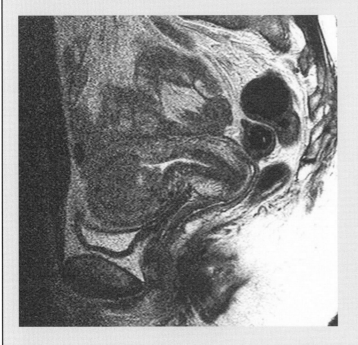

Case 19.3 T2-weighted sagittal image showing a bulky endometrial tumour invading most of the myometrium.

CERVICAL CANCER

Cervical cancer is a common female malignancy. The most common histological type, found in 85–90% of cases, is squamous cell carcinoma, while adenocarcinoma accounts for 5–10%. Most tumours arise from the squamocolumnar junction (SCJ). The SCJ is a transitional zone at the junction of the squamous epithelium of the vaginal portion of the cervix and the columnar epithelium of the endocervical canal. With advancing age, the SCJ moves proximally, and as a result cervical cancer in younger women tends to be exophytic since the SCJ is located outside the external os. On the other hand, cervical cancer in older women tends to involve the endocervical canal. The role of MRI is to assess the size of the primary tumour and locoregional spread.

Key sequences

- T2-weighted FSE coronal and axial through the pelvis with a large FOV and a slice thickness of 5 mm
- T1-weighted SE coronal and axial through the abdomen and pelvis with a large FOV and a slice thickness of 5 mm
- T2-weighted SE sagittal and oblique axial (perpendicular to the long axis of the cervix and tumour) with a small FOV and a slice thickness of 3 mm
- T1-weighted FS sagittal and oblique axial through the cervix with a small FOV and a slice thickness less than 3 mm

Imaging findings

Cervical cancer is hyperintense on T2-weighted and hypointense on T1-weighted images.

The dark stromal ring of the cervix should be carefully investigated for any breach by the tumour, since this would upstage the tumour from stage Ib to stage II and will change treatment options.

Look for hypointense tumour strands extending into hypointense upper third of the vagina (stage IIa) on T2-weighted images and into hyperintense parametrial fat on T1-weighted images (stage IIb).

Examine for any suggestions of extension into the pelvic sidewall or lower vagina (stage III) or into the rectal or bladder wall for (stage IV).

Hints and tips

Look for hydronephrosis due to tumour encasing the ureter in parametrial invasion.

Look for lymphadenopathy in the pelvis and upper abdomen and in the groin.

Metastases may present with ascites, subcapsular liver deposits, abdominopelvic soft tissue masses or omental infiltration.

Further reading

Hulse PA, ed. *Handbook of MRI Staging of Pelvic Cancer*. London: Informa Healthcare, 2003.

Husband JE, ed. *Imaging in Oncology*. London: Informa Healthcare, 2004.

Case 20: Cervical cancer

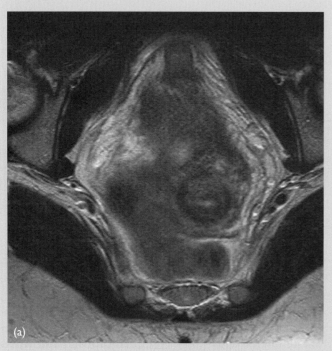 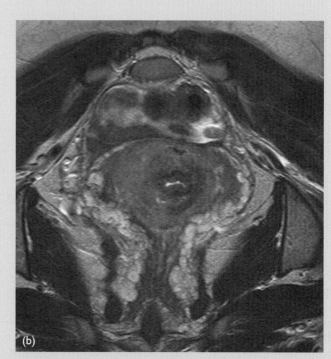

Case 20.1 (a) T2-weighted image illustrating a stage I tumour that has not breached the dark stromal ring. (b) An intermediate-signal tumour breaching the stromal ring: stage II disease – in this example, tumour can be seen extending into the parametrium (stage IIb).

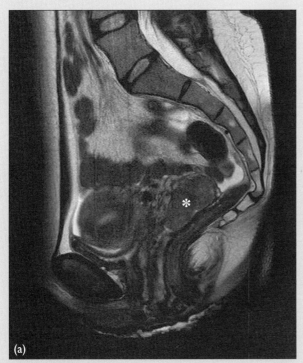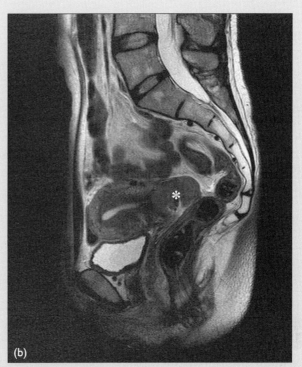

Case 20.2 (a, b) T2-weighted sagittal images showing two different cases of stage IIb cervical tumour (asterisk) occupying the upper vagina.

VULVAL CANCER

Primary vulval cancer is rare and, together with vaginal cancer, accounts for 7% of gynaecological primary cancers in the UK. Vulval cancer incidence is highest among women aged 65 and above. Unlike other gynaecological cancers, the risk of vulval cancer is not related to reproductive factors or use of exogenous hormones. Human papillomavirus and smoking are strong causative factors. Squamous cell carcinoma accounts for about 90% of vulval cancers, while the other 10% include melanoma, sarcoma, basal cell carcinoma and adenocarcinoma. The role of MRI is to identify deep tumour invasion and local lymph node involvement, and should be performed in all proven carcinoma of the vulva.

Key sequences

- T2-weighted FSE axial through the pelvis with a large FOV and a slice thickness of 5 mm
- T1-weighted SE coronal through the abdomen and pelvis with a large FOV and a slice thickness of 5 mm
- T2-weighted SE and short-tau inversion recovery (STIR) coronal and axial through the perineum with a small FOV and a slice thickness of 3 mm
- T1-weighted axial and coronal through the perineum with a small FOV and a slice thickness of 3 mm

Imaging findings

Large-FOV imaging is to identify any evidence of pelvic or abdominal lymphadenopathy or disease deposits.

On T2-weighted images, the tumour is intermediate signal, i.e. higher than muscle and lower than fat. The extent of tumour invasion through the low-signal vaginal introitus and the anorectal sphincter mechanism should be identified. The relationship of the tumour to the clitoris, urethra, vagina and anus is important both for treatment and prognosis.

Lymph node involvement is best assessed morphologically (for size, shape and fat content) on T1-weighted images, while tissue characterization is best done on T2-weighted and STIR images. High signal in lymph nodes on these later sequences is suspicious for malignant involvement.

Hints and tips

In cases of recurrence, assessment can be difficult owing to inflammatory changes and anatomic distortion, particularly in the early postoperative period.

T2-weighted imaging is also important for assessing the other genital tract organs, since metastatic vulvovaginal tumours from cervical, endometrial or ovarian carcinomas are more common than primary cancer.

Further reading

Hulse PA, ed. *Handbook of MRI Staging of Pelvic Cancer.* London: Informa Healthcare, 2003.

Husband JE, ed. *Imaging in Oncology.* London: Informa Healthcare, 2004.

Case 21: Vulval cancer

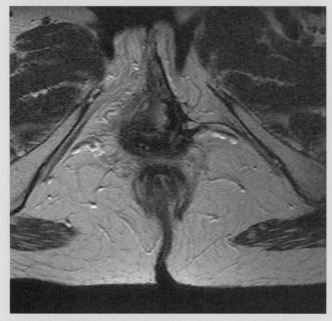

Case 21.1 T2-weighted axial image of the perineum showing an intermediate-signal vulvovaginal tumour.

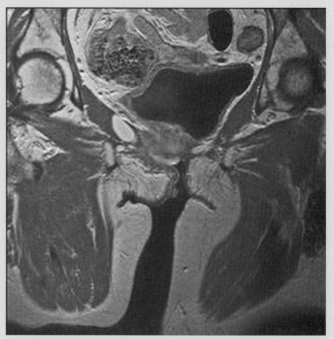

Case 21.3 Post-Gd T1-weighted coronal image showing an enhancing right vulval tumour involving the urethra.

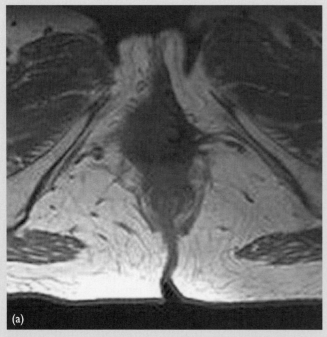

(a)

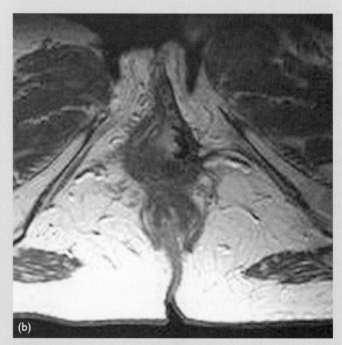

(b)

Case 21.2 (a, b) T1-weighted and post-Gd T1-weighted axial images of the perineum showing enhancement of the tumour.

BLADDER CANCER

Bladder cancer has a rising incidence in men from the sixth decade onwards. The most common histological subtype is transitional cell cancer, while other types are squamous cell and adenocarcinoma, the latter usually being seen in urachal remnants. The role of MRI in bladder cancer is to achieve local staging in cases considered suitable for curative resection. Post-biopsy changes can lead to upstaging of the cancer – hence MRI should be performed with a 2-week delay post-biopsy in these cases.

Key sequences

- T2-weighted FSE axial through the abdomen with a large FOV and a slice thickness of 5 mm
- T1-weighted SE axial through the pelvis with a large FOV and a slice thickness of 5 mm
- FS T1-weighted GRE axial and coronal through the pelvis before and immediately after Gd with a small FOV and a slice thickness less than 3 mm
- T2-weighted SE axial and coronal through the bladder with a small FOV and a slice thickness less than 3 mm

Imaging findings

On T2-weighted images, the bladder shows hyperintensity of urine against hypointensity of the bladder muscle wall. Bladder tumours are seen as intermediate- to low-signal masses or plaques. T2-weighted imaging is particularly useful in determining the depth of tumour infiltration into and beyond the bladder wall.

T1-weighted imaging is useful to establish the extent of hypointense tumour beyond the bladder wall into hyperintense fat. Lymphadenopathy and bone marrow infiltration can also be assessed on these images.

Gd-enhanced images can be helpful in defining the tumour and its extent in equivocal cases

Large-FOV T2-weighted images are useful to assess associated findings such as hydronephrosis, ascites and extent of lymph node involvement.

Hints and tips

Look carefully for involvement of seminal vesicles, rectal or uterine wall, and urethral encasement.

Infiltration into the corpus spongiosum at the base of the penis may lead to priapism.

Look for synchronous carcinoma in the bladder and upper renal tract.

Further reading

Hulse PA, ed. *Handbook of MRI Staging of Pelvic Cancer.* London: Informa Healthcare, 2003.
Husband JE, ed. *Imaging in Oncology.* London: Informa Healthcare, 2004.

Case 22: Bladder cancer

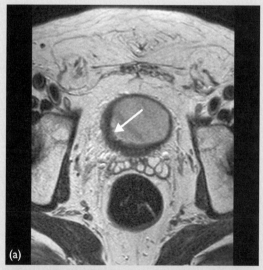
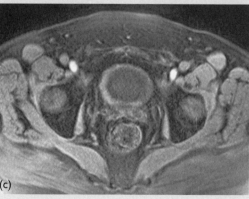
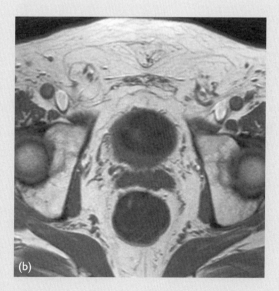

Case 22.1 (a, b) T2-weighted axial images showing intermediate-signal tumour against hypointense detrusor. No breach is seen through the muscle layer. (c) Post-Gd, the tumour shows intense enhancement of thickened bladder wall.

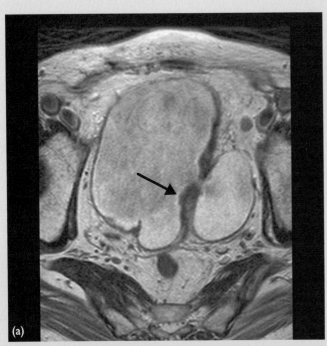
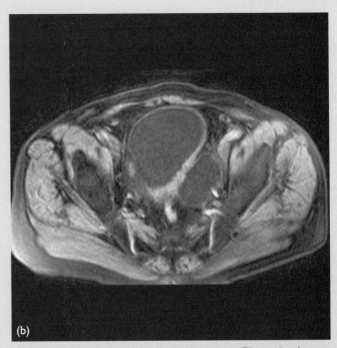

Case 22.2 (a, b) Another example of stage T2 disease with tumour at the mouth of a giant bladder diverticulum on a T2-weighted image that enhances post-Gd.

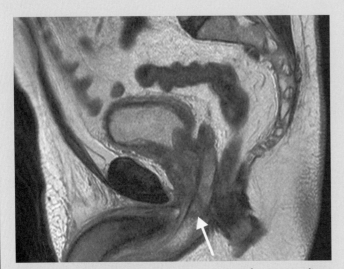
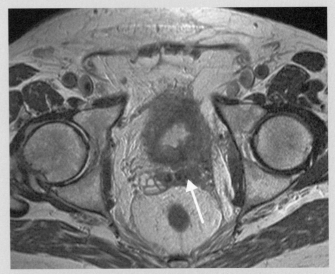

Case 22.3 T2-weighted image showing invasion of an intermediate-signal stage T3 tumour into the prostate and corpus spongiosum (arrow).

Case 22.4 T2-weighted image showing an intermediate-signal stage T3 tumour replacing the normally bright seminal vesicle.

PROSTATE CANCER

Prostate cancer is the most common cancer in men in the UK and is the second most common cause of cancer death in UK men. Prostate cancer is frequently multifocal within the gland. While 70% of prostate cancers occur in the peripheral zone, approximately 20% are found in the transition zone and 10% in the central zone. MRI should be used in patients with prostate-specific antigen (PSA) greater than 12 ng/mL, a Gleason score of 8 or more and a clinical stage T3 or T4 disease. MRI is essential when radical treatment is under consideration.

Key sequences

- T2-weighted FSE axial through the abdomen with a large FOV and a slice thickness of 5 mm

- T1-weighted SE axial through the pelvis with a large FOV and a slice thickness of 5 mm
- T1-weighted SE axial through the prostate with a small FOV and a slice thickness less than 3 mm
- T2-weighted SE axial and coronal through the prostate with a small FOV and a slice thickness less than 3 mm

Imaging findings

On T1-weighted small-FOV images, look for the outline of the dark gland against periprostatic bright fat. These are also good images on which to look for intraprostatic blood: this is common if imaging is performed after transrectal ultrasound (TRUS) biopsy. On larger-FOV images, look for nodal enlargement and particularly loss of nodal sinus fat. This also provides a free view of the bone marrow fat for loss of fat signal in cases of metastasis.

On T2-weighted small-FOV images, the prostate cancer appears as an area of low signal in the hyperintense peripheral zone. Look for involvement of the bladder base, obliteration of the rectoprostatic angle, invasion through the capsule into bright periprostatic fat and hyperintense seminal vesicles. On larger-FOV images, look for nodal involvement and renal obstruction.

Hints and tips

Low signal on T2-weighted images in the peripheral zone can also be seen in several benign conditions, such as haemorrhage and prostatitis and following radiation therapy.

MR spectroscopy (MRS) along with MRI increases diagnostic value. MRS provides metabolic information about prostatic tissue by displaying the relative concentrations of chemical compounds within a small voxel of interest. Using the classification described by Kurhanewicz et al, a voxel can be classified as normal, suspicious for cancer or very suspicious for cancer. Voxels that show an increase in choline–creatinine ratio and a marked decrease in or absence of citrate are suspicious for malignancy.

Further reading

Hulse PA, ed. *Handbook of MRI Staging of Pelvic Cancer.* London: Informa Healthcare, 2003.

Husband JE, ed. *Imaging in Oncology.* London: Informa Healthcare, 2004.

Case 23: Prostate cancer

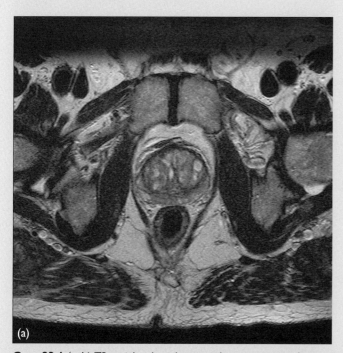 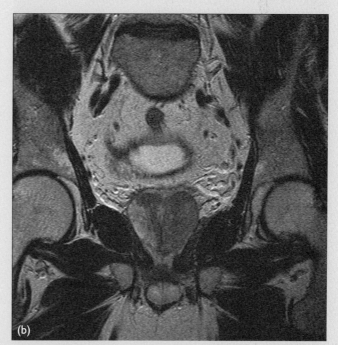

Case 23.1 (a, b) T2-weighted axial images showing intermediate-signal tumour against hypointense detrusor. No breach is seen through the muscle layer. (c) Post-Gd, the tumour shows intense enhancement of thickened bladder wall.

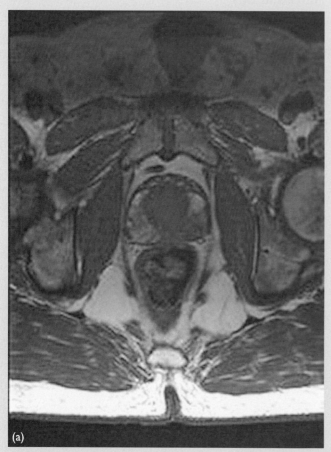

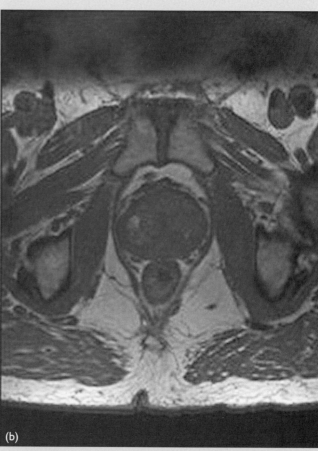

Case 23.2 (a, b) T1-weighted axial images in two different cases depicting hyperintense foci of haemorrhage within the prostate gland. This is commonly seen, since MRI scans are often performed after prostate biopsy, which causes the haemorrhage in the gland.

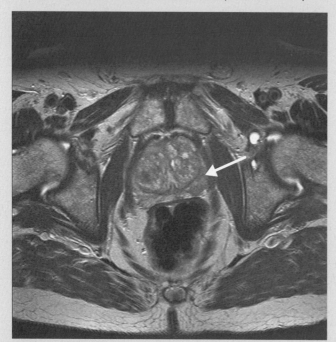

Case 23.3 T2-weighted axial image showing hypointense tumour breaching the capsule (arrow), making this stage T3a disease.

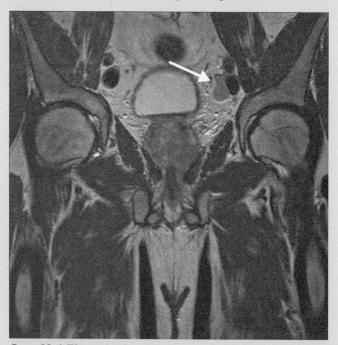

Case 23.4 T2-weighted coronal image showing tumour involving both lobes and breaching the capsule near the left apex. Note the enlarged left iliac lymph node, which shows signal intensity similar to that of the tumour. Hence, this is stage T3N1 disease.

URETHRAL DIVERTICULUM

Urethral diverticulum is a relatively uncommon condition, but is becoming more prevalent in clinical practice. Urethral diverticulum is seen more often in women, commonly between 30 and 60 years of age. The obstructed and/or infected paraurethral glands (Skene's glands) form an abscess and rupture into the urethra, forming the diverticulum. Other aetiologies include obstetric trauma and perineal surgery. Diverticula can be single or multiple and simple or complex.

Key sequences

- T2-weighted SE sagittal through the pelvis with a large FOV and a slice thickness of 5 mm
- FST2-weighted FSE axial and coronal or sagittal through the bladder and urethra with a small FOV and a slice thickness of 3 mm
- T1-weighted GRE axial and coronal through the area under investigation. Gd-enhanced FS imaging in the same plane may be necessary.

Imaging findings

The diverticulum wraps around the urethra like a 'saddle bag' and is located in the middle third of the urethra. In 95% of cases, it is situated posterolaterally between the 3 o'clock and 9 o'clock positions.

On T2-weighted images, the fluid within the diverticular sac is hyperintense and the extent and size of the diverticulum is best seen on FS T2-weighted sequences. On T1-weighted images, fluid in dependent portions may be bright if it contains blood or pus.

Contrast-enhanced images can be useful in identifying associated infection or malignant changes.

Hints and tips

Look for calculus within the diverticulum.

In cases of repeated infections, hypointense fibrosis may be seen around the diverticulum on T2-weighted images; this enhances on post-contrast T1-weighted images. Similarly, a fluid–fluid level within the diverticulum on T2-weighted images raises the possibility of recurrent infections.

Periurethral collagen injections performed for bladder neck dysfunction can mimic a diverticulum.

Rarely adenocarcinoma or transitional cell or squamous cell carcinoma may develop within the diverticulum, presenting as a low- to intermediate-signal soft tissue mass projecting within the hyperintense fluid of diverticulum on T2-weighted images. Use T1-weighted Gd enhancement to confirm.

Further reading

Chou CP, Levenson RB, Elsayes KM et al. Imaging of female urethral diverticulum: an update. *Radiographics* 2008; **28**: 1917–30.

Case 24: Urethral diverticulum

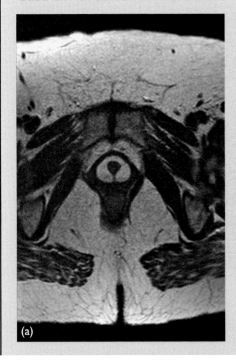 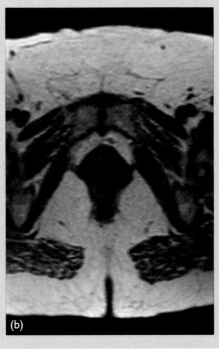

Case 24.1 (a, b) T2- and T1-weighted axial images through the urethral diverticulum. The diverticulum wraps around the urethra like a 'saddle bag'. It is of fluid intensity and contains urine in this case.

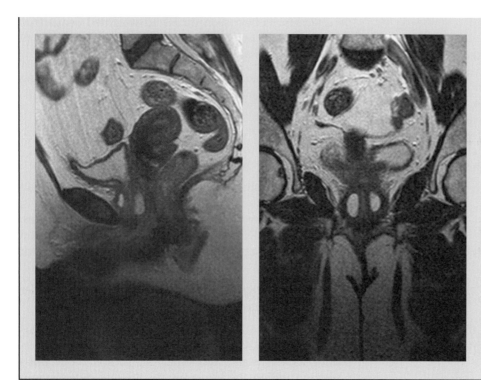

Case 24.2 (a, b) T2-weighted sagittal and coronal images showing high signal in the diverticulum in the posterolateral position.

UNIT IV

Cardiothoracic MRI

Edward TD Hoey, SK Bobby Agrawal

1 KEY SEQUENCES

BLACK BLOOD (FIGURE 1.1)

Typically, this is a spin echo sequence that is acquired in diastole. The signal from blood is suppressed by using a double-inversion preparation technique. Images can be acquired with T1 or T2 weighting, with or without additional fat suppression. Black blood imaging is used for anatomic assessment and tissue characterization.

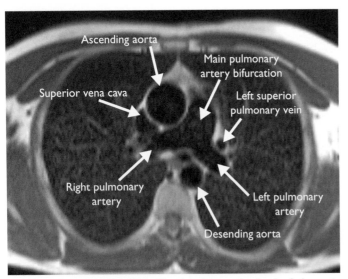

Figure 1.1 Transverse black blood image at the level of the main pulmonary artery bifurcation.

STEADY-STATE FREE-PRECESSION (SSFP) (FIGURES 1.2–1.4)

This is a fast gradient echo sequence acquired throughout the cardiac cycle with time references to the ECG, which enables depiction of heart and valvular motion from 'cine' images. Moving blood appears bright (so-called 'bright blood imaging') and myocardium appears dark owing to their different ratios of T2/T1 contrast. Acquisition of SSFP images through the left ventricle in a short axis view enables calculation of ejection fraction and other functional parameters.

MYOCARDIAL TAGGING

This technique employs spatially selective presaturation pulses to produce geometric grids across the myocardium. Dynamic images are acquired and contractile abnormalities are depicted as a lack of grid deformation during the cardiac cycle. Tagging is especially useful for detecting subtle wall motion abnormalities in cases of suspected cardiomyopathy.

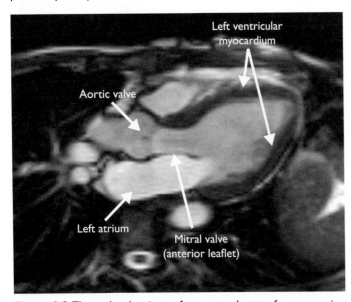

Figure 1.2 Three-chamber image from a steady-state free-precession (SSFP) sequence in diastole.

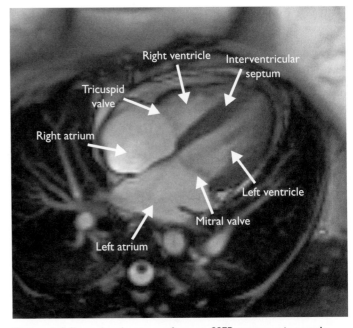

Figure 1.3 Four-chamber image from an SSFP sequence in systole.

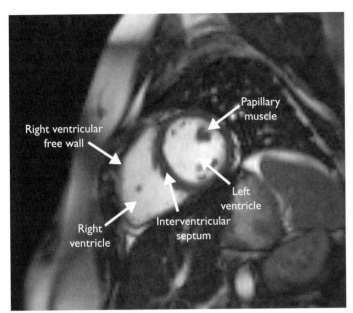

Figure 1.4 Short-axis mid left ventricular image from an SSFP sequence.

VELOCITY-ENCODED PHASE CONTRAST

This gradient echo technique is used to quantify the direction and velocity of blood flow by measuring the phase shift that occurs as spinning protons pass through a magnetic field. To ensure accurate estimation of flow, the acquisition plane must be placed perpendicular to the vessel of interest. Phase contrast imaging can be used to assess valvular regurgitant fraction, severity of valvular stenosis and diastolic dysfunction (transmitral flow), as well as for quantification of intracardiac shunts (pulmonary flow/ systemic flow ratio Q_p/Q_s).

DELAYED MYOCARDIAL ENHANCEMENT

This is a T1-weighted inversion recovery fast gradient echo sequence, usually performed 10 minutes or more following intravenous administration of a gadolinium (Gd)-based contrast medium. Gd accumulates in scar tissue and gives a high signal owing to its T1-shortening effects. In order to maximize contrast between scar tissue and normal myocardium, the operator selects an appropriate inversion time that will null normal myocardial signal. Delayed enhancement is used principally in the assessment of myocardial viability, but can also be of value for characterizing cardiomyopathies and a suspected cardiac mass by demonstration of regional variations in washout kinetics.

MYOCARDIAL PERFUSION IMAGING

This is a gradient echo technique that is performed under stress following administration of a Gd-based contrast medium in conjunction with pharmacological agents such as adenosine (a coronary artery vasodilator) or dobutamine (a positive inotropic agent). Images are reviewed as a cine loop and used to assess regional abnormalities in the perfusion of Gd through the myocardium as an indicator of inducible myocardial ischaemia. Perfusion imaging may also be applied to the assessment of cardiac masses.

2 CARDIOVASCULAR PATHOLOGIES

MYOCARDIAL ISCHAEMIA

Cardiac MRI is an established means of assessing ischaemic myocardium. The subendocardium is the region most vulnerable to injury, since it lies remote from the epicardial coronary arteries. The degree of myocardial injury depends on the extent and duration of ischaemia. Prolonged ischaemia causes necrosis that extends transmurally towards the epicardium. Hibernating myocardium is defined as viable but dysfunctional myocardium that improves in function after revascularization, and its identification is key to the selection of patients who would benefit from revascularization.

Key sequences

- Steady-state free precession (SSFP) sequences through the left ventricle in the short-axis plane
- Delayed myocardial enhancement imaging
- Adenosine or dobutamine stress imaging

Imaging findings

The following features are suggestive of myocardial ischaemia:
- regional wall motion abnormality corresponding to a coronary artery territory
- impaired left ventricular ejection fraction (<55%)
- delayed myocardial enhancement
- inducible (seen on stress only) perfusion defect on adenosine perfusion imaging

- inducible wall motion abnormality on high-dose dobutamine imaging

The following features are suggestive of myocardial viability:
- transient improvement in regional wall motion on low-dose dobutamine imaging
- delayed myocardial enhancement ≤ 25% transmural extent

Hints and tips

Myocardial necrosis shows delayed gadolinium (Gd) enhancement, but viable myocardium does not.

The transmural extent of enhancement predicts the likelihood of functional recovery following revascularization:
- < 25% transmural extent: high likelihood of functional improvement
- >75% transmural extent: low likelihood of functional improvement

Susceptibility artifact can mimic a subendocardial defect on adenosine perfusion imaging. In favour of artefact are that its appearance coincides exactly with arrival of the Gd bolus in the left ventricular cavity. A true perfusion defect tends to appear slightly later.

Further reading

Kim RJ, Wu E, Rafael A et al. The use of contrast-enhanced magnetic resonance imaging to identify reversible myocardial dysfunction. *N Engl J Med* 2000; **343**: 1445–53.

Case 1: Myocardial ischaemia

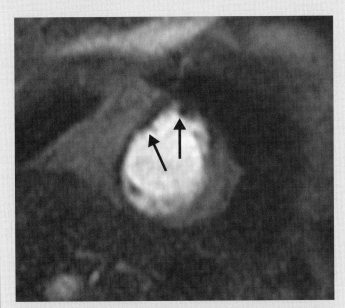

Case 1.1 Short-axis mid left ventricular image from a dynamic adenosine perfusion study. A perfusion defect (arrows) is demonstrated in the left anterior descending (LAD) coronary artery territory.

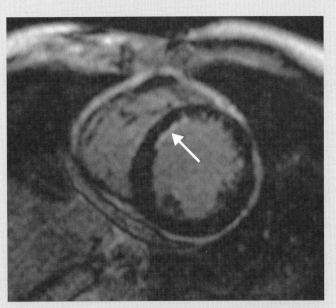

Case 1.2 Short-axis mid left ventricular image from a delayed myocardial enhancement sequence demonstrating <25% thickness subendocardial infarction (arrow) in the LAD coronary artery territory.

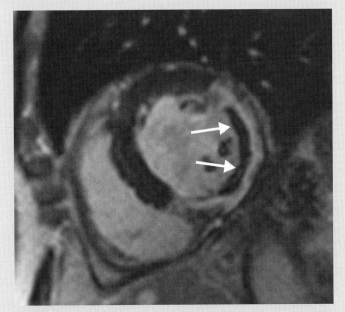

Case 1.3 Short-axis mid left ventricular image from a delayed myocardial enhancement sequence demonstrating transmural infarction in the circumflex coronary artery territory with associated left ventricular mural thrombus formation (arrows).

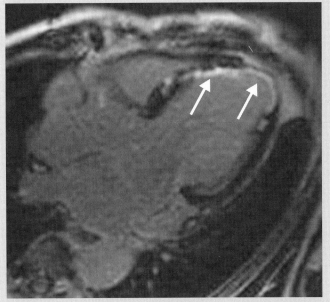

Case 1.4 Four-chamber mid left ventricular image from a delayed myocardial enhancement sequence demonstrating approximately 50% transmural infarction (arrows) in the LAD coronary artery territory.

HYPERTROPHIC CARDIOMYOPATHY (HCM)

HCM is a primary disease of the cardiac sarcomere with an autosomal dominant inheritance pattern. There is abnormal myocardial thickening without systemic hypertension, aortic stenosis or other identifiable cause. HCM is the most common cause of sudden cardiac death in young people, with a prevalence estimated at 1 in 500. MRI enables a comprehensive evaluation, including accurate measurement of myocardial mass and depiction of regional wall motion abnormalities and foci of fibrosis.

Key sequences

- SSFP sequences through the left ventricle in the short-axis plane
- Myocardial tagging
- Delayed myocardial enhancement imaging

Imaging findings

Focal hypertrophy of the interventricular septum is the most frequently encountered pattern; there may be associated systolic anterior motion (SAM) of the mitral valve (leaflet displacement into the left ventricular outflow tract).

Other patterns include symmetric HCM, apical HCM, midventricular HCM and focal 'mass-like' ventricular thickening.

Subtle regional wall motion abnormalities may be evident in hypertrophied regions, and are more readily visualized on tagged sequences.

There may be normal or increased left ventricular ejection fraction.

Patchy mid-myocardial delayed enhancement in abnormally thickened regions is characteristic (80% of cases).

Hints and tips

Increased myocardial mass is a typical feature; however, measurements may remain within normal limits, particularly with an asymmetric disease pattern.

The extent of delayed enhancement correlates with episodes of ventricular arrhythmia and risk of sudden cardiac death.

Differential diagnosis of symmetric HCM includes athlete's heart, amyloidosis, aortic stenosis and hypertensive heart disease:

- A diastolic wall thickness/left ventricular end-diastolic volume ratio of <0.15 has been shown to be a reliable cut-off for athlete's heart.
- Amyloidosis is suggested by a global subendocardial enhancement pattern and/or difficulty selecting an inversion time for delayed enhancement imaging.
- Aortic stenosis is suggested by restricted leaflet opening and flow acceleration on SSFP sequences. Stenosis can be quantified by performing phase contrast imaging.
- Hypertensive heart disease is a diagnosis of exclusion, and requires clinical correlation.

Further reading

Hansen MW, Merchant N. MRI of hypertrophic cardiomyopathy: Part I, MRI appearances. *AJR Am J Roentgenol* 2007; **189**: 1335–43.

Hansen MW, Merchant N. MRI of hypertrophic cardiomyopathy: Part 2, Differential diagnosis, risk stratification, and posttreatment MRI appearances. *AJR Am J Roentgenol* 2007; **189**: 1344–52.

Case 2: Hypertrophic cardiomyopathy (HCM)

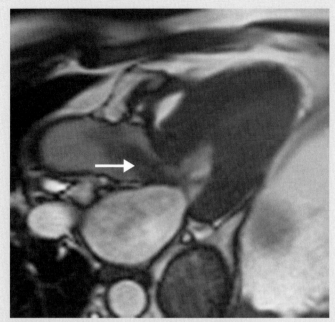

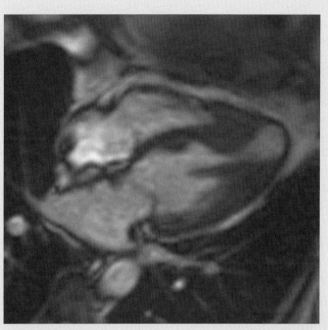

Case 2.1 Three-chamber view in end-systole from an SSFP sequence. There is global left ventricular hypertrophy with obliteration of the ventricular cavity. Flow acceleration is seen in the left ventricular outflow tract (arrow), in keeping with outflow obstruction secondary to SAM.

Case 2.2 Four-chamber image in early systole from an SSFP sequence showing midventricular HCM. There is thinning of the left ventricular apex, which is a recognized association of this form of the disease.

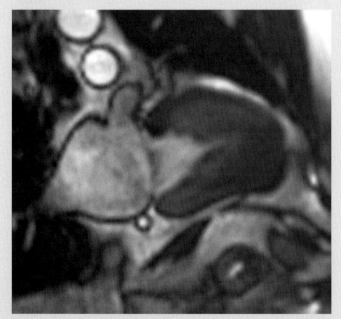

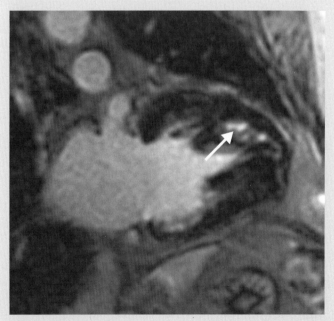

Case 2.3 Two-chamber view in end-systole from an SSFP sequence showing pronounced hypertrophy of the mid and apical left ventricular segments in keeping with 'apical' HCM.

Case 2.4 Two-chamber view from a delayed myocardial enhancement sequence in the same patient as in Case 2.3 showing patchy areas of delayed hyperenhancement (arrow), in keeping with foci of fibrosis, an adverse prognostic sign.

DILATED CARDIOMYOPATHY (DCM)

The most common causes of DCM are ischaemic, idiopathic, postviral and alcohol-induced. MRI is valuable in the assessment of left ventricular functional parameters and is especially useful in helping distinguish ischaemic DCM from non-ischaemic causes. Those patients with ischaemia may potentially benefit from revascularization, either surgical or catheter-directed, whereas the other group will not. Treatment options for non-ischaemic DCM depend upon the clinical severity score and include pharmacological therapy, ventricular assist devices and transplantation.

Key sequences

- SSFP sequences through the left ventricle in the short-axis plane
- Delayed myocardial enhancement imaging

Imaging findings

There is a globally dilated left ventricle (the right ventricle may also be involved) with wall motion abnormalities.

Ischaemic DCM usually shows delayed enhancement, which may be subendocardial or transmural.

Non-ischaemic aetiologies may show mid-wall enhancement, most often in the mid-interventricular septum and thought to be due to replacement fibrosis.

Hints and tips

The presence of delayed contrast enhancement is an adverse prognostic indicator.

Further reading

Vogel-Claussen J, Rochitte CE, Wu KC et al. Delayed enhancement MR imaging: utility in myocardial assessment. *Radiographics* 2006; **26**: 795–810.

Cummings KW, Bhalla S, Javidan-Nejad C et al. A pattern-based approach to assessment of delayed enhancement in nonischemic cardiomyopathy at MR imaging. *Radiographics* 2009; **29**: 89–103.

Case 3: Dilated cardiomyopathy (DCM)

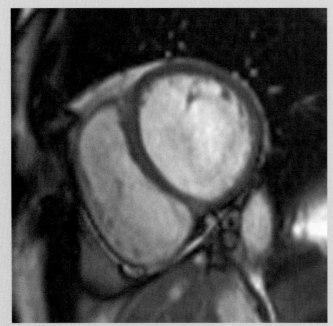

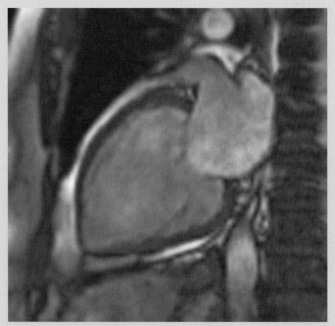

Case 3.1 Short-axis mid left ventricular image in end-systole from an SSFP sequence showing dilatation of the left ventricle, which was noted to be globally hypokinetic on cine imaging.

Case 3.2 Two-chamber view in end-diastole from an SSFP sequence showing global left ventricular dilatation that has a spherical geometry.

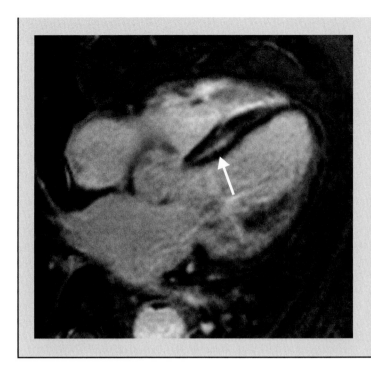

Case 3.3 Four-chamber mid left ventricular image from a delayed myocardial enhancement sequence demonstrating linear mid-myocardial enhancement in the interventricular septum (arrow), which is a characteristic feature of DCM.

LEFT VENTRICULAR NON-COMPACTION (LVNC)

LVNC is a rare congenital cardiomyopathy that is thought to be caused by an arrest of endomyocardial morphogenesis. The subepicardial myocardium is thin and normally compacted, with a thicker non-compacted subendocardial layer. Prompt recognition of LVNC is mandatory because of its clinical manifestations, which include heart failure, thromboembolic events and ventricular arrhythmias. MRI provides clear delineation of the extent of non-compaction and also helps distinguish pathological LVNC from lesser degrees of trabeculation that may be seen in healthy subjects.

Key sequences

- SSFP sequences through the left ventricle in the short-axis plane.
- Myocardial tagging
- Delayed myocardial enhancement imaging

Imaging findings

There is a dilated hypocontractile left ventricle with prominent trabeculations and deep interventricular recesses that produce a 'two-layered' appearance.

Apical and mid left ventricular segments are most commonly involved.

A ratio of non-compacted to compacted myocardium of >2.3 : 1 is considered diagnostic.

There is impaired ventricular systolic function (with a left ventricular ejection fraction of <55%).

Delayed contrast enhancement within areas of non-compaction is an occasional finding.

Hints and tips

The compacted/non-compacted ratio should be measured in the end-diastolic phase and on SSFP sequences.

A ratio cutoff of 2.3 has been shown to have a higher diagnostic accuracy for distinguishing pathological LVNC from lesser degrees of non-compaction observed in healthy, dilated and hypertrophied hearts.

Further reading

Petersen SE, Selvanayagam JB, Wiesmann FR et al. Left ventricular non-compaction: insights from cardiovascular magnetic resonance imaging. *J Am Coll Cardiol* 2005; **46**: 101–5.

Case 4: Left ventricular non-compaction (LVNC)

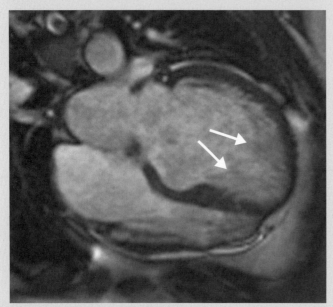

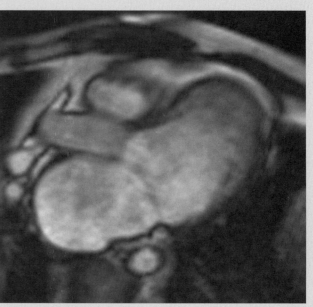

Case 4.1 Four-chamber image in end-diastole from an SSFP sequence showing dilatation of the left ventricle, which has a two-layered wall composed of an outer layer of normally compacted myocardium and an inner non-compacted layer. Note the deep intertrabecular recesses (arrows).

Case 4.2 Three-chamber image in mid-systole from an SSFP sequence showing LVNC. Note the distribution of disease, which predominantly involves the apex and mid left ventricular segments.

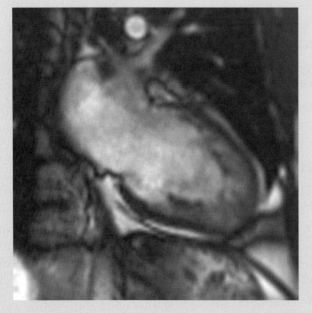

Case 4.3 Two-chamber image in early diastole from an SSFP sequence showing LVNC.

ARRHYTHMOGENIC RIGHT VENTRICULAR CARDIOMYOPATHY (ARVC)

ARVC is characterized by progressive fibrous or fibrofatty replacement of normal right ventricular myocardium. This can lead to electrical instability with resultant dysrhythmias, including ventricular fibrillation. Diagnostic criteria are based upon the Task Force recommendations, and include a combination of imaging findings, electrophysiological abnormalities and family history.

Key sequences

- SSFP sequences through the right ventricle and outflow tract in the transverse plane

- T1-weighted black blood imaging (short axis through the right ventricle)
- T1-weighted fat-suppressed black blood imaging
- Delayed myocardial enhancement imaging

Imaging findings

There is right ventricular wall motion abnormality (dyskinesis or aneurysm).

The right ventricle shows wall thinning and signs of fatty infiltration.

Delayed myocardial enhancement may sometimes be present.

Right ventricular ejection fraction is impaired (<45%).

Fatty replacement may also involve the left ventricular myocardium

Hints and tips

Right ventricular wall motion abnormalities are considered more sensitive than black blood imaging signs of fat infiltration.

An inversion time for delayed enhancement imaging should be chosen according to the right ventricular myocardium and may be different from that of the left.

The insertion point of the moderator band into the right ventricular free wall can normally appear hypokinetic – this should not be mistaken for ARVC.

The presence of intramyocardial fat is not pathognomonic for ARVC, since small fatty foci may sometimes be seen in normal myocardium.

A normal MRI appearance does not exclude a diagnosis of ARVC, and this should be stated in the report.

Further reading

Castillo E, Tandri H, Rodriguez R et al. Arrhythmogenic right ventricular dysplasia: ex vivo and in vivo fat detection with black-blood MR imaging. *Radiology* 2004; **232**: 38–48.

Kayser HWM, de Roos A, Schalij MJ et al. Usefulness of magnetic resonance imaging in diagnosis of arrhythmogenic right ventricular dysplasia and agreement with electrocardiographic criteria. *Am J Cardiol* 2003; **91**: 365–7.

Case 5: Arrhythmogenic right ventricular cardiomyopathy (ARVC)

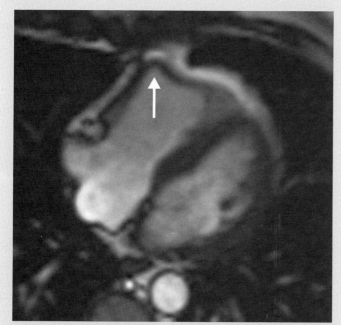

Case 5.1 Four-chamber image in end-diastole from an SSFP sequence showing a focal aneurysm of the right ventricular free wall (arrow).

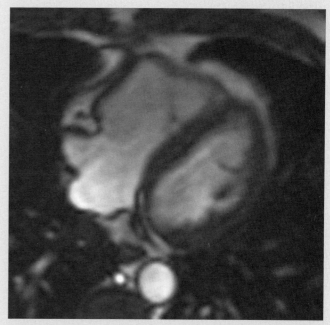

Case 5.2 Four-chamber image in early systole from an SSFP sequence in the same patient as in Case 5.1, again showing focal aneurysmal dilatation of the right ventricular free wall.

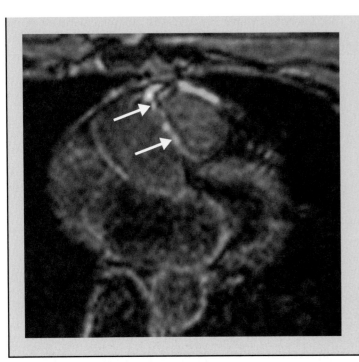

Case 5.3 Transverse image through the right ventricular outflow tract from a delayed myocardial enhancement sequence demonstrating myocardial enhancement (arrows).

SARCOID HEART DISEASE

Sarcoidosis is an idiopathic multisystem disease characterized by widespread development of non-caseating epithelioid granulomas. Cardiac involvement occurs in around 20% of patients, of whom around 5% have clinical manifestations. In early-stage disease, the clinical picture is usually that of a restrictive pattern. Postinflammatory scarring may eventually lead to wall thinning and a dilated cardiomyopathy. Sarcoidosis has a predilection to involve the cardiac conduction system, and patients may develop heart block and other arrhythmias.

Key sequences

- T2-weighted black blood imaging
- SSFP sequences through the left ventricle in the short-axis plane
- Delayed myocardial enhancement imaging

Imaging findings

Focal areas of high T2 signal are seen in the acute phase.

There is myocardial infiltration (thickening), with a predilection for the basal interventricular septum and lateral wall.

Nodular areas of mid-wall delayed myocardial enhancement correspond to the areas of wall motion abnormality/thickening.

In late-phase disease, the left ventricle may be dilated and thin-walled.

Hints and tips

Delayed enhancement may occasionally be subendocardial or transmural and mimic the pattern of myocardial infarction.

Delayed myocardial enhancement may be used as an accurate guide for obtaining an endomyocardial biopsy.

Further reading

Jackson E, Bellenger N, Seddon M et al. Ischaemic and non-ischaemic cardiomyopathies – cardiac MRI appearances with delayed enhancement. *Clin Radiol* 2007; **62**: 395–403.

Dubrey A, Bell A, Mittal TK. Sarcoid heart disease. *Postgrad Med J* 2007; **83**: 618–23.

Case 6: Sarcoid heart disease

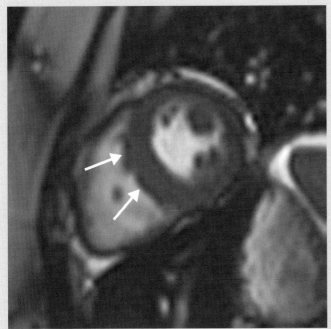

Case 6.1 Short-axis mid left ventricular image in end-diastole from an SSFP sequence in a patient with known pulmonary sarcoidosis. There is subtle thickening of the interventricular septum (arrows).

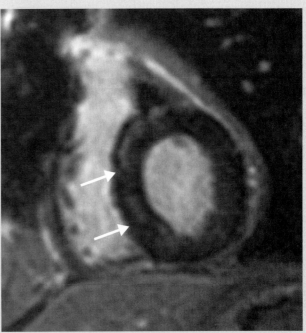

Case 6.2 Corresponding image from a delayed myocardial enhancement sequence in the same patient as in Case 6.1 demonstrating nodular areas of mid-myocardial enhancement (arrows).

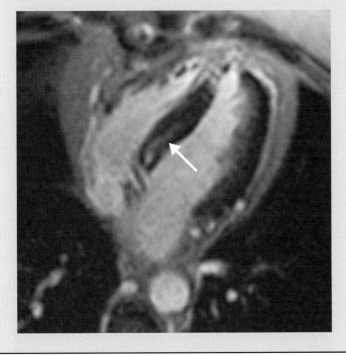

Case 6.3 Four-chamber mid left ventricular image from a delayed myocardial enhancement sequence in the same patient as in Cases 6.1 and 6.2 demonstrating mid-myocardial enhancement along the interventricular septum (arrows).

ATRIAL SEPTAL DEFECT (ASD)

ASD is the most common form of congenital heart disease presenting in adulthood and is an important cause of morbidity and mortality. Clinical manifestations include atrial arrhythmias, stroke (from paradoxical embolism) and pulmonary arterial hypertension. Small ASDs (<1 cm in diameter) are usually not haemodynamically significant and may remain clinically silent. A left-to-right shunt with a pulmonary flow/systemic flow ratio Q_p/Q_s of >1.5/1.0 or causing right heart dilatation is considered significant.

Key sequences

- Velocity-encoded phase contrast imaging through the proximal ascending aorta and main pulmonary artery (shunt quantification).
- Gd-enhanced pulmonary angiography
- SSFP sequences through the left ventricle in the short-axis plane and through the right ventricle in the transverse plane

Imaging findings

Secundum ASD involves the midportion of the atrial septum in the region of the fossa ovalis.

Primum ASD involves the lower portion of the septum and is often associated with ventricular septal defect and anomalies of the mitral valve.

Sinus venosus ASD lies outside the confines of the fossa ovalis, most often in a superior location at the superior vena/cava right atrial junction. There is a frequent association with anomalous pulmonary venous drainage (80–90%).

Hints and tips

The normally thinned tissue in the fossa ovalis may exhibit little or no signal intensity and may therefore be mistaken for a secundum ASD. The following clues help in avoiding this pitfall:

- An intact septum thins gradually toward the site of signal intensity absence.
- The septum at the edge of a secundum ASD usually appears thickened.

Careful review of transverse black blood images is essential to detect anomalous pulmonary venous drainage, which may not be readily apparent on the smaller field of view in SSFP sequences.

Look for signs of secondary pulmonary arterial hypertension: a main pulmonary artery diameter of >3 cm (measured at its bifurcation), right ventricular hypertrophy (a free-wall thickness of >3 mm) and tricuspid regurgitation (with a flow jet extending into the right atrium).

Further reading

Wang ZJ, Reddy GP, Gotway MB et al. Cardiovascular shunts: MR imaging evaluation. *Radiographics* 2003; **23**: S181–94.

Case 7: Atrial septal defect (ASD)

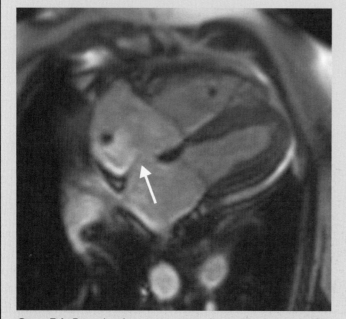

Case 7.1 Four-chamber image in early systole from an SSFP sequence showing a large defect in the midportion of the interatrial septum (secundum-type ASD, arrow).

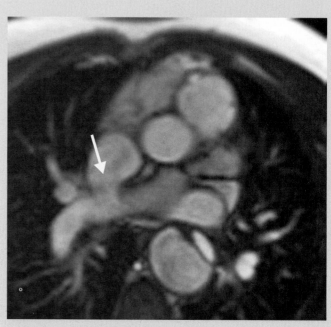

Case 7.2 Transverse image from an SSFP sequence at the level of the pulmonary outflow tract showing a superior sinus venosus ASD (arrow).

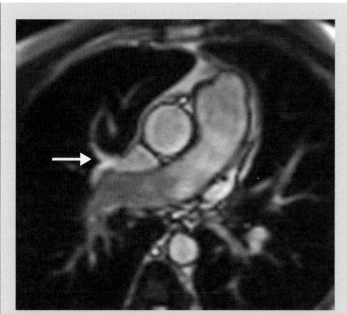

Case 7.3 Transverse image from an SSFP sequence at the level of the right main pulmonary artery showing anomalous venous drainage of the right superior pulmonary vein into the superior vena cava (arrow).

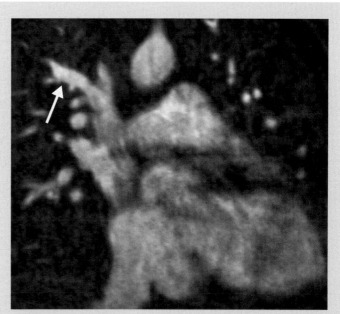

Case 7.4 Coronal image from a Gd-enhanced pulmonary angiogram in the same patient as in Case 7.3, again showing the anomalous pulmonary venous anatomy (arrow).

CONGENITALLY CORRECTED TRANSPOSITION

Congenitally corrected transposition is characterized by double discordance (atrioventricular and ventriculo-arterial). The right atrium connects to the morphological left ventricle, which supplies the lungs. The left atrium connects to the morphological right ventricle, which supplies the systemic circulation. The heart is physiologically normal in terms of connections, but the majority of patients eventually develop systemic ventricular failure. Associated anomalies are fairly common and include pulmonary stenosis, Ebstein's anomaly and ventricular septal defect.

Key sequences

- Transverse black blood images
- SSFP sequences through the systemic ventricle in the short axis plane

Imaging findings

The aorta arises in an anterior position with respect to the pulmonary trunk.

The systemic ventricle is morphlogically right (it has a moderator band, septophilic mitral valve and muscular conus).

There are signs of systemic ventricular failure (hypokinesia and reduced ejection fraction).

Hints and tips

The main role of MRI is to quantify the function of the systemic ventricle and to make an assessment of any associated anomalies.

Further reading

Kellenberger CJ, Yoo SJ, Valsangiacomo Büchel ER. Cardiovascular MR imaging in neonates and infants with congenital heart disease. *Radiographics* 2007; **27**: 5–18.

Case 8: Congenitally corrected transposition

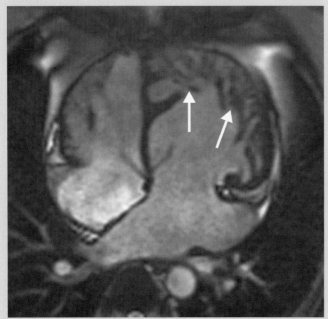

Case 8.1 Four-chamber image in diastole from an SSFP sequence showing a dilated, heavily trabeculated systemic ventricle that is the morphological right ventricle (arrows).

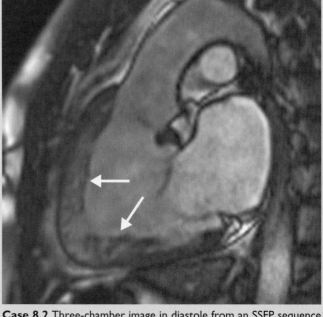

Case 8.2 Three-chamber image in diastole from an SSFP sequence showing the left atrium opening through the mitral valve into a dilated, trabeculated, systemic ventricle (arrows) that connects to the aorta.

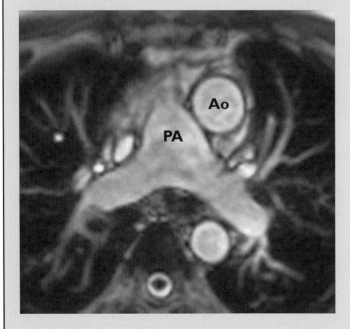

Case 8.3 Transverse image from an SSFP sequence at the level of the main pulmonary artery bifurcation showing the anterior position of the aorta (Ao) with respect to the pulmonary artery (PA).

INTRACARDIAC THROMBUS

The most common sites for thrombus formation are the left atrium and ventricle. Atrial fibrillation is the major predisposing factor for development of left atrial thrombus secondary to impaired mechanical function and decreased flow velocity. Left ventricular thrombus is usually associated with left ventricular dysfunction (e.g. dilated cardiomyopathy). Thrombus within the left heart chambers has the potential for systemic embolization and stroke. MRI appearances vary with age, and care must be taken not to mistake thrombus for a cardiac neoplasm and vice versa.

Key sequences

- Two- and four-chamber SSFP cine imaging
- Transverse and coronal T1-weighted black blood imaging
- Transverse and coronal T2-weighted black blood imaging
- Transverse fat-saturation T1-weighted black blood imaging
- Gd-enhanced T1-weighted black blood imaging (dynamic perfusion and 5 minutes delayed)

Imaging findings

Acute thrombus is bright on T1- and T2-weighted images.

Subacute thrombus is bright on T1-weighted and low signal on T2-weighted images.

Thrombus does not enhance following administration of Gd.

Thrombus does not show signal inversion with increasing inversion times.

Hints and tips

Typical location and absence of contrast enhancement are the most useful discriminators of thrombus versus a cardiac neoplasm.

Very occasionally, thrombus may display a thin rim of surface enhancement (tumours do not show this pattern).

Further reading

Sparrow PJ, Kurian JB, Jones TR et al. MR imaging of cardiac tumours. *Radiographics* 2005; **25**: 1255–76.

Case 9: Intracardiac thrombus

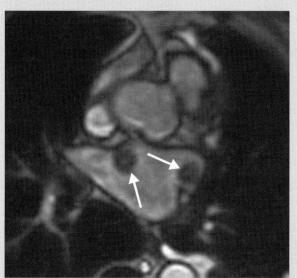

Case 9.1 Transverse image through the body of the left atrium from an SSFP sequence showing two well-circumscribed low-signal foci (arrows).

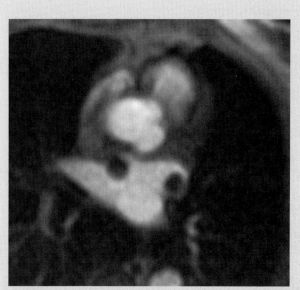

Case 9.2 Transverse image through the body of the left atrium from a dynamic Gd perfusion study in the same patient as in Case 9.1 showing absence of enhancement in the low-signal lesions, in keeping with left atrial thrombus.

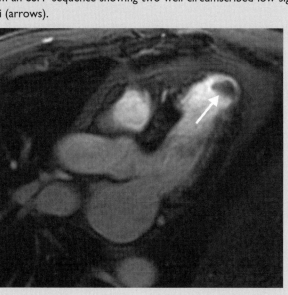

Case 9.3 Three-chamber image from a delayed myocardial enhancement sequence demonstrating transmural infarction at the left ventricular apex. There is an associated well-demarcated low-signal focus in this region, which has the typical appearance of intraventricular thrombus (arrow).

CARDIAC TUMOURS

Metastatic involvement of the heart and pericardium accounts for the majority of cases of cardiac neoplasia. Primary cardiac tumours are rare; most are benign, with myxomas, lipomas and fibromas accounting for the majority. Malignant primary cardiac tumours are mostly sarcomatous in nature. Clinical presentation is varied and may be due to arrhythmias or symptoms relating to pericardial tamponade or valvular obstruction. MRI is the modality of choice for the assessment of a cardiac mass, since it can provide a comprehensive evaluation of lesion morphology, extent and relationships.

Key sequences

- Two- and four-chamber SSFP cine imaging
- Transverse (also sagittal/coronal/oblique as required) T1-weighted imaging
- Transverse (also sagittal/coronal/oblique as required) T2-weighted imaging
- Transverse fat-saturation T1-weighted imaging
- Gd-enhanced T1-weighted imaging (dynamic perfusion and 5 minutes delayed)

Imaging findings

Signal characteristics vary widely and depend upon tumour vascularity, the presence of necrosis/haemorrhage and water/fat content.

The following are relatively specific findings:

- Lipomas are sharply marginated and display homogeneous high signal on T1- and T2-weighted images, with signal suppression on fat-saturated sequences.
- Myxomas usually manifest as a lobulated mass in the left atrium with a narrow attachment point at the fossa ovalis. They demonstrate heterogeneous signal intensity on T1- and T2-weighted images owing to areas of myxoid change and haemorrhage. Large lesions may be seen to prolapse through the mitral valve orifice in diastole.
- Sarcomas are usually large infiltrative masses with heterogeneous contrast medium enhancement and variable signal intensity on T1- and T2-weighted images. Patchy areas of delayed enhancement are typical and reflect regional variations in tumour vascularity with differential washout kinetics.
- Malignant pericardial deposits are in general low signal on T1-weighted images and high signal on T2-weighted images and display varying degrees of contrast medium enhancement. Typically, there is an associated haemorrhagic pericardial effusion.

Hints and tips

Tumours must be distinguished from thrombus, which tends to occur in typical locations (left atrial appendage and left ventricular apex) and does not enhance following intravenous contrast medium.

Further reading

Sparrow PJ, Kurian JB, Jones TR et al. MR imaging of cardiac tumours. *Radiographics* 2005; **25**: 1255–76.

Case 10: Cardiac tumours

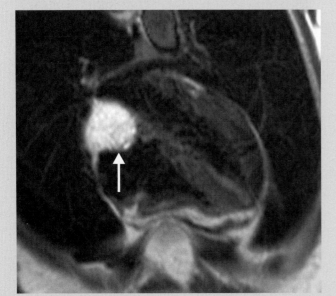

Case 10.1 Four-chamber image from a T2-weighted sequence showing a well-circumscribed high-signal lesion in the interatrial septum (arrow).

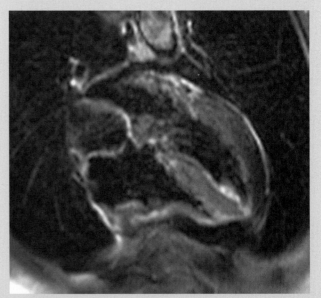

Case 10.2 Four-chamber image from a T2-weighted fat-suppressed sequence in the same patient as in Case 10.1 showing uniform signal suppression in the inter atrial lesion, in keeping with a lipoma.

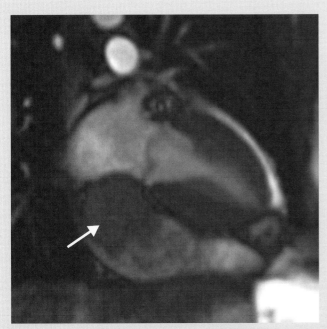

Case 10.3 Two-chamber image from an SSFP sequence showing a pericardial mass (arrow) indenting the undersurface of the left atrium and an associated pericardial effusion.

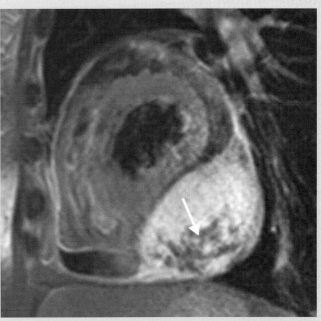

Case 10.4 Short-axis mid left ventricular image from a delayed myocardial enhancement sequence in the same patient as in Case 10.3 showing avid enhancement of the pericardial mass with central low-signal regions (arrow), in keeping with areas of necrosis. Appearances are in keeping with a malignant pericardial mass, and, following resection, this lesion proved to be metastatic adenocarcinoma.

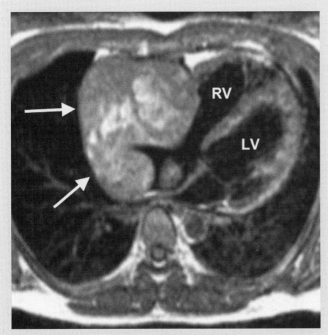

Case 10.5 Axial image from a T1-weighted sequence showing a large, infiltrative mixed-signal intensity mass centred on the right atrial free wall. This proved to be an angiosarcoma.

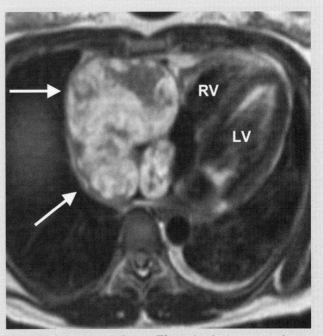

Case 10.6 Axial image from a T2-weighted sequence in the same patient as in case 10.5. The large angiosarcoma is seen to have areas of high signal intensity consistent with a high water content, which is typical of a malignant tumour.

PERICARDITIS

Pericarditis (inflammation of the pericardium) may occur in isolation or in association with inflammation of the underlying myocardium (myocarditis). It may be caused by a variety of conditions, including viral infections, rheumatic fever, connective tissue disorders and uraemia. Clinically, it can mimic angina, and MRI is a useful problem solving tool. With longstanding or recurrent episodes, there may be progression to pericardial constriction, with the formation of dense adhesive bands and pericardial calcification.

Key sequences

- SSFP sequences through the left ventricle in the short-axis plane
- T2-weighted black blood imaging
- Delayed myocardial enhancement imaging

Imaging findings

A pericardial thickness of >4 mm is considered abnormal.

Pericarditis is invariably associated with a pericardial effusion. Simple effusions have low T1 and high T2 signal. Haemorrhagic, infective or malignant effusions have variable signal characteristics and may contain septations and/or solid components.

There may be epi-myocardial delayed enhancement (associated myocarditis).

Hints and tips

The pericardium is most readily identified on transverse T1-weighted black blood images.

A thin black line is sometimes seen along the outer edge of the myocardium, at its interface with epicardial fat. This is caused by chemical shift artefact and should not be mistaken for pericardium.

Smooth pericardial enhancement is characteristic of pericarditis, whereas irregular or nodular thickening suggests a malignant pericardial process.

Further reading

Wang ZJ, Reddy GP, Gotway MB et al. CT and MR imaging of pericardial disease. *Radiographics* 2003; **23**: S167–80.

Case 11: Pericarditis

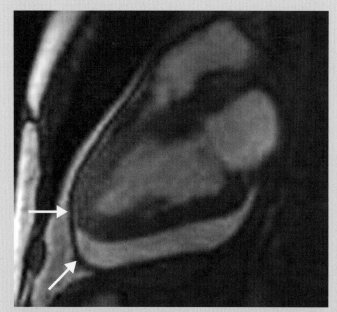

Case 11.1 Two-chamber image from an SSFP sequence showing diffuse smooth pericardial thickening (arrows) and an associated pericardial effusion.

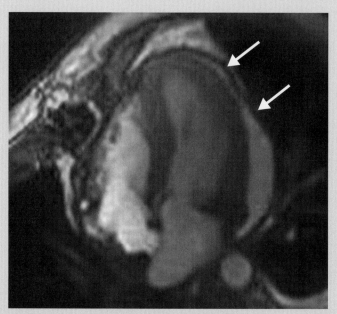

Case 11.2 Four-chamber image from an SSFP sequence in the same patient as in Case 11.2 showing smooth pericardial thickening (arrows), an associated pericardial effusion and small bilateral pleural effusions.

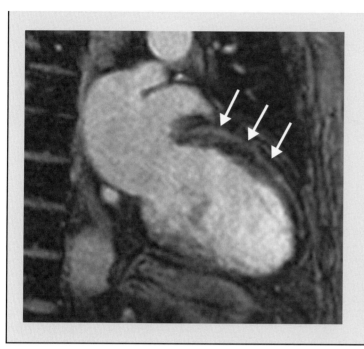

Case 11.3 Two-chamber image from a delayed myocardial enhancement sequence showing epi-myocardial enhancement along the anterior wall of the left ventricle, in keeping with recent peri-myocarditis (arrows).

CONSTRICTIVE PERICARDITIS

Pericardial constriction occurs when diastolic filling of the heart is limited by decreased pericardial compliance and adhesions. Restricted ventricular filling causes increased diastolic pressure in all four cardiac chambers and equalization of atrial and ventricular pressures. Causes include mediastinal irradiation, connective tissue diseases and infections (particularly tuberculous). Constrictive pericarditis may be impossible to distinguish from restrictive cardiomyopathy on clinical grounds, since they present with similar symptoms. MRI is especially useful for differentiating between these two conditions.

Key sequences

- Transverse T1- and T2-weighted black blood imaging
- Four-chamber and left ventricular short-axis SSFP sequences
- Short-axis free-breathing 'real-time' SSFP sequences
- Delayed myocardial enhancement imaging

Imaging findings

Pericardial calcification appears as signal void.

With right ventricular constriction, the ventricle may assume a sigmoid shape.

With left ventricular constriction, the left ventricle may appear flattened.

Dilated vena cava, hepatic veins and coronary sinus are ancillary findings.

Pericardial fibrosis may show delayed Gd enhancement.

With constrictive physiology, the ventricular septum shows 'reverse bowing' on early inspiration (deviation towards the left ventricle).

Hints and tips

The ventricular septum deviates to the left on inspiration in cases of pericardial constriction, because the stiffened pericardium prevents the right ventricular free wall from expanding when right-sided filling pressures rise.

Computed tomography should be considered as a complementary imaging test, since it is the modality of choice for depicting the extent and distribution of pericardial calcification.

Further reading

Wang ZJ, Reddy GP, Gotway MB et al. CT and MR imaging of pericardial disease. *Radiographics* 2003; **23**: S167–80.

Case 12: Constrictive pericarditis

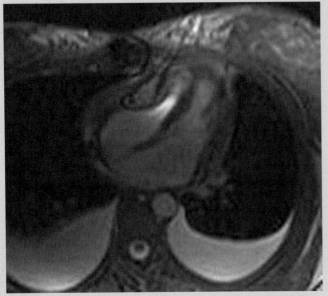

Case 12.1 Transverse image from a T2-weighted fat-suppressed sequence showing right ventricular compression (sigmoid morphology) with moderate-sized bilateral pleural effusions in a patient with pericardial constriction.

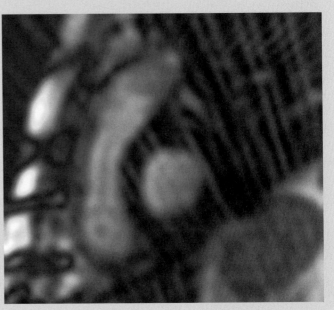

Case 12.2 Short-axis mid left ventricular image from a real-time SSFP sequence in end-expiration (note the elevated left hemidiaphragm) showing normal left ventricular morphology.

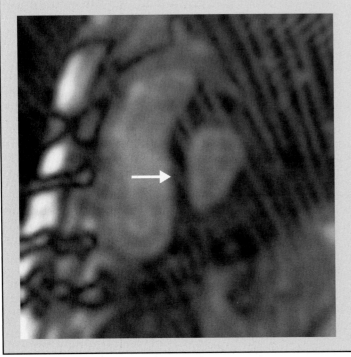

Case 12.3 Short-axis mid left ventricular image from a real-time SSFP sequence in early inspiration (note the depressed left hemidiaphragm) showing reverse bowing of the interventricular septum (arrow) indicative of pericardial constriction.

AORTIC STENOSIS

Valvular aortic stenosis most often occurs as a result of degeneration of a morphologically normal (trileaflet) valve. It may also occur as a complication of congenital valvular disease (e.g. bicuspid valve) or following rheumatic fever. The normal aortic valve orifice measures >2 cm^2. Stenosis is considered critical with a valve area of <0.8 cm^2 and/or a peak transvalvular gradient of >50 mmHg. Cardiac MRI can be used to assess stenosis severity, aetiology and secondary effects such as the degree of left ventricular hypertrophy.

Key sequences

- Sagittal black blood imaging to profile the aortic long axis
- SSFP images paralleling the left ventricular outflow tract
- SSFP images perpendicular to the outflow tract and aortic valve
- Velocity-encoded phase contrast imaging through the proximal ascending aorta (just beyond the valve)
- SSFP sequences through the left ventricle in the short-axis plane to quantify left ventricular mass and function

Imaging findings

Flow acceleration is seen in the proximal ascending aorta.

There is post-stenotic aortic dilatation.

There is concentric left ventricular hypertrophy.

The pressure gradient can be calculated using the modified Bernoulli equation: pressure = 4 × (peak transvalvular velocity)^2.

A bicuspid aortic valve has a characteristic 'fishmouth' opening appearance, assuming an ellipsoid configuration in systole.

Hints and tips

Valvular calcifications appear as signal void on all MRI sequences.

In cases of severe stenosis, the velocity-encoded setting should be adjusted appropriately (with a 2 m/s starting point and increased in gradual increments as required to 4 m/s) to avoid aliasing artefact.

Always review the aortic arch carefully for any associated coarctation.

Further reading

Glockner JF, Johnston DL, McGee KP. Evaluation of cardiac valvular disease with MR imaging: qualitative and quantitative techniques. *Radiographics* 2003; **23**: e9.

Case 13: Aortic stenosis

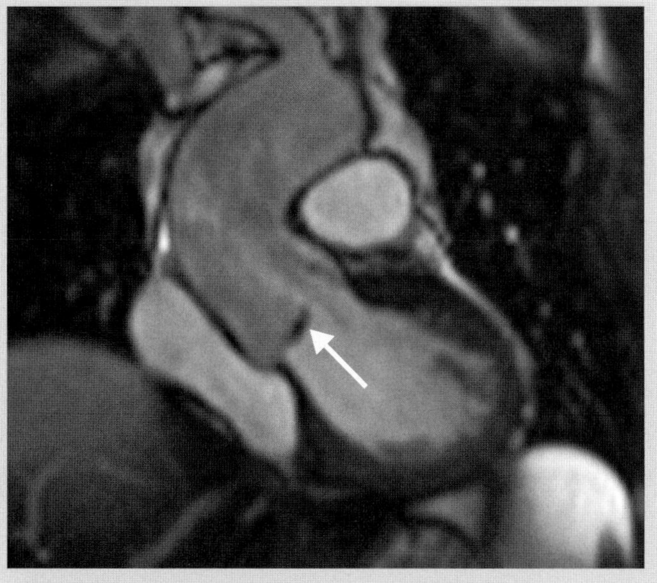

Case 13.1 Coronal oblique image through the left ventricular outflow tract from an SSFP sequence in systole showing restricted opening and thickening of the aortic valve leaflet (arrow) with associated flow acceleration.

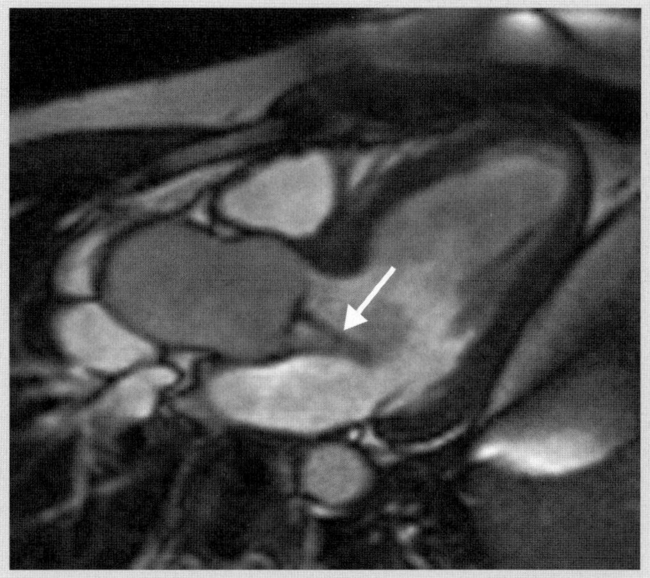

Case 13.2 Three-chamber image from an SSFP sequence in diastole in the same patient as in Case 13.1 showing a central regurgitant jet (arrow), in keeping with mixed aortic valve disease (combined stenosis and regurgitation).

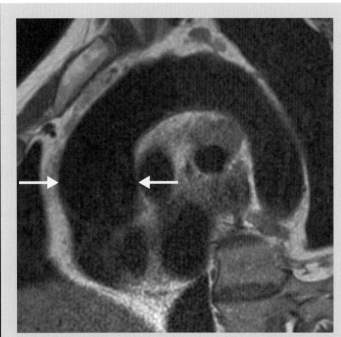

Case 13.3 Sagittal oblique black blood image in a patient with severe aortic stenosis showing dilatation of the proximal ascending thoracic aorta (arrows).

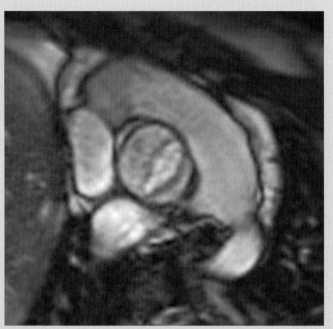

Case 13.4 Transverse oblique image through the aortic valve from an SSFP sequence in systole showing the characteristic 'fishmouth' appearance of a bicuspid aortic valve.

AORTIC DISSECTION

Aortic dissection is a cardiovascular emergency that requires prompt diagnosis. Multidetector computed tomography is the modality of choice in the acute setting, but MRI is a useful means of following up patients who have undergone surgical repair. The Stanford classification divides dissections into type A (involving the ascending aorta or aortic arch) and type B (involving the aorta distal to the origin of the left subclavian artery). Patients with type A dissection usually undergo surgical repair with root or ascending aortic replacement using a Dacron graft (interposition or inclusion technique). The aim of surgical repair is to close entry to the false lumen and prevent extension of dissection. Complications following repair include anastomotic stenosis, perigraft haematoma, pseudoaneurysm formation and progressive enlargement of the false lumen.

Key sequences

- Transverse black blood imaging from just above the aortic arch to the level of the common iliac arteries
- Sagittal oblique black blood imaging, profiling the aortic long axis
- Gd-enhanced MR angiography (MRA)

Imaging findings

The intimal flap appears as a hypointense line with a linear or 'S' shape in the transverse plane.

The true lumen is usually smaller than the false lumen and appears thin or flat in the transverse plane.

Concentric perigraft thickening (up to 10 mm thick) is an expected postsurgical appearance.

Perigraft haematoma usually appears asymmetric with a heterogeneous signal on black blood images.

Pseudoaneurysm results from partial dehiscence of either the proximal or distal suture line and appears as a focal contrast-medium-filled outpouching on angiographic images.

Hints and tips

The false lumen may demonstrate persistent blood flow due to distal intimal tears or communication with principal **aortic** branch vessels.

Measurements should be taken perpendicular to the aorta at stated levels to enable reproducibility on serial studies. Both the true and false lumen diameters should be stated in the report.

A patent false lumen can lead to progressive dilatation, followed by collapse of the true lumen and, potentially, late aortic rupture.

Further reading

García A, Ferreirós J, Santamaría M et al. MR angiographic evaluation of complications in surgically treated type A aortic dissection. *Radiographics* 2006; **26**: 981–92.

Case 14: Aortic dissection

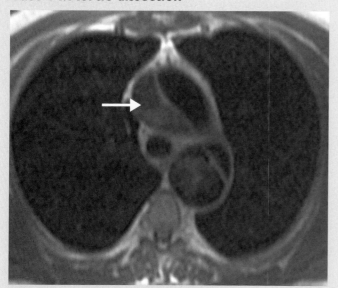

Case 14.1 Transverse black blood image through the aortic arch showing a dissection flap with slow flow (high signal) in the false lumen (arrow).

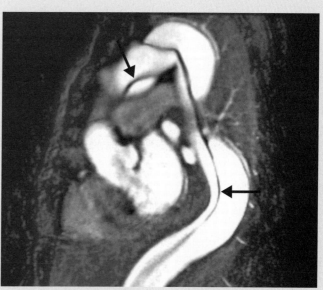

Case 14.2 Maximum-intensity projection (MIP) image from a Gd-enhanced angiogram in the same patient as in Case 14.1 showing a dissection flap that extends from the level of the aortic valve and along the entire length of the thoracic aorta (arrows), in keeping with a type A dissection.

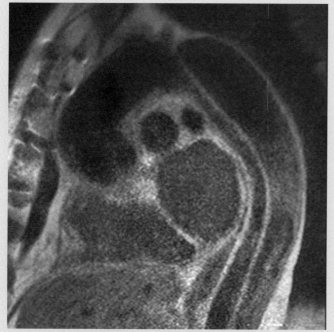

Case 14.3 Sagittal oblique black blood image showing a dissection flap that begins just distal to the left subclavian artery and extends along the descending thoracic aorta (a type B dissection).

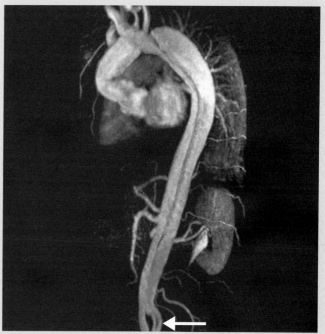

Case 14.4 MIP image from a Gd-enhanced angiogram in the same patient as in Case 14.3 showing the type B dissection, which extends into the left common iliac artery (arrow).

MARFAN'S SYNDROME

Marfan's syndrome is an autosomal dominant disorder in which degeneration of elastic tissue fibres leads to progressive aortic root dilatation. This process begins in the sinuses of Valsalva and progresses to involve the sinotubular junction and aortic valve annulus. Aneurysm rupture and dissection account for the majority of deaths in these patients, who require serial imaging studies to determine the timing of surgical intervention. The most important risk factor for sudden death is the degree of root dilatation.

Key sequences

- Sagittal oblique black blood imaging profiling the aortic long axis
- Velocity-encoded phase contrast imaging through the proximal ascending aorta
- SSFP sequences through the left ventricle in the short-axis plane

Imaging findings

The characteristic appearance of Marfan's syndrome is loss of normal 'waisting' at the sinotubular junction.

Upper limits of normal for sinus of Valsalva diameter are 40 mm in men and 36 mm in women.

Aortic regurgitation is a frequent sequel of root dilatation.

Hints and tips

Surgical repair is indicated when the sinus of Valsalva diameter exceeds 5 cm.

Further reading

Russo V, Renzulli M, La Palombara C et al. Congenital diseases of the thoracic aorta. Role of MRI and MRA. *Eur Radiol* 2006; **16**: 676–84.

Judge DP, Dietz HC. Marfan's syndrome. *Lancet* 2005; **366**: 1965–76.

Case 15: Marfan's syndrome

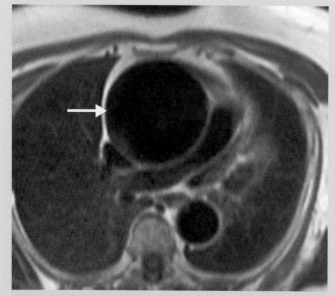

Case 15.1 Transverse black blood image through the aortic root showing pronounced dilatation at the level of the sinuses of Valsalva (arrow).

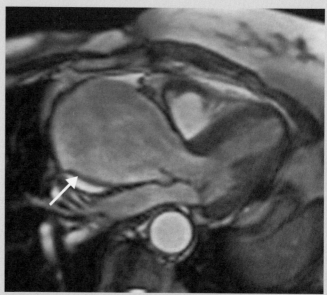

Case 15.2 Three-chamber image from an SSFP sequence in systole in the same patient as in Case 15.1 showing dilatation of the sinuses of Valsalva and loss of normal 'waisting' at the sinotubular junction (arrow).

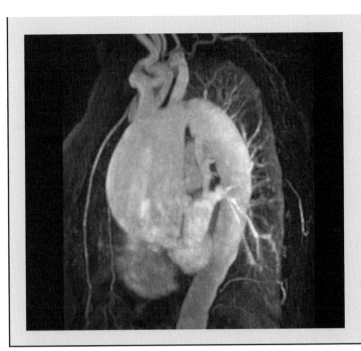

Case 15.3 MIP image from a Gd-enhanced angiogram in the same patient as in Cases 15.1 and 15.2 showing fusiform dilatation of the aortic root and ascending thoracic aorta with loss of 'waisting' at the sinotubular junction.

COARCTATION OF THE AORTA

Aortic coarctation is a discrete narrowing of the aortic arch, just distal to the left subclavian artery. It may occur in isolation or in association with other structural disease such as bicuspid aortic valve, atrial septal defect and patent ductus arteriosus. Haemodynamically significant stenosis leads to the development of prominent collateral vessels that bypass the affected segment. MRI permits evaluation of haemodynamic severity and is also used in the follow-up of patients who have undergone prior surgical or catheter-based intervention.

Key sequences

- Sagittal oblique black blood imaging to profile the aortic long axis
- Velocity-encoded phase contrast imaging:
  - through the proximal ascending aorta
  - just proximal to the narrowed segment
  - just distal to the narrowed segment
  - at the level of the diaphragm
- Gd-enhanced three-dimensional MRA

Imaging findings

There is a localized segment of aortic narrowing.

Haemodynamically significant narrowing is characterized by extensive collateralization and a pressure gradient of >20 mmHg.

Those patients who have undergone prior subclavian flap aortoplasty or patch repair are prone to aneurysm formation and restenosis.

Hints and tips

The amount of collateral flow and its effect on blood volume increase (measured at two points – one just distal to the lesion and the other at the level of the diaphragm) reflects the haemodynamic severity of obstruction.

Adequate repair, either surgical or catheter-based, is represented by a return to normalcy of aortic flow patterns.

Pseudocoarctation may appear similar on black blood imaging, but the degree of collateralization is typically less severe and the pressure gradient is not significant

Further reading

Hom JJ, Ordovas K, Reddy GP. Velocity-encoded cine MR imaging in aortic coarctation: functional assessment of hemodynamic events. *Radiographics* 2008; **28**: 407–16.

Case 16: Coarctation of the aorta

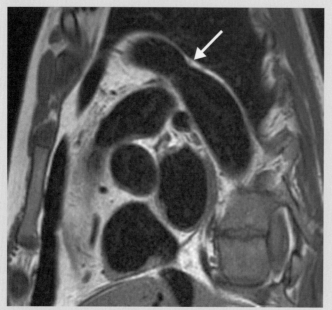

Case 16.1 Sagittal oblique black blood image showing a focal narrowing in the proximal descending thoracic aorta (arrow).

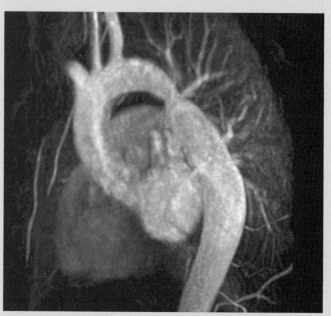

Case 16.2 MIP image from a Gd-enhanced angiogram in the same patient as in Case 16.1 showing the coarctation. Note the prominent intercostal collateral vessels that serve to bypass the stenotic segment.

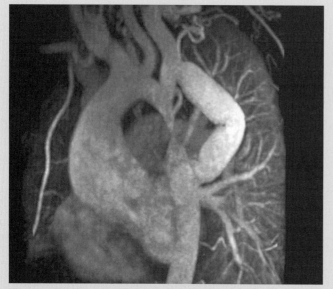

Case 16.3 MIP image from a Gd-enhanced angiogram in a patient under follow-up following the creation of a conduit from the left subclavian artery to the aorta.

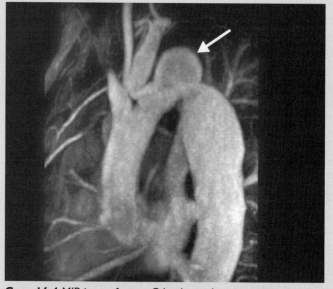

Case 16.4 MIP image from a Gd-enhanced angiogram in a patient under follow-up following flap repair of aortic coarctation. An aneurysm (arrow) has formed at the site of surgical repair.

PULMONARY HYPERTENSION

Pulmonary hypertension is defined as a mean pulmonary artery pressure of >25 mmHg at rest or >30 mmHg with exercise. Causes are diverse, ranging from chronic thromboembolic disease to intracardiac shunts. A multimodality imaging approach is usually employed to investigate these patients, and typically includes echocardiography and computed tomographic pulmonary angiography. Cardiac MRI is the modality of choice for assessing right ventricular function, and also permits assessment and quantification of intracardiac shunts. Magnetic resonance angiography (MRA) is an emerging technique for non-invasive assessment of the pulmonary arterial tree.

Key sequences

- Transverse black blood imaging covering the entire thorax
- SSFP sequences through the right ventricle in the transverse plane
- Gd-enhanced pulmonary angiography

Imaging findings

The main pulmonary artery diameter (measured at its bifurcation) is >30 mm.

There is right ventricular dilatation (>45 mm) with hypertrophy of its free wall (>3 mm).

Right ventricular ejection fraction is impaired (<45%).

There is tricuspid regurgitation (with a flow jet extending into the right atrium).

Pulmonary arterial occlusions, stenoses, webs and aneurysms may be seen in cases of proximal chronic thromboembolic disease on MRA.

Hints and tips

Congenital systemic-to-pulmonary shunts can lead to pulmonary hypertension and may be overlooked on initial echocardiographic assessment (especially sinus venosus atrial septal defect, anomalous pulmonary venous drainage and patent ductus arteriosus). It is therefore important to look specifically for these defects, which may be best appreciated on transverse black blood images.

Further reading

Coulden R. State-of-the-art imaging techniques in chronic thromboembolic pulmonary hypertension. *Proc Am Thorac Soc* 2006; **3**: 577–83.

Case 17: Pulmonary hypertension

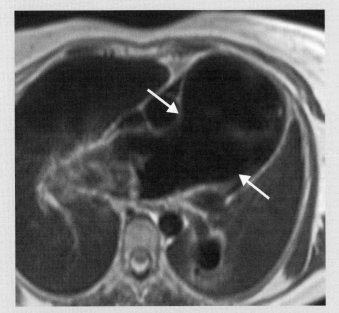

Case 17.1 Transverse black blood image at the level of the main pulmonary artery bifurcation, which is markedly dilated (arrows). This patient had pulmonary hypertension secondary to chronic thromboembolic disease.

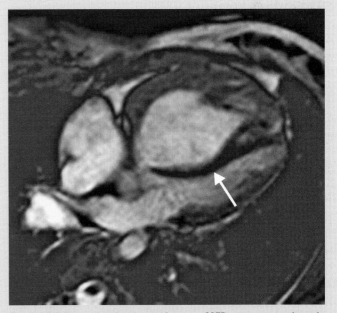

Case 17.2 Four-chamber image from an SSFP sequence in diastole in the same patient as in Case 17.1 showing right ventricular dilatation, reverse bowing of the interventricular septum (arrow) and right ventricular hypertrophy.

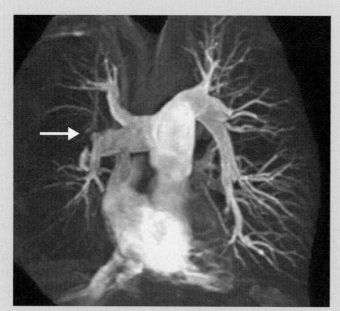

Case 17.3 MIP image from a Gd-enhanced pulmonary angiogram in the same patient as in Cases 17.1 and 17.2 showing truncation of the proximal pulmonary vasculature, especially involving the segmental arteries supplying the right lower lobe at the origin of the middle lobe vessels (arrow).

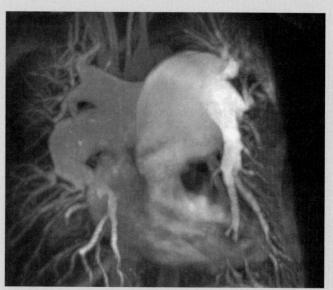

Case 17.4 MIP image from a Gd-enhanced pulmonary angiogram in a patient with a longstanding secundum-type atrial septal defect. The main, left and right pulmonary arteries are markedly dilated, with pruning of the more distal vasculature.

PULMONARY ARTERIOVENOUS MALFORMATION (AVM)

Pulmonary AVM is a direct communication between a pulmonary artery and pulmonary vein that permits right-to-left shunting. It may occur in isolation or as part of a systemic process in hereditary haemorrhagic telangiectasia. Pulmonary AVMs may be single or multiple, and usually manifest as fragile thin-walled aneurysms. The absence of a filtering capillary bed offers the potential for paradoxical embolism, with an attendant risk of stroke, cerebral abscess formation and seizures. MRI is able to provide precise information on the number, location, complexity and haemodynamic significance of pulmonary AVMs. Treatment options include transarterial coil embolization, especially for lesions with a feeding vessel diameter of >3 mm.

Key sequences

- Velocity-encoded phase contrast imaging through the proximal aorta and main pulmonary artery (right-to-left shunt quantification)
- SSFP sequences through the left ventricle in the short-axis oblique plane
- Gd-enhanced pulmonary angiography

Imaging findings

There is a septated aneurysm sac with an enlarged feeding artery and draining vein.

Small pulmonary AVMs are often peripheral in location. Larger AVMs tend to be located more centrally.

Hints and tips

Feeding vessel diameter may be difficult to measure precisely on the MR pulmonary angiography images, especially with small lesions. A maximal AVM dimension exceeding 5 mm serves as a useful guide when assessing suitability for embolization therapy.

Maximum-intensity projection (MIP) reconstructions from the raw data of pulmonary angiography are useful for visualizing the course of the feeding vessels when planning embolization therapy.

Further reading

Schneider G, Uder M, Koehler M et al. MR angiography for detection of pulmonary arteriovenous malformations in patients with hereditary hemorrhagic telangiectasia. *AJR Am J Roentgenol* 2008; **190**: 892–901.

Case 18: Pulmonary arteriovenous malformation (AVM)

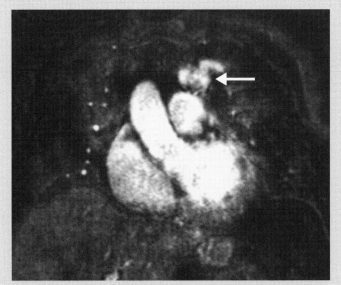

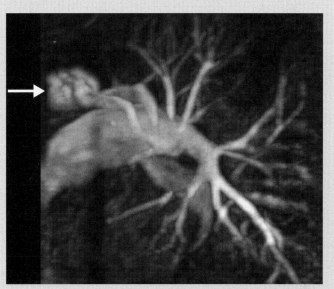

Case 18.1 Coronal source image from a Gd-enhanced pulmonary angiogram showing a serpinginous vascular lesion in the left upper lobe (arrow).

Case 18.2 MIP image from a Gd-enhanced pulmonary angiogram in the same patient as in Case 18.1 showing a pulmonary AVM. The aneurysm sac (arrow), feeding vessel and draining vein are clearly demonstrated.

THORACIC TUMOURS

A variety of tumours can arise in the thorax, of which bronchogenic carcinomas (small cell and non-small cell varieties) account for the vast majority. Less common tumour types include those arising from the pleura or chest wall (malignant mesothelioma, solitary fibrous tumour and sarcomas) and those with a neurogenic origin (ganglioneuroma). Computed tomography and positron emission tomography form the mainstay of imaging evaluation; however, MRI can be a useful complementary test for assessing the extent of local invasion prior to surgical resection and for tissue characterization owing to its superior soft tissue resolution.

Key sequences

- Respiratory-gated T1-weighted, T2-weighted, fat-suppressed and Gd-enhanced black blood imaging in the transverse, coronal and sagittal planes
- Cardiac gating with SSFP and myocardial tagged sequences are especially useful for assessing pericardial invasion.

Imaging findings

Signal characteristics vary widely and depend upon tumour vascularity, the presence of necrosis/haemorrhage and water/fat content.

The following findings are relatively specific:
- Circumferential nodular pleural thickening that is isointense on T1-weighted images and moderately high signal on T2-weighted images and displays avid contrast medium enhancement is suggestive of mesothelioma.

- A large soft tissue mass with heterogeneous signal intensity on T1-weighted images, central high signal on T2-weighted images and a heterogeneous pattern of contrast medium enhancement is suggestive of a solitary fibrous tumour. These primary pleural neoplasms are mostly benign, but malignant degeneration with invasion of diaphragm/chest wall is recognized
- An ovoid sharply marginated paravertebral mass with smooth internal septations is characteristic of a ganglioneuroma (a benign tumour arising from sympathetic ganglia).

Hints and tips

For a lesion that contains fatty elements, incomplete signal suppression on fat-saturated sequences is suggestive of liposarcoma rather than lipoma.

Ill-defined mediastinal fat planes and >50% tumoral encasement of a mediastinal structure is suggestive of local invasion.

A smooth interface between tumour and pericardium with unrestricted motion on SSFP sequences suggests absence of pericardial invasion.

Further reading

Tateishi U, Gladish GW, Kusumoto M et al. Chest wall tumors: radiologic findings and pathologic correlation. *Radiographics* 2003; **23**: 1477–90.

Rosado-de-Christenson ML, Abbott GF, McAdams HP et al. From the Archives of the AFIP: Localized fibrous tumors of the pleura. *Radiographics* 2003; **23**: 759–83.

Case 19: Thoracic tumours

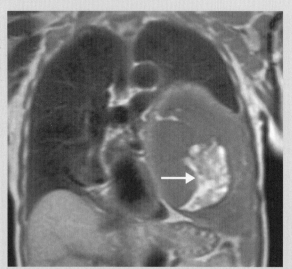

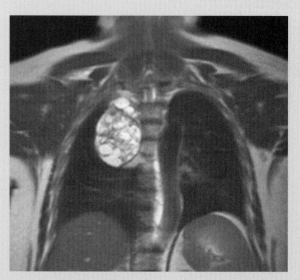

Case 19.1 Coronal image from a T2-weighted sequence showing a large mass occupying much of the left hemithorax and causing a mediastinal shift to the right. The lesion has well-circumscribed margins, contains central areas of high signal (arrow) and shows no signs of chest wall or diaphragmatic invasion. Appearances are typical of a solitary fibrous tumour.

Case 19.2 Coronal image from a T2-weighted sequence showing a well-circumscribed high-signal right paraspinal mass that contains multiple internal septations. Following surgical resection, this lesion proved to be a ganglioneuroma.

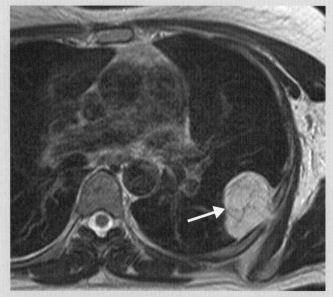

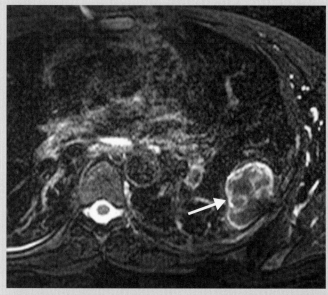

Case 19.3 Transverse image from a T2-weighted sequence showing a well-circumscribed high-signal mass arising from the pleura of the left posterior chest wall (arrow).

Case 19.4 Transverse image from a T2-weighted fat-suppressed sequence in the same patient as in Case 19.3 showing incomplete signal suppression. Following surgical resection, this lesion proved to be a liposarcoma.

UNIT V

Vascular MRI

Sapna Puppala

1 TECHNIQUE AND SEQUENCES

Vascular imaging has evolved over the last decade, moving away from invasive angiography to non-invasive imaging utilizing magnetic resonance angiography (MRA), Doppler ultrasound and computed tomography angiography (CTA). Doppler is operator-dependent and is less accurate with calcified runoff vessels. Calcification also causes blooming artefact on CTA, making it less accurate. MRA is safer than CT in terms of contrast reaction and does not involve radiation. MRA does, however, overestimate the degree of stenosis.

There are two basic types of MRA sequences: contrast-enhanced MRA (CEMRA) and non-contrast MRA.

CONTRAST-ENHANCED MRA

The three-dimensional (3D) CEMRA technique is based on the acquisition of heavily T1-weighted 3D gradient echo datasets (fast imaging with steady-state precession: FISP) with ultrashort echo time (<2 ms) and repetition time (<5 ms) during the arterial phase of an intravenously injected bolus of a T1-shortening paramagnetic agent such as gadolinium (Gd). It has improved sensitivity and specificity compared with non-contrast sequences. Time-resolved imaging of contrast kinetics (TRICKS) has improved temporal resolution, with real-time acquisition of images as contrast flows through the vessels.

Standard CEMRA can also be used to image veins. Delayed imaging can generate an image of the venous system called a magnetic resonance venogram (MRV). The advent of blood pool contrast agents has improved venous imaging further.

Further reading

Ersoy H, Rybicki FJ. MR angiography of the lower extremities. *AJR Am J Roentgenol* 2008; **190**: 1675–84.

Zhang H, Maki JH, Prince MR. 3D contrast-enhanced MR angiography. *J Magn Reson Imaging* 2007; **25**: 13–25.

Case 1: Contrast-enhanced MRA

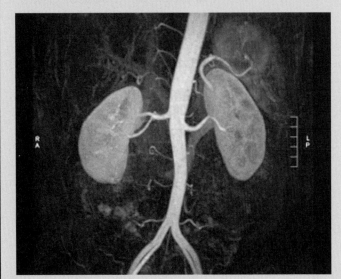

Case 1.1 3D–CEMRA coronal maximum-intensity projection (MIP) showing the normal abdominal aorta and branches.

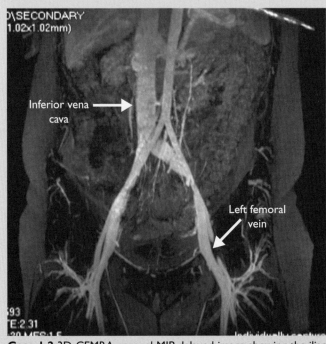

Case 1.2 3D-CEMRA coronal MIP delayed image showing the iliac veins and inferior vena cava.

NON-CONTRAST MRA SEQUENCES

Here the flow dynamics is utilized in producing the image. 3D time of flight (TOF) and black and white blood techniques are non-contrast MRA sequences. The 3D-TOF technique is largely used in intracranial imaging. 2D-TOF suffers from artefacts in most regions and is only used as localizer prior to CEMRA. The black and white blood imaging techniques are often gated acquisitions used in assessment of the heart and aorta. The occurrence of nephrogenic systemic fibrosis has led to renewed interest in non-contrast MRA.

Further reading

Ersoy H, Rybicki FJ. MR angiography of the lower extremities. *AJR Am J Roentgenol* 2008; **190**: 1675–84.

Kaufman JA, McCarter D, Geller SC, Waltman AC. Two-dimensional time-of-flight MR angiography of the lower extremities: artefacts and pitfalls. *AJR Am J Roentgenol* 1998; **171**: 129–35.

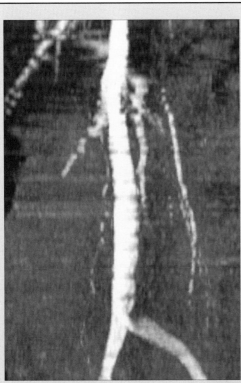

Case 2.1 2D-TOF image of the abdominal aorta showing degradation of image quality due to step artefact.

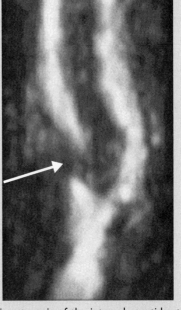

Stenosis of origin of internal carotid artery

Case 2.2 3D-TOF showing stenosis of the internal carotid artery origin. Note the poor quality of the image.

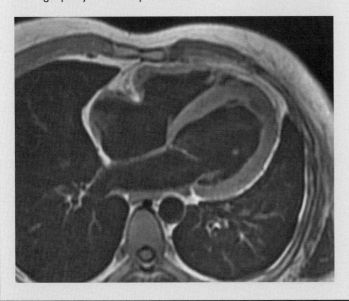

Case 2.3 Gated black blood (spin echo) image of the heart and descending aorta. This sequence is useful to assess the walls of the vessels and the myocardium.

VASCULAR PSEUDO-OCCLUSION

With any form of imaging, it is important to be aware of common pitfalls and avoid misinterpretation of the images. MRA is no exception. An important technical artefact that can be encountered is pseudo-occlusion, often of the pelvic vessels. Peripheral MRA is a 3D volume acquisition in the coronal plane. If the coronal slab or extent of imaging is not wide enough to include the depth of the pelvis, the posterior vessels or segments are not included in the field of view (FOV), thus leading to a false appearance of occlusion of the iliac vessels or their branches.

Imaging findings

There is symmetrical and abrupt cutoff of vessels or their branches.

Hints and tips

Review the raw data, which will show that images of the non-visualized portions were not acquired.

Rotate the maximum-intensity projections and view in the sagittal plane, which will show the posterior extent of the FOV.

Further reading

Ersoy H, Zhang H, Prince MR. Peripheral MR angiography. *J Cardiovasc Magn Reson* 2006; **8**: 517–28.

Case 3: Vascular pseudo-occlusion

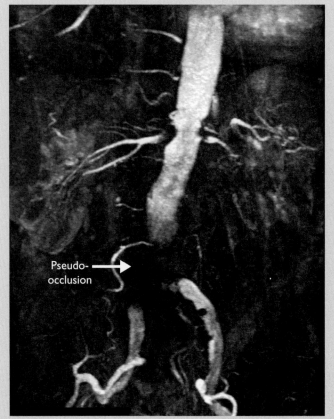

Case 3.1 CEMRA coronal MIP showing abrupt symmetrical exclusion of both common iliac arteries.

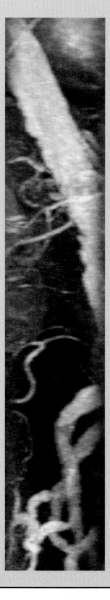

Case 3.2 Sagittal view showing that the FOV never included this part of the vessels and they were not imaged.

2 VASCULAR PATHOLOGIES

ATHEROSCLEROTIC PERIPHERAL VASCULAR DISEASE

Atherosclerosis is the most common vascular pathology, leading to various symptoms. It affects all vessels, from coronary arteries to the periphery. The atherosclerotic plaques commonly cause stenosis and occlusions, but equally atherosclerosis is the most common cause of aneurysm formation. The same individual can manifest both vascular stenosis and aneurysms affecting more than one vessel at a time. Peripheral vascular atherosclerotic disease is a common cause of claudication, rest pain and ulceration. Contrast-enhanced magnetic resonance angiography (CEMRA) is a non-invasive method of assessing the whole peripheral vascular system without the risk of ionizing radiation and contrast nephropathy. However, while CEMRA provides reliable diagnostic accuracy in the aorta and the proximal sections of its branches, small peripheral arteries cannot be assessed accurately.

Key sequences

- 3D-CEMRA performed from diaphragm to feet; stepping-table or three-stations imaging with generous overlap
- TRICKS (time-resolved imaging of contrast kinetics) for runoff vessels

Imaging findings

There are focal, multifocal or diffuse stenosis or occlusions, which may be unilateral or bilateral and with involvement of more than one vessel.

There may be associated aneurysms – review the raw data.

Dissection flaps and false lumens may be present.

Hints and tips

Always review raw data, since maximum-intensity projections (MIPs) can overestimate stenosis.

Review raw data for thrombosed aneurysm sacs, walls and thrombosed false lumens.

The presence of metallic stents can cause a drop in signal, giving the appearance of stenosis or occlusions.

Always look for incidental pathology.

Further reading

Low G, Mizzi A, Ong K, Lau PF, McKinstery J. Technical inadequacies of peripheral contrast-enhanced magnetic resonance angiography: incidence, causes and management strategies. *Clin Radiol* 2006; **61**: 937–45.

Mell M, Tefera G, Thornton F et al. Clinical utility of time-resolved imaging of contrast kinetics (TRICKS) magnetic resonance angiography for infrageniculate arterial occlusive disease. *J Vasc Surg* 2007; **45**: 543–8; discussion 548.

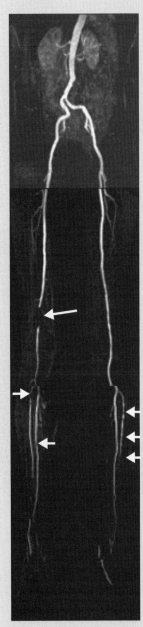

Case 4: Atherosclerotic peripheral vascular disease

Case 4.1 3D-CEMRA for peripheral vascular disease: three-station examination. The coronal MIPs have been put together after postprocessing. There is a short occlusion in the right femoral artery (long arrow), long occlusions in the posterior tibial arteries bilaterally, and multifocal stenosis in the anterior tibial and peroneal vessels bilaterally (short arrows).

POPLITEAL ARTERY ANEURYSM

Popliteal artery aneurysms are the most common peripheral artery aneurysms, accounting for 70% of the total aneurysms in the periphery. More than 95% occur in men, and the average age of patients at presentation is 65 years. Atherosclerosis is the most common aetiology, being seen in more than 90% of cases. Most popliteal artery aneurysms are fusiform, they are bilateral in 25% of cases and they are associated with abdominal aortic aneurysms in 20–40% of cases. Although the standard treatment of popliteal artery aneurysms has been open repair, there are an increasing number of reports in the literature of endovascular management.

Key sequences

- 3D-CEMRA, including the region from the abdominal aorta to the ankles because of the possibility of associated aortic aneurysms
- T2-weighted axial through the knee to assess the contents of the aneurysm sac

Imaging findings

When an aneurysm of the popliteal artery is seen, if it is ectatic, it should be compared with the superficial femoral artery above (twice the size).

The aneurysm may be thrombosed and, if it is acute, there may be no popliteal or runoff flow.

Look for the presence of bilateral aneurysms or aneurysms at other sites.

Hints and tips

Always review the raw data and axial images, since the luminogram or MRA MIPs will only reveal the patent lumen, which can be normal or even reduced in size.

Always assess the other vessels, especially the contralateral popliteal artery and aorta.

An important differential diagnosis is cystic adventitial disease, which occurs in the wall of the vessel. Ultrasound is better than MRI at differentiating the two.

Further reading

Holden A, Merilees S, Mitchell N, Hill A. Magnetic resonance imaging of popliteal artery pathologies. *Eur J Radiol* 2008; **67**: 159–68.

Case 5: Popliteal artery aneurysm

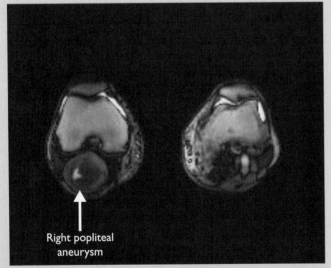

Case 5.1 T2-weighted axial image showing the heterogeneous contents of the aneurysm sac of a popliteal artery aneurysm.

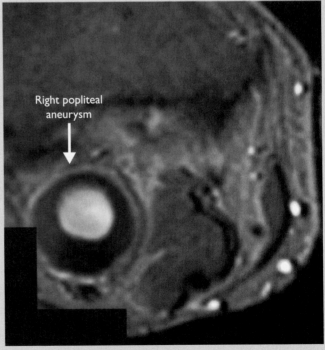

Case 5.2 Reviewing postcontrast T1-weighted raw data as an axial scan through the knee shows the extent of the aneurysm as compared with the CEMRA MIP, which only reveals the lumen.

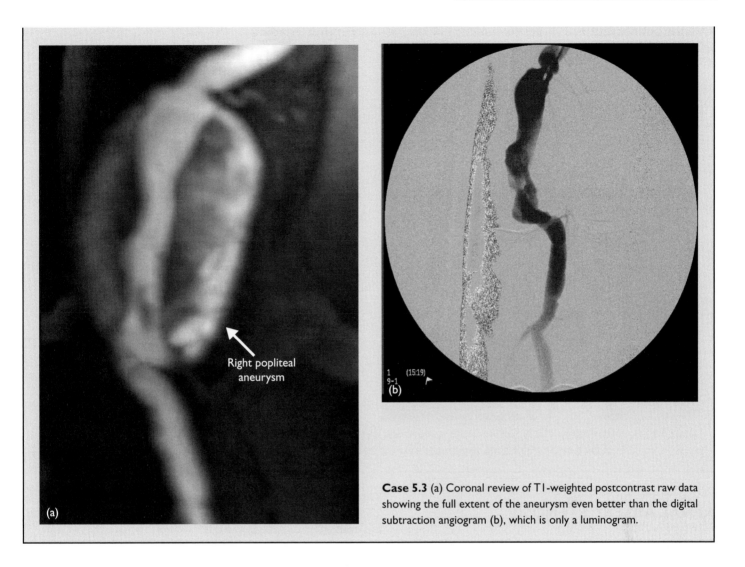

Case 5.3 (a) Coronal review of T1-weighted postcontrast raw data showing the full extent of the aneurysm even better than the digital subtraction angiogram (b), which is only a luminogram.

SUBCLAVIAN ARTERY OCCLUSIVE DISEASE

Stenoses and occlusion of the subclavian artery (SCA) can lead to distal ischaemia and embolization, and when they affect the vertebrobasilar territory, they can evoke serious disturbances, including ischaemic stroke. CEMRA is a non-invasive, robust technique for imaging subclavian pathologies with high diagnostic performance. Sensitivity and specificity are 90% and 95%, respectively, in detecting steno-occlusive disease (including functional and arterial stenoses), and 100% for other vascular pathologies (dilatation, kinking, anomalous origin and arteriovenous malformations).

Key sequences

- 3D-CEMRA is the main sequence performed in the neutral position for atherosclerotic lesions.
- If thoracic outlet syndrome is suspected then perform imaging with the arms in a neutral and abducted and extended position.

- T2-weighted axial and/or high-resolution T1-weighted axial sequences are useful to assess the vessel wall, post-stenotic aneurysms and extrinsic compressions.

Imaging findings

There is focal narrowing or occlusion of the SCA. Eighty-five percent of atherosclerotic lesions occur near the left SCA origin and are proximal to the origin of the vertebral artery.

There may be poststenotic dilatation if the condition is severe.

Long, smooth tapering stenosis is suggestive of vasculitis or dissection.

Hints and tips

Atherosclerosis affects the origin and is proximal to the vertebral arteries.

Thoracic outlet syndrome shows compression of the vessels at the thoracic outlet, with or without poststenotic dilatation.

Vasculitis can affect anywhere, but has a predilection for the distal SCA and the axillary artery.

Further reading

Cosottini M, Zampa V, Petruzzi P et al. Contrast-enhanced three-dimensional MR angiography in the assessment of subclavian artery diseases. *Eur Radiol* 2000; **10**: 1737–44.

Case 6: Subclavian artery occlusive disease

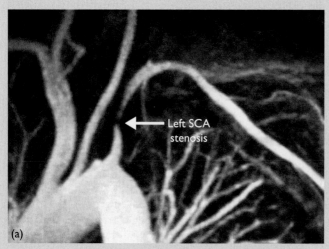

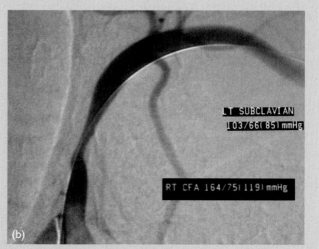

Case 6.1 (a) Oblique sagittal MIP of CEMRA showing short focal stenosis of the SCA close to its origin, in keeping with atherosclerotic stenosis. (b) DSA of the same, confirming the stenosis and showing the haemodynamic significance.

RENAL ARTERY STENOSIS

This is narrowing of the renal artery due to various causes, leading to renal ischaemia and thus reducing renal function or causing hypertension. Ultrasound, computed tomography angiography and MRA have all been used to assess the renal artery. MRA has the advantage of not involving iodinated contrast. However, it is poor at assessing the vessels at the hilum and beyond. Post-transplant assessment of the renal artery can also be done with MRA if time permits, but obtaining an MRA should not delay intervention if ultrasound has already revealed the abnormality.

Key sequences

- Native renal artery: CEMRA coronal acquisition and review of axial reformats for origin of disease and renal vessel tortuosity
- Transplant renal artery: CEMRA coronal acquisition, with the field of view based on the site of transplant (i.e. pelvis, lower abdomen, etc.)

Imaging findings

There is focal or multifocal narrowing of the renal arteries, unilaterally or bilaterally.

Post-stenostic dilatation is seen.

Web-like lesions or a beaded appearance suggest fibromuscular dysplasia (FMD).

There may be a reduction in the size of the kidneys, especially if the renal artery is nearly or fully occluded.

Hints and tips

Stenosis is graded as <50%, >50% and >70% reduction of diameter. A reduction of >50% is haemodynamically significant. If it is >70% then it is likely to cause hypertension and/or ischaemia.

Atherosclerosis affects the origin and FMD affects the distal renal artery and branches. FMD is often multifocal.

Always look out for accessory vessels, which may be stenosed even though the main renal artery is normal.

Transplant renal artery stenosis is usually at the anastomosis, but can be distal.

Further reading

Law YM, Tay KH, Gan YU et al. Gadolinium-enhanced magnetic resonance angiography in renal artery stenosis: comparison with digital subtraction angiography. *Hong Kong Med J* 2008; **14**: 136–41.

Case 7: Renal artery stenosis

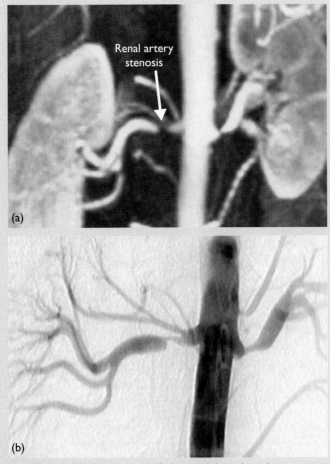

(a)

(b)

Case 7.1 (a) CEMRA coronal MIP showing bilateral renal artery origin stenosis in an elderly patient with atherosclerosis. (b) Digital subtraction angiogram in the same patient, confirming the MRA findings.

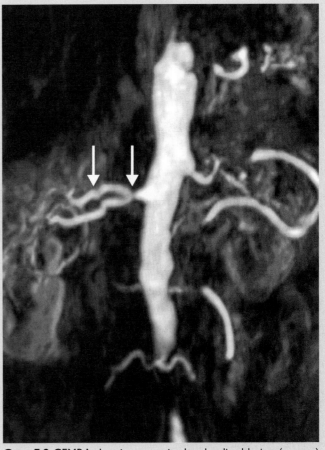

Case 7.2 CEMRA showing a proximal and a distal lesion (arrows) in proven FMD.

MESENTERIC OCCLUSIVE DISEASE

By definition, this condition involves stenosis or occlusion of the coeliac artery and/or the superior mesenteric artery, possibly causing mesenteric ischaemia. An acute occlusion of one vessel can lead to acute mesenteric ischaemia. In chronic mesenteric occlusive disease, patients are symptomatic when two out of three vessels are involved. Imaging for chronic mesenteric ischaemia can be undertaken with ultrasound, computed tomography angiography (CTA) or MRA, all of which are accurate and have 85–95% sensitivity. In acute mesenteric ischaemia, computed tomography angiography is better and preferable.

Key sequences

- CEMRA with image acquisition in the coronal plane

Imaging findings

There is stenosis or occlusion of one or more vessels at or close to their origin, with poststenotic dilatation.

Hypertrophied collaterals are present.

Hints and tips

Review of sagittal reformats is essential to assess these vessels.

An important differential diagnosis is median arcuate ligament compression of coeliac origin. Here the coeliac origin is compressed by the arcuate ligament in expiration, and imaging should therefore be performed in both inspiration and expiration.

Further reading

Shih MC, Hagspiel KD. CTA and MRA in mesenteric ischemia: Part 1, Role in diagnosis and differential diagnosis *AJR Am J Roentgenol* 2007; **188**: 452–61.

Case 8: Mesenteric occlusive disease

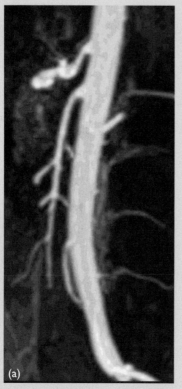 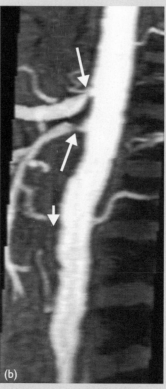

Case 8.1 (a) Normal aorta, coeliac artery, and superior and inferior mesenteric arteries. (b) Stenosis of the origins of the coeliac and superior mesenteric arteries (arrows). The origin of the inferior mesenteric artery is occluded (arrowhead). Note the poststenotic dilatation and background diseased aorta.

ABDOMINAL AORTIC ANEURYSM

Abdominal aortic aneurysms continue to be a major cause of mortality because of their potential for rupture. The incidence is around 4% in men over the age of 64, rising to 7–14% of those with both hypertension and peripheral vascular disease, and 11–28% of those with a first-degree relative with abdominal aortic aneurysm. Contrast-enhanced MRA can be an accurate and reliable method for arterial evaluation of the abdominal aorta and peripheral vessels. The basic issues relate to proper synchronization of imaging with peak arterial enhancement.

Key sequences

- 3D-CEMRA in the coronal plane from diaphragm to groins
- T2-weighted axial for assessing the sac
- TRICKS if assessing for endoleaks

Imaging findings

There is fusiform or saccular dilatation of the infrarenal, juxtarenal or suprarenal aorta.

Patent or thrombosed contents of the sac are seen with varying signal depending on the time of thrombus formation.

There may be associated aneurysms of the iliac arteries.

Hints and tips

Look for associated aneurysms.

Avoid reporting from the postprocessed MIPs. Review the raw data.

Perform delayed imaging for endoleaks.

Further reading

Michaely HJ, Attenberger UI, Kramer H et al. Abdominal and pelvic MR angiography. *Magn Reson Imaging Clin N Am* 2007; **15**: 301–14, v–vi.

Case 9: Abdominal aortic aneurysm

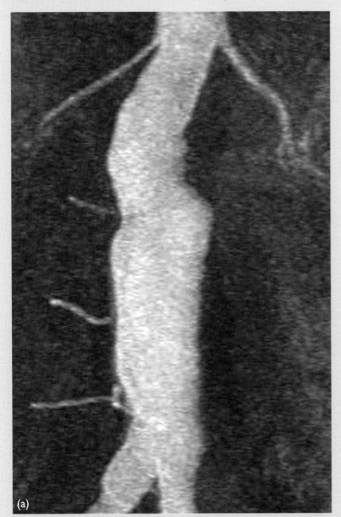 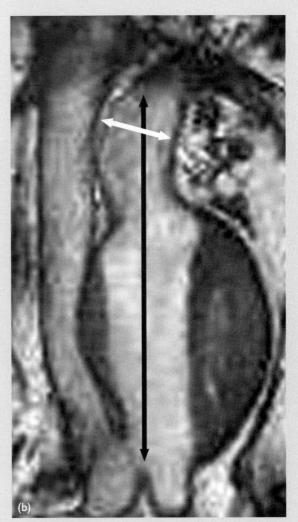

Case 9.1 (a) 3D-CEMRA coronal MIP showing the enhanced lumen and giving an impression of ectatic aorta only. (b) Review of the raw data clearly depicts the extent of the aneurysm of the infrarenal aorta.

OVARIAN VEIN CONGESTION

Chronic pelvic pain is a common and disabling condition affecting women of childbearing age and is a common cause of gynaecological referral. It can occur as a result of ovarian vein incompetence leading to pelvic congestion. 3D contrast-enhanced magnetic resonance venography (CEMRV) is now routinely used to confirm the clinical diagnosis prior to intervention. The sensitivity and specificity of CEMRV reach 88% and 67% for ovarian veins.

Key sequences

- CEMRA of the abdomen, pelvis and upper thighs, preferably using a blood pool contrast agent (e.g. Vasovist)
- CEMRV or delayed-phase imaging

- High-resolution coronal sequences (e.g. volumetric interpolated breath-hold examination: VIBE)

Imaging findings

The veins of the pelvis are prominent or dilated.

Ovarian vein(s), especially the left ovarian vein, are dilated.

There are vulval varices.

Arteries are normal.

Hints and tips

Ensure patency of the inferior vena cava and iliac veins, which may be the cause of pelvic congestion rather than ovarian vein incompetence.

Compression of the iliac vein by the iliac artery (May–Thurner syndrome) can also lead to congestion of iliac vein branches.

Identifying the above two differential diagnoses is important, since management is different.

Further reading

Asciutto G, Mumme A, Marpe B et al. MR venography in the detection of pelvic venous congestion. *Eur J Vasc Endovasc Surg* 2008; **36**: 491–6.

Case 10: Ovarian vein congestion

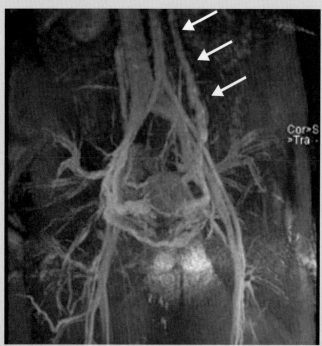

Case 10.1 Coronal MIP of CEMRV or delayed-phase imaging showing contrast in artery and veins. Note the prominent pelvic veins and the dilated draining left ovarian vein (arrows).

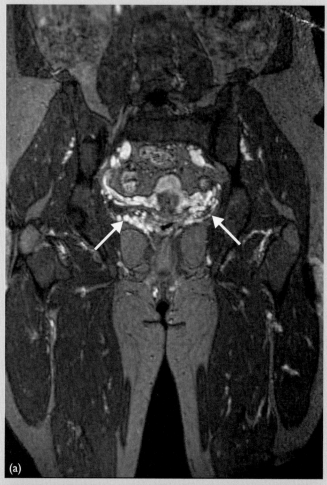

(a)

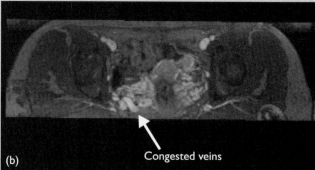

(b) Congested veins

Case 10.2 (a, b) Coronal and axial slices of a high-resolution sequence (VIBE) showing the congested dilated pelvic veins (arrows).

UNIT VI

Breast MRI

Nisha Sharma, Barbara JG Dall

1 TECHNIQUE

TIME

The total examination time should be less than 30 minutes.

ORIENTATION

Both breasts should be examined. This can be achieved by scanning in the axial or coronal plane or using an interleaved sagittal approach. The scanning plane depends on viewing preference and resolution optimization (see below).

RESOLUTION

Spatial resolution

High spatial resolution is required to assess lesion morphology. The slice thickness (as defined by the actual slice profile) should be 2 mm or less. The in-plane resolution (as defined by the actual resolution) should be less than 1.0 mm.

Temporal resolution

High temporal resolution is required for dynamic sequences to assess lesion kinetics. The dynamic scan time should be less than 120 s. The dynamic scan should be repeated out to 5–7 minutes post-contrast.

Optimization

Spatial and temporal resolution should be optimized. If parallel imaging is available, it should be used (the direction of parallel imaging may dictate the scanning orientation). Time-saving techniques, such as reducing the field of view in the phase-encoding direction when scanning in the coronal plane, should be used.

SEQUENCES

T2-weighted fast spin echo

This provides high resolution for characterizing lesions and improves specificity. Fat suppression should not be employed.

T1-weighted spoiled gradient echo

A dynamic set of sequences is obtained before contrast injection and then repeated as rapidly as possible for 5–7 minutes after a rapid intravenous bolus of a gadolinium-containing contrast agent.

3D or 2D (multislice) techniques can be employed.

A fat-suppression technique should be used to improve lesion conspicuousness. This can be done either by integral frequency-based fat suppression (e.g. frequency-selective fat saturation or water excitation) of the dynamic sequence or by using a subtraction technique. If integral frequency-based fat suppression is applied, the sequence may optionally be run without fat suppression before the dynamic set in order to help characterize lesions.

The option of applying 3D non-rigid registration to minimize artefacts in the subtraction images due to patient motion during the examination may be helpful.

T1-weighted spoiled gradient echo with fat suppression

This is an ultrahigh-resolution post-contrast scan for assessing lesion morphology. It should have a 50% improvement in voxel size compared with the dynamic scan (unless this is already achieving an in-plane resolution of 0.6 mm).

It can be used with an integral frequency-based fat-suppression technique such as frequency-selective fat saturation or water excitation.

HORMONAL FACTORS: TIMING OF EXAMINATION

The examination should be carried out in the mid-portion of the menstrual cycle to reduce normal parenchymal tissue enhancement. It should be timed to days 6–16 of the menstrual cycle.

2 ROLE OF MRI IN BREAST IMAGING

Breast MRI is playing an increasingly important role not only in the diagnosis of breast cancer but also in its management.

The following are the key clinical indications for MRI:
- as a problem solver when complete triple assessment (clinical, imaging and pathology) is inconclusive
- for evaluation of patients with metastatic axillary nodal disease with negative imaging (i.e. mammography and ultrasound) and clinical findings
- to monitor the response of patients with known breast cancer who are receiving neoadjuvant chemotherapy
- for breast cancer screening of patients with a high risk of breast cancer
- to examine implants

MRI is not indicated routinely in assessing the local extent of newly diagnosed breast cancer. There are, however, specific indications where it has been proven to be of benefit if breast conservation is being considered:
- lobular cancer on histology
- assessment of tumour size when there is clinical and radiological discordance about the size of the known tumour
- Paget's disease of the nipple

Its usefulness is still being assessed in patients with dense breast tissue and a family history of breast cancer that is not high-risk.

INVASIVE LOBULAR CANCER (ILC)

ILC accounts for less than 10% of all breast cancers. These tumours can be very subtle and difficult to identify on conventional imaging because of their diffusely infiltrating nature. MRI is established as a useful tool in determining the extent of involvement when compared with conventional imaging. Studies have shown that MRI is likely to identify additional disease in a significant number of patients and therefore aid the surgeon in deciding the best operative procedure for the patient.

Imaging findings

The following features are suggestive of ILC, although it should be noted that appearances can be variable.

The most common finding is a mass with or without rim enhancement. This mass can be focal. It will often have low or heterogenous signal on T1- and T2-weighted images. The margins are often irregular or spiculate in nature.

There can be multifocal masses. This is often evident on T1- and T2-weighted images, with either several irregular masses or one dominant mass with adjacent or distant satellites.

There can be an area of enhancement that resembles normal glandular patterns. T1- and T2-weighted images will essentially be normal, since there is no solid component visible. Following intravenous contrast administration, there will be an area of enhancement, which may be focal or more extensive and exhibiting a more infiltrative picture.

Enhancement curves are variable for ILC, reflecting tumour histology. They can vary from a typical malignant type III curve with rapid uptake and washout to an apparently benign type I curve (Figure 2.1). The reason for this latter appearance is that ILCs may infiltrate and grow without significant angiogenesis and/or neovascularity.

Hints and tips

MRI must only be reported in conjunction with the current mammogram and ultrasound, particularly when appearances can be subtle.

If additional disease is found, this must be confirmed by a further needle biopsy – either ultrasound- or MRI-guided.

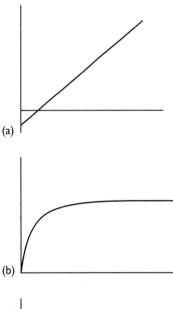
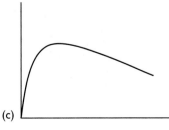

Figure 2.1 Typical shapes of enhancement curves: (a) type I (benign); (b) type II (suspicious); (c) type III (malignant).

Case 1: Invasive lobular cancer

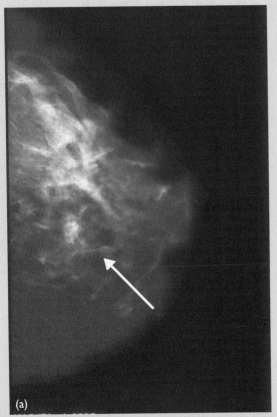

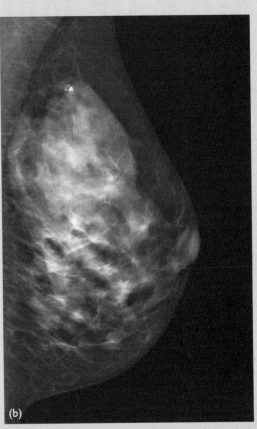

Case 1.1 (a) Left craniocaudal mammogram showing a subtle area of increased density in the inner half of the left breast (arrow). (b) The mediolateral-oblique view is unremarkable.

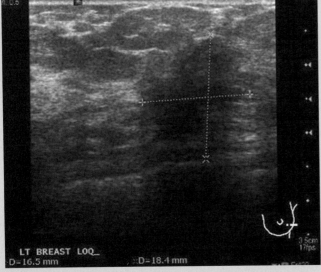

Case 1.2 Ultrasound showing a 16 mm irregular mass.

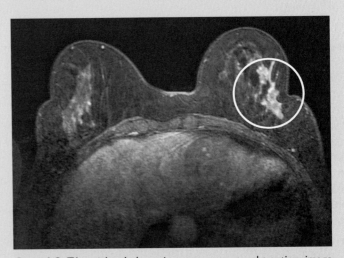

Case 1.3 T1-weighted dynamic post-contrast subtraction image showing the extensive nature of the tumour – measuring 55 mm in maximum diameter.

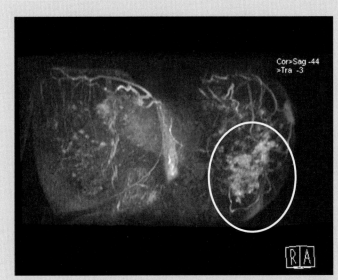

Case 1.4 A 3D reconstruction of the early subtraction dynamic sequence.

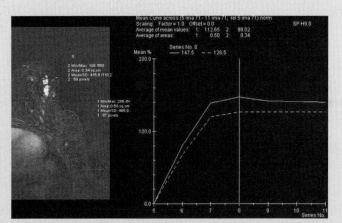

Case 1.5 The enhancement curve is of type II, i.e. suspicious.

NEOADJUVANT CHEMOTHERAPY (NACT)

NACT has been proven to be just as good as adjuvant chemotherapy, and may have additional benefit in reducing the amount of surgery.

The role of MRI is to evaluate the response of the tumour to the chemotherapy regime.

Patients suitable for NACT are those who are young, have a high-grade tumour, a large tumour or metastatic involvement of the axillary lymph nodes.

A baseline MRI scan is performed and the tumour extent and enhancement profile are assessed.

Following two cycles of chemotherapy, the patient has a repeat MRI scan. The tumour extent and enhancement profile are reassessed (Table 2.1):
• If the tumour is responding well, the findings are discussed with the oncologists, and the patient continues with their current treatment.
• If the response is considered to be none or minimal, the chemotherapy regime is altered. The patient will then have a further scan after a further two cycles.

Imaging findings

Tumours can respond either by concentric reduction or fragmentation – where the bulk is reduced but the extent is similar.

If the tumour is responding concentrically then the insertion of a marker clip should be considered, since there may

Table 2.1 Action following assessment of response to chemotherapy

Response[a]	Action
Progression Stable disease Minimal response	Consider changing treatment
Partial response[b] Almost complete response	Continue treatment

[a]The criteria for assessing response are tumour extent, tumour bulk and tumour activity (increased, static or decreased in each case).

[b]A partial response is defined by a greater than 50% reduction in the diameter of the main mass or a 25–50% reduction in the main mass plus an improvement in the enhancement curve.

be a complete MRI response (this also aids the pathologist at the time of surgery).

Enhancement profiles also show improvement, since cytotoxic agents affect tumour vascularization and vascular wall permeability.

Hints and tips

MRI is useful in documenting the initial extent of the disease.

The second scan is a good time to plan surgery.

A type I ('benign') enhancement curve (see Figure 2.1a) indicates response to treatment but not absence of tumour.

Case 2: Neoadjuvant chemotherapy (NACT)

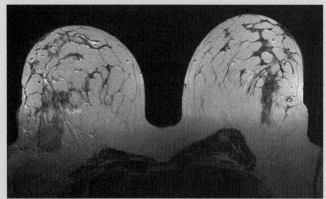

Case 2.1 T2-weighted axial image showing a 40 mm solid, irregular mass in the upper outer quadrant of the right breast.

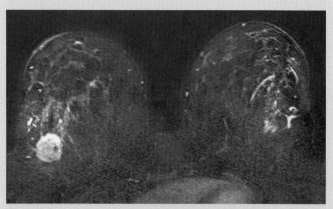

Case 2.2 A T1-weighted dynamic post-subtraction image shows the mass to be enhancing.

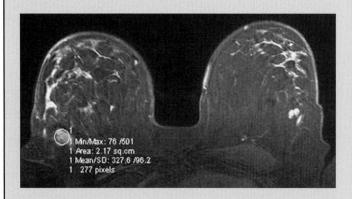

Case 2.3 The enhancement profile shows a type III (malignant) curve.

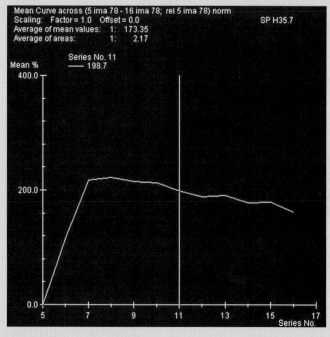

Case 2.4 Following two cycles of chemotherapy, a T2-weighted axial image shows that the tumour has decreased in size, now measuring 25 mm.

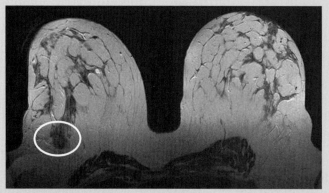

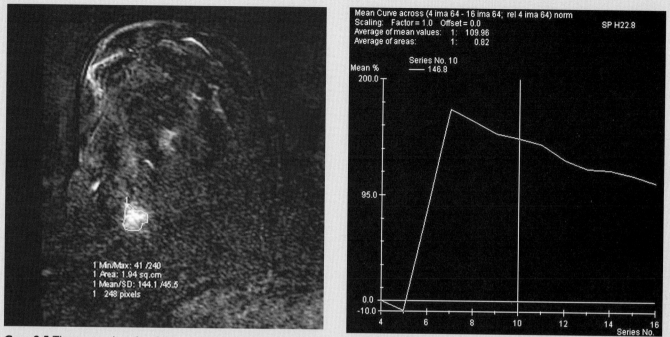

Mean Curve across (4 ima 64 - 16 ima 64; rel 4 ima 64) norm
Scaling: Factor = 1.0   Offset = 0.0
Average of mean values: 1:   109.96
Average of areas: 1:   0.82

SP H22.8

1 Min/Max: 41 /240
1 Area: 1.94 sq.cm
1 Mean/SD: 144.1 /46.5
1   248 pixels

Case 2.5 The tumour has also shown an improvement in the enhancement curve, although it still remains type III. This would be considered a partial response to NACT, since there has been both a reduction in tumour bulk and an improvement in the enhancement curve.

UNIT VII
Head and Neck MRI

Amit Roy, Kshitij Mankad

1 HEAD AND NECK MRI

INTRODUCTION

Diagnostic imaging is fundamentally important in the investigation of head and neck pathology as there is poor accessibility of certain anatomical areas to clinical examination and direct visualisation.

Although ultrasound is unparalleled in the evaluation of thyroid and salivary gland lesions (due to its coupling with fine needle aspiration techniques) and computed tomography is unquestionably the modality of choice for the investigation of sinonasal and petromastoid anatomy, magnetic resonance imaging currently provides the greatest contrast resolution for soft tissues. It is the modality of greatest utility in the investigation of the soft tissue spaces of the neck; particularly those that are inaccessible on ultrasound, such as the skull base and parapharyngeal regions.

Basic sequences

As elsewhere in the body, T1-weighted images provide excellent anatomical resolution, while T2-weighted images are generally superior in delineating abnormal tissues such as those harbouring infection, inflammation or malignancy. T1-weighted images are useful in establishing bony disease as loss of normal marrow signal is sensitive for marrow replacement. T1-weighted images are also useful in determining cartilaginous involvement of the larynx in laryngeal malignancy, an observation that is important both in terms of management and prognostication. T2-based sequences are particularly advantageous in the elucidation of cystic abnormalities or those in which necrosis occurs on account of the high inherent T2 signal of water.

Gadolinium is the most common contrast agent used in MR imaging. T1-weighted contrasted images are used to demonstrate an augmentation of signal, or enhancement, which can be a feature of various pathological entities.

Fat-suppressed sequences such as STIR (short-tau inverse recovery) improve conspicuity of pathological processes such as oedema where the high signal of fat may obscure the boundaries of a pathological process.

FLAIR can also be useful, for example in removing CSF signal to improve conspicuity of skull base lesions.

Other techniques such as FIESTA/CISS sequencing, angiographic time-of-flight (TOF) imaging and gradient echo (GRE) imaging have been discussed elsewhere and are of relevance particularly in the evaluation of cerebello-pontine angle lesions, vascular abnormalities and haemorrhagic abnormalities respectively.

Diffusion-weighted imaging (DWI) has been discussed previously and utilises the principle that the signals generated by protons in water molecules differ depending on whether free diffusion is occurring. Intrinsic T2-weighted information is contained when creating a DWI. Arithmetic processing is required to create the so-called ADC map, which eliminates T2 contribution. The diffusion characteristics of a number of pathological processes are reproducible and this thus aids in narrowing the differential diagnosis.

DWI has been an emerging technique in recent years. There are a number of scenarios in which its utility is clear in the head and neck perspective. One of these situations is in the differentiation of residual or recurrent disease from post-treatment changes, which can be exceedingly difficult with conventional imaging techniques. Some studies have demonstrated its high sensitivity and specificity in distinguishing malignant from benign involvement of cervical lymph nodes in squamous cell carcinoma.

Protocols

Table 1.1 summarises some of the key protocols often utilised in head and neck imaging.

The list is not intended to be exhaustive or comprehensive, merely demonstrating which sequences may be used to highlight particular clinical entities.

Further reading

Mack MG, Vogl TJ. MR imaging of the head and neck. *Eur Radiol* 1999; **9**(7):1247–51.

BASIC ANATOMY

Surgical anatomy of the neck makes reference to a number of 'triangles' in relation to which the walls, floor, roof and contents are described. Although clearly useful, radiological reports instead generally make reference to the fascial spaces of the neck – potential spaces lined by the deep cervical fascia which 'divide' the neck into a number of compartments. Indeed, knowledge of these anatomical compartments and understanding patterns of spread and how these spaces may distort in the face of various

Table 1.1 Some key protocols

Protocol (indication)	Sequence
Neck (tumour, infection)	T1-coronal T1-axial T2-axial fat-suppressed T1-sagittal fat-suppressed + gadolinium T1-axial fat-suppressed + gadolinium T1-coronal fat-suppressed + gadolinium DWI-axial
Neck MRA (carotid/vertebral vessel disease) Arch to circle of Willis	2D time of flight-axial T1-axial fat-suppressed (if dissection suspected) 3D time of flight-coronal 3D time of flight-sag/oblique +/- brain protocol if required
Face (tumour, infection, sinonasal lesion)	T1-coronal T1-axial T2-axial fat-suppressed T2-coronal fat-suppressed T1-sagittal fat-suppressed + gadolinium T1-axial fat-suppressed + gadolinium T1-coronal fat-suppressed + gadolinium DWI-axial
Skull base (tumour, infection)	T1-axial Fluid attenuated inversion recovery (FLAIR)-axial T2-axial fat-suppressed T2-coronal T1-axial fat-suppressed + gadolinium T1-coronal fat-suppressed + gadolinium T1-sagittal fat-suppressed + gadolinium GRE-axial DWI-axial
Orbit	T2-axial T2-coronal fat-suppressed T1-axial T1-axial fat-suppressed + gadolinium T1-coronal fat-suppressed + gadolinium +/- brain if field/cranial nerve deficit
Internal auditory meatus (CP angle lesion, sensorineural hearing loss, facial nerve palsy, etc.)	T1-sagittal T2-coronal T2-axial T1-axial GRE FIESTA-axial T1-axial fat-suppressed + gadolinium T1-coronal fat-suppressed + gadolinium

pathological entities aids differential diagnosis significantly. Indeed, the various layers form natural physical boundaries to the dissemination of neoplastic or infective processes.

The superficial cervical fascia is a subdermal layer that envelops the head and neck, continuing inferiorly into the thorax.

The deep fascia has a number of components:
- The superficial or investing layer, which envelops all of the deeper structures excluding the cervical lymph nodes and platysma
- The middle layer, which lies anterior to the strap muscles, surrounding the thyroid gland and encircling the trachea and oesophagus
- The deep layer, which invests the vertebral elements and paraspinal muscles

The carotid sheath has contributions from all three of the above and invests the common carotid artery, internal jugular vein, vagus nerve and deep cervical lymph nodes.

The supra-hyoid neck can be further subdivided into lateral compartments as follows:
- The parapharyngeal space (which can be further subdivided into pre- and post-styloid compartments)
- The masticator space
- The parotid space

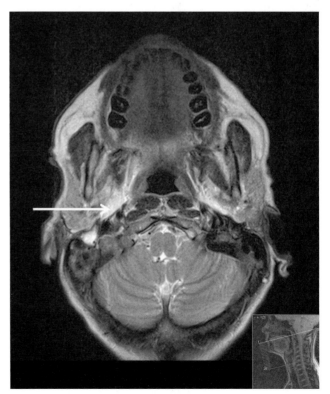

Figure 1.1 Arrow denotes pre-styloid parapharyngeal space.

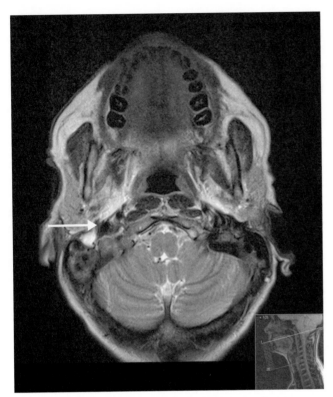

Figure 1.2 Arrow denotes post-styloid parapharyngeal space.

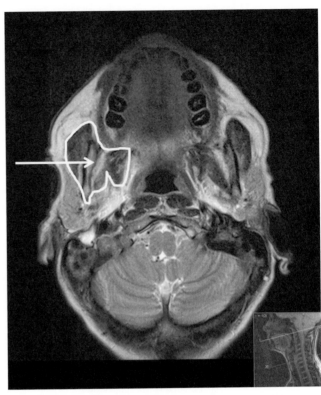

Figure 1.3 Arrow denotes masticator space.

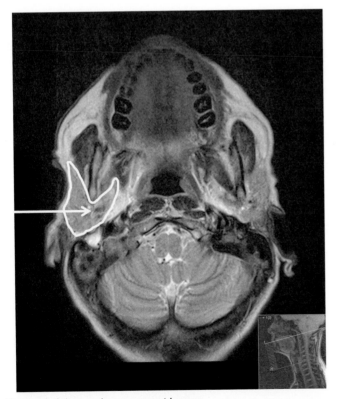

Figure 1.4 Arrow denotes parotid space.

Midline compartments of the supra-hyoid neck include:
- The pharyngeal mucosal space
- The retropharyngeal space
- The peri-vertebral and danger spaces – so-called due to the absence of distinct midline and inferior boundaries allowing infection to spread not only across the midline but also inferiorly into the thorax

The parapharyngeal space

This is divided into pre- and post-styloid compartments. Contents include the internal maxillary and ascending pharyngeal arteries, pharyngeal venous plexus, minor salivary gland rests and small branches of the mandibular trigeminal nerve division in its pre-styloid component. The post-styloid space contains the internal carotid artery, internal jugular vein, cranial nerves IX–XII and the accompanying sympathetic nervous plexus.

The masticator space

This contains the mandibular ramus and body; pterygoid, masseter and temporalis muscles; branches of the mandibular division of the trigeminal nerve; and the inferior alveolar artery and vein.

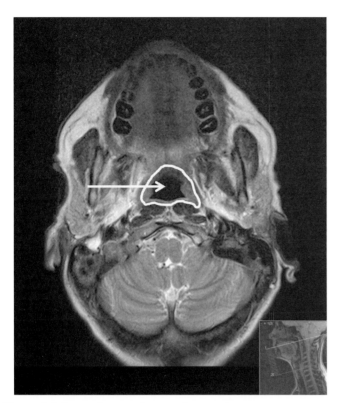

Figure 1.5 Arrow denotes pharyngeal mucosal space.

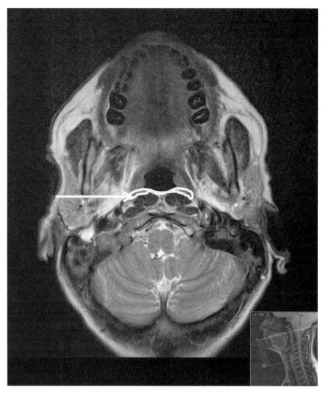

Figure 1.6 Arrow denotes retropharyngeal space.

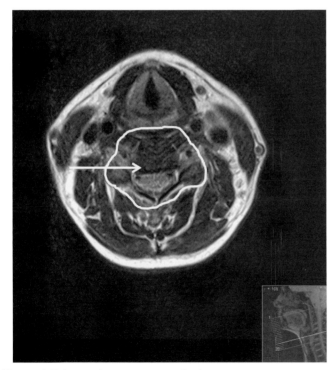

Figure 1.7 Arrow denotes peri-vertebral space.

The parotid space

This contains the parotid gland; facial nerve; external carotid and internal maxillary arteries; retromandibular vein and lymph nodes.

The pharyngeal mucosal space

This space contains pharyngeal mucosa; Waldeyer's ring of reticulo-endothelial tissue; minor salivary glands and muscles including the superior and middle pharyngeal constrictors: palatopharyngeus and salpingopharyngeus.

The retropharyngeal space

This is a potential space normally containing merely fat and retropharyngeal nodes.

The pre-vertebral (and danger) spaces

This is subdivided into pre-vertebral and paraspinal components. The former contains the vertebral bodies, vertebral vessels, longus and scalene muscles and brachial plexus. The latter portion contains the paraspinal muscles and posterior vertebral elements. The danger space is so-called on account of the absence of distinct midline and inferior boundaries allowing infection to spread, not only across the midline, but also inferiorly into the thorax.

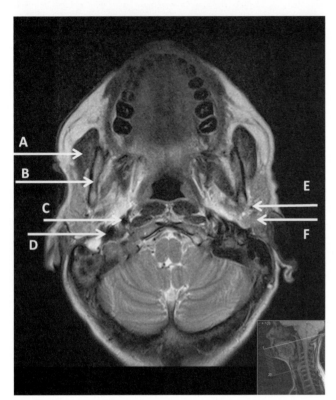

Figure 1.8 A, masseter muscle; B, mandibular ramus; C, internal carotid artery; D, internal jugular vein; E, external carotid artery; F, parotid gland.

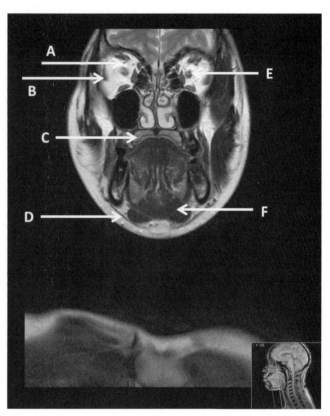

Figure 1.9 A, superior ophthalmic vein; B, lateral rectus muscle; C, hard palate; D, platysma muscle; E, optic nerve; F, mylohyoid muscle.

CASE STUDIES

The following cases illustrate a number of the scanning techniques and protocols mentioned earlier in the chapter. The selection of cases is not intended to be a comprehensive account of the range of pathologies one may encounter in this complex anatomical area, merely a collection that demonstrates some of the aforementioned technical and anatomical principles.

SQUAMOUS CELL CARCINOMA OF THE ORAL CAVITY

Introduction

The overwhelming majority of oral cavity tumours are malignant, although benign lesions arising from epithelial, salivary and connective tissue origin do occasionally occur. The majority of malignant lesions are squamous cell carcinomas, with the remainder comprising malignant salivary neoplasms, melanomas and sarcomas.

Although imaging is not strictly required for the small minority of superficial lesions that are readily accessible,

precise anatomical tumour mapping is an invaluable resource for the remaining majority of lesions. Imaging plays an important role in treatment planning and can, for example, demonstrate vascular or neural invasion, which may profoundly impact management decisions. In addition to permitting accurate visualisation of the primary lesion, MRI can be invaluable in detecting the presence of nodal disease.

Key sequences

- T1-axial, coronal
- T2-axial
- STIR-axial
- T1 fat-suppressed post contrast – axial, coronal, sagittal
- DWI (nodal assessment) – axial from skull base to thoracic inlet

Imaging findings

The most common imaging appearance for a malignant oral cavity lesion is that of an enhancing, invasive soft tissue mass of low T1, high T2 and high STIR signal. Post-contrast enhancement may be variable and some lesions may demonstrate internal necrosis with the appearance of peripheral enhancement, making discrimination from infection difficult in these situations. MRI is also useful in the assessment of nodal disease, with the most frequent appearance of involved nodes being heterogeneously enhancing low T1- and high T2-signal lesions with internal foci of necrosis.

Hints and tips

Involvement of mandibular bone by the disease process may be determined by assessing marrow signal on T1.

The differential diagnosis for oral cavity neoplastic lesions includes abscesses and infective lesions. The latter should,

however, be associated with considerable cellulitis of the surrounding and overlying soft tissues. A rare lesion such as a lingual thyroid may also mimic an oral cavity neoplasm; in this case enhancement characteristics should follow that of normal thyroid tissue.

As mentioned earlier in the chapter, diffusion-weighting may have a role in distinguishing benign from malignant nodes in difficult cases.

Further reading

Shah GV, Wesolowski JR, Ansari SA, Mukherji SK. New directions in head and neck imaging. *J Surg Oncol* 2008; **97**(8):644–8.

Case 1.1 Squamous cell carcinoma of the oral cavity

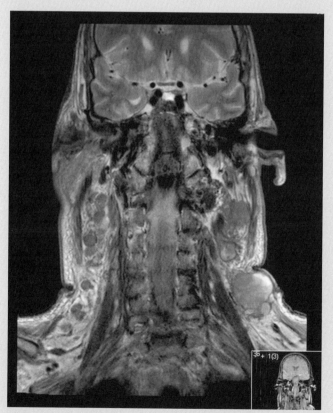

Case 1.1 T2-coronal image demonstrating multiple abnormal enlarged cervical lymph nodes at all levels.

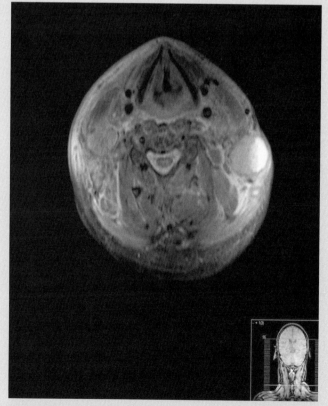

Case 1.2 Axial STIR image demonstrating multiple abnormal enlarged lymph nodes, the largest on the left. Intermediate signal within both internal jugular veins is in keeping with thrombosis.

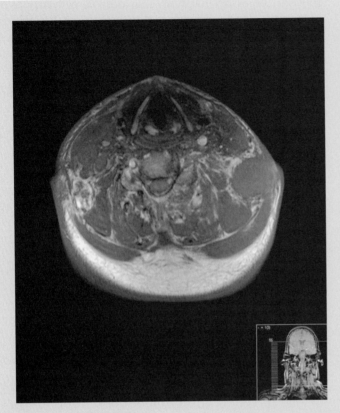

Case 1.3 T1-axial image.

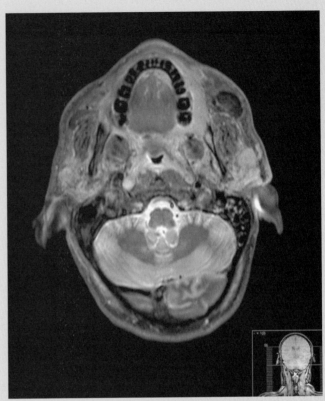

Case 1.4 Axial STIR image demonstrating a 4cm lesion of high signal in the left buccal sulcus, in keeping with the primary tumour.

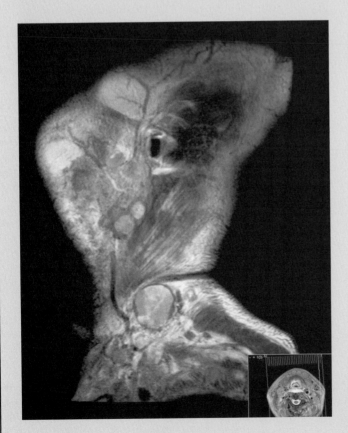

Case 1.5 T2-sagittal image through the left side of the neck again demonstrates enlarged nodes. Internal high T2 signal is in keeping with necrosis.

SOFT TISSUE TUMOUR OF THE FACE

Introduction

Soft tissue lesions are frequently encountered in clinical practice and characterisation can be extremely difficult despite recent advances in modern imaging techniques.

The range of possible underlying diagnoses is vast, comprising a range of benign and malignant pathological entities. The World Health Organisation (WHO) classification of soft tissue tumours includes nine categories of lesion depending upon the tissue of origin and includes entities such as lipomas, haemangiomas, neurofibromas and sarcomas.

Key sequences

- T1- axial, coronal
- T2- axial
- T1 fat-suppressed post contrast – axial, coronal, sagittal
- STIR- axial
- MRA/MRV if AVM suspected
- DWI- axial
- GRE- axial

Imaging findings

MRI is the modality of choice – owing to its intrinsically high soft-tissue contrast – and allows tumour staging, assessment of neurovascular invasion and pre-operative planning. Imaging protocols generally involve T1, T2 and fat-suppressed sequences at a minimum. Additional sequences such as T2* gradient echo can be particularly helpful in assessing the presence of haemosiderin, which causes magnetic susceptibility effects giving rise to the so-called 'blooming' artefact. This can be useful in diagnosing haematomas and haemangiomas. The use of post-contrast imaging can be useful in the differentiation of solid from cystic structures and knowledge of the patterns of contrast enhancement can aid the distinguishing of benign from malignant lesions.

Hints and Tips

Lymphangiomas (or lymphatic malformations) are best evaluated on T2-weighted imaging and are generally hyperintense throughout, often with multiple internal septations. Areas of enhancement are uncommon and may suggest alternate pathology. Foci of high T1-weighted signal may represent internal haemorrhage.

The hallmark of vascular malformations is the presence of phleboliths, which manifest as rounded signal voids on MR. Flow voids are also a characteristic feature. Enhancement may be variable, ranging from avid to mild.

Further reading

Wu JS, Hochman MG. Soft-tissue tumors and tumor-like lesions: a systematic imaging approach. *Radiology* 2009; **253**(2):297–316.

Case 2 Soft tissue tumour of the face

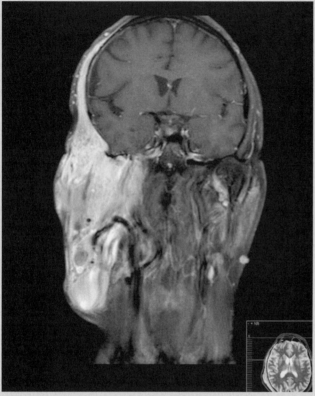

Case 2.1 T1-coronal SPIR post-Gad image demonstrating an extensive complex soft tissue mass involving the superficial and deep fascial layers of the right face.

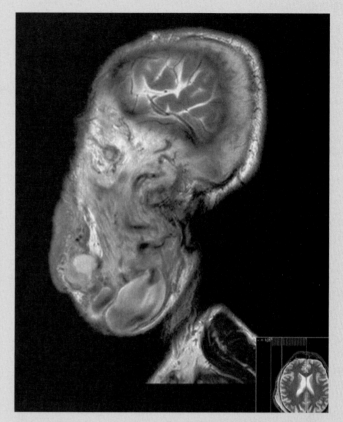

Case 2.2 T2-sagittal image demonstrating the same features.

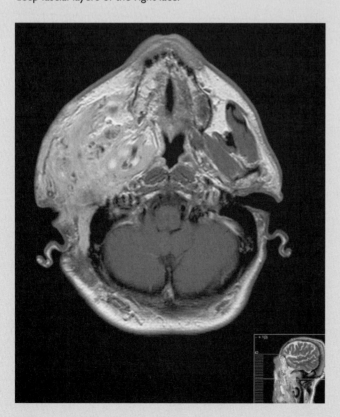

Case 2.3 T1-axial post-Gad image in the same patient demonstrating an avidly enhancing lesion with internal flow voids centred on the masticator space with replacement of the temporalis, masseter and pterygoid muscles. The lesion was a complex plexiform neurofibroma.

SKULL BASE LESION

Introduction

Familiarity with the complex anatomy of the skull base is a requisite for the correct diagnosis of skull base lesions. Imaging plays a crucial role in the diagnosis and management of such lesions, not least due to the relative inaccessibility of this complex anatomical area. CT and MR imaging are complementary and are almost invariably used in conjunction to map the full disease process.

The skull base can be divided into anterior, middle and posterior compartments and the range of pathological entities differs depending upon the region concerned. Commonly encountered pathologies include congenital/developmental lesions such as cephaloceles; benign neoplasms, such as angiofibroma and meningioma; and aggressive lesions, such as nasopharyngral carcinoma, chordoma and chondrosarcoma.

Key sequences

- T1-axial, coronal
- T2-axial
- FLAIR-axial
- T1 fat-suppressed post-contrast axial, coronal, sagittal
- GRE-axial
- DWI-axial

Imaging findings

As mentioned above, the differential diagnosis for neoplastic lesions in this area is extensive. Meningiomata characteristically demonstrate a durally-based 'tail' on post-contrast T1 imaging. Focal cystic and haemorrhagic change is not uncommon. Calcification may give rise to 'blooming' artefact on GRE imaging.

Chordomas classically demonstrate high T2 signal with foci of haemorrhage on GRE imaging.

Other differential diagnoses include chondrosarcomas, nasopharyngeal carcinomas, plasmacytomas and giant cell tumours. No unique imaging features or signal characteristics are demonstrated, highlighting the difficulty faced in confidently making a diagnosis.

Hints and tips

CT is often employed concurrently to assess bony involvement.

The utility of MRI is highlighted by its ability to detect perineural spread at an earlier stage than other modalities.

Further reading

Borges A. Imaging of the central skull base. *Neuroimaging Clin N Am* 2009; **19**(4):669–96.

Case 3 Skull base lesion

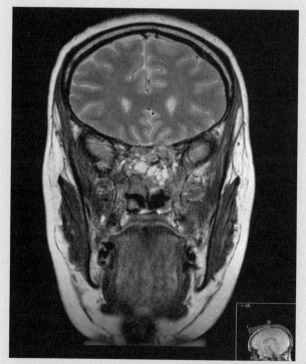

Case 3.1 T2-coronal image demonstrating a large central skull base tumour. Biopsy revealed an angiosarcoma. The patient had previously undergone radiotherapy to the skull base.

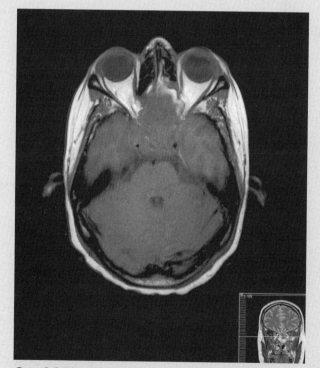

Case 3.2 T1-axial image demonstrating the same lesion.

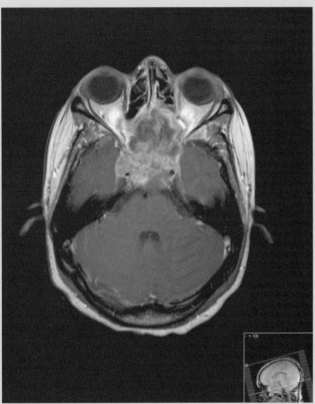

Case 3.3 T1-axial post-Gad image demonstrating avid post-contrast enhancement of the complex skull base mass with extension into the cavernous sinuses and filling of the pituitary fossa.

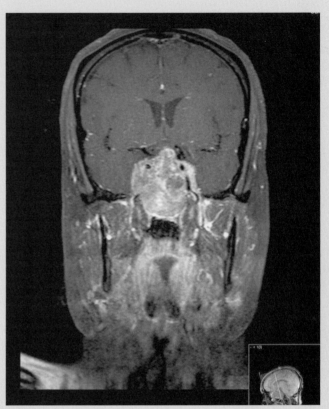

Case 3.4 T1-coronal post-Gad image demonstrating suprasellar extension of the lesion and displacement of the optic chiasm.

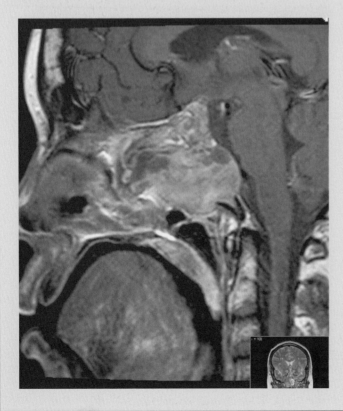

Case 3.5 T1-sagittal post-Gad image demonstrating the same features.

NEUROENDOCRINE TUMOURS

Paragangliomas are rare neuroendocrine neoplasms that may develop at a number of sites within the body, including the head and neck. They derive from chromaffin cells in paraganglia or glomus cells derived from the neural crest.

Although a relatively small minority of these tumours occur in the head and neck, they are most likely to be symptomatic in this region. Examples include carotid body tumours (chemodectomas), glomus jugulare, tympanicum and vagale tumours.

Although the majority are sporadic, a significant proportion of these rare lesions are either directly heritable or occur as part of a syndrome such as the Carney triad or Neurofibromatosis type 1.

Key sequences

- T1-axial, coronal
- T2-axial
- FLAIR-axial
- T1 fat-suppressed post-contrast axial, coronal, sagittal
- GRE-axial
- MRA/MRV

Imaging findings

Glomus jugulare/vagale/tympanicum and carotid body paragangliomas demonstrate a characteristic 'salt and pepper' appearance on MR; the former relates to T1-weighted hyperintensities caused by microhaemorrhagic foci while the latter refers to small serpiginous flow voids due to vessels in larger lesions. Avid post-contrast enhancement is the norm for these rare lesions.

Hints and tips

The differential diagnosis for these lesions includes jugular foramen meningiomata, schwannomata and metastases. For carotid body paragangliomas, a characteristic feature is splaying of the carotid bifurcation by the soft tissue mass.

Further reading

Mendenhall W M, Amdur R J, Vaysberg M, Mendenhall C M, Werning J W. Head and neck paragangliomas report of 175 patients (1989–2010). *Head & Neck* 2011 [Epub ahead of print].

Case 4 Neuroendocrine tumours

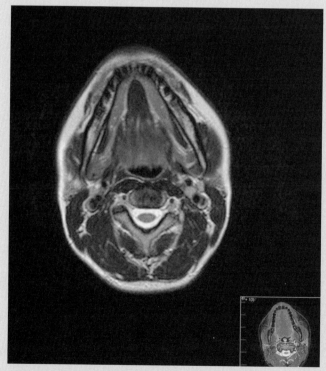

Case 4.1 T2-axial image demonstrating an 8mm lesion of intermediate signal intensity at the bifurcation of the left common carotid artery. The mass represented a chemodectoma (or carotid body tumour) occurring as part of the Carney Triad in this patient.

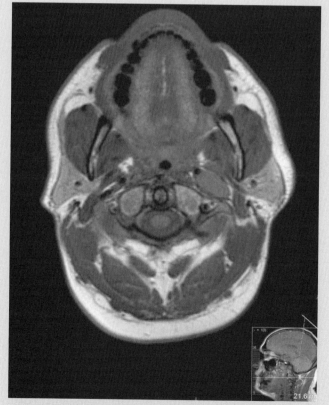

Case 4.2 T1-axial image demonstrating an intermediate-signal mass in the left parapharyngeal space.

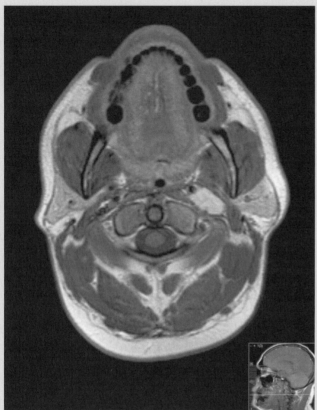

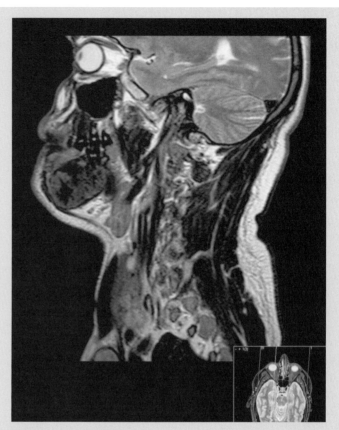

Case 4.3 T1-axial post-Gad image in the same patient demonstrates avid enhancement. The mass represents a carotid sheath paraganglioma.

Case 4.4 T2-sagittal image in the same patient demonstrates a large low signal mandibular lesion in keeping with a fibroma. The patient had Hyperparathyroidism-jaw tumour (HPT-JT) syndrome.

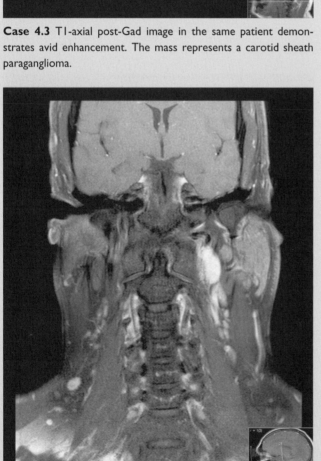

Case 4.5 T1-coronal post-Gad image in the same patient again demonstrates the avidly-enhancing left upper carotid sheath paraganglioma.

THYROID LESION

While ultrasound is the modality of choice for the initial evaluation of the thyroid gland (not least due to its coupling with diagnostic FNA) MR imaging can provide a useful adjunctive role.

Malignant thyroid neoplasms can take many forms, but a useful starting point is the division between differentiated (such as papillary and follicular) and undifferentiated (anaplastic) forms.

If cross-sectional imaging is considered, MRI is preferable to CT as iodinated contrast media are contraindicated if treatment with radioactive iodine is being considered.

Key sequences

- T1-axial, coronal +/- fat-suppression
- T2-axial
- T1 post-contrast +/- fat-suppression; axial, coronal, sagittal

Imaging findings

Features of differentiated lesions include a heterogeneously enhancing mixed-signal mass, distinguished from a benign entity by the presence of invasive margins. Anaplastic lesions are frankly invasive and more likely to demonstrate calcification, haemorrhage and necrosis, giving rise to a more heterogeneous appearance.

Hints and Tips

Imaging cannot reliably distinguish malignant from benign disease, but when the diagnosis has been established or is suspected cytologically, MRI is the modality of choice for staging.

Imaging from the skull base to the carina is indicated to exclude mediastinal extension, extracapsular spread and nodal metastasis.

Further reading

Weber AL, Randolph G, Aksoy FG. The thyroid and parathyroid glands: CT and MR imaging and correlation with pathology and clinical findings. *Radiol Clin North Am* 2000; **38**(5):1105–29.

Case 5 Thyroid lesion

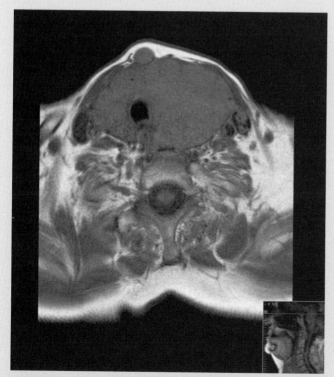

Case 5.1 T1-axial image demonstrating a large thyroid mass with tracheal displacement and distortion of the surrounding fascial planes.

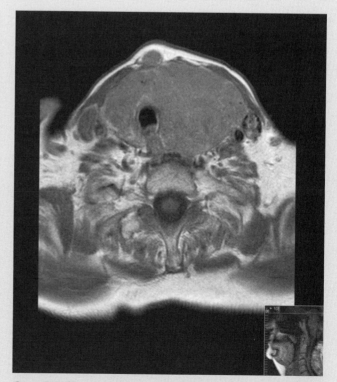

Case 5.2 T1-axial post-Gad image demonstrating a heterogeneously enhancing thyroid mass, which proved to be Hurtle cell carcinoma. Intermediate-signal material within the left internal jugular vein lumen is in keeping with thrombus.

THYROID OPHTHALMOPATHY/ ORBITOPATHY

Thyroid orbitopathy, often referred to as Graves' ophthalmopathy, is an autoimmune process affecting the orbit and peri-orbital tissues, thyroid gland, pre-tibial skin and digital soft tissues. Although Graves' disease is the most common associated thyroid abnormality, other disorders such as Hashimoto's thyroiditis and even thyroid carcinoma can be associated. Approximately 40% of patients with Graves' disease develop thyroid orbitopathy.

Key sequences

- T1-axial and coronal-demonstrating isointense extra-ocular muscle enlargement
- T2-axial and coronal
- STIR-axial
- T1 fat-suppressed post-contrast: axial, coronal +/- sagittal

Imaging findings

Enlargement of the extra-ocular muscles is the most sensitive imaging manifestation of this condition. Classically, the inferior and medial rectus muscles are affected earliest and most severely. Approximately 85% of cases show bilateral disease.

In the acute stage, T2 signal may be increased within the extra-ocular muscles. Progressively over time, however, signal may diminish due to repeat episodes of inflammation and fibrosis. STIR imaging is useful as signal from orbital fat is suppressed, and post-contrast imaging generally reveals greater enhancement within affected muscles when compared with uninvolved counterparts.

Hints and tips

Radiologically, enlargement of the bellies of the extra-ocular muscles with relative sparing of the tendinous insertions is the hallmark of this condition. This can help in distinguishing this entity from other causes of extra-ocular muscle enlargement such as infection, sarcoidosis and idiopathic orbital pseudotumour.

Multiplanar imaging is essential in establishing the extent of muscular involvement and the involvement of other orbital structures, such as the optic nerve.

Further reading

Hoang JK, Eastwood JD, Glastonbury CM. What's in a name? Eponyms in head and neck imaging. *Clin Radiol* 2010; **65**(3):237–45.

Case 6 Thyroid ophthalmopathy/orbitopathy

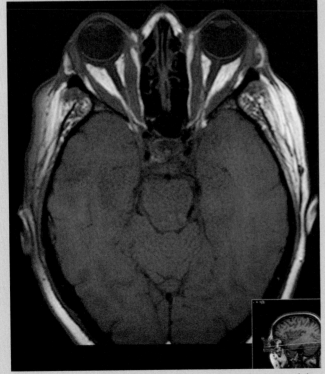

Case 6.1 T1-axial image through the orbits demonstrating bilateral, almost symmetrical enlargement of the extra-ocular muscles.

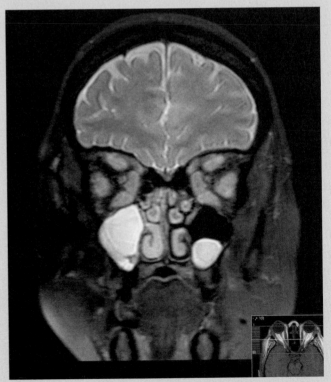

Case 6.2 T2-3D SPIR coronal image demonstrating fusiform expansion of the extra-ocular muscles bilaterally.

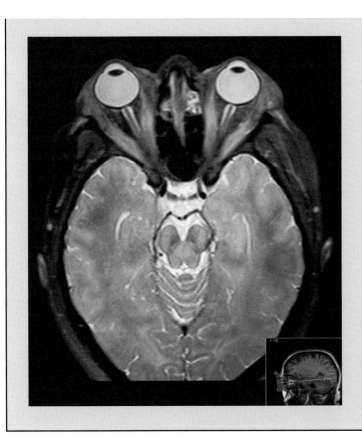

Case 6.3 T2-3D SPIR axial image demonstrating extrinsic compression of both optic nerves by the swollen extra-ocular muscles bilaterally.

ORBITAL TRAUMA

Orbital contents are vulnerable to injury despite the bony protection afforded by the osseous orbit. Orbital fractures are common and CT is the modality of choice given its ready availability and efficacy in detecting bony injury. A number of patterns of injury to the globe itself may also occur, including globe rupture, lens dislocation, vitreous and subretinal haemorrhage. In such cases, MR is more sensitive than CT owing to superior soft tissue contrast resolution.

The utility of MR imaging in the detection of haemorrhage of differing age has been dealt with elsewhere.

Key imaging sequences

- T1-axial and coronal
- STIR-axial
- T2 with fat saturation
- T1 fat-suppressed post-contrast: axial, coronal +/- sagittal

Imaging features

Imaging features of globe rupture include loss of normal globe contour and volume, intra-ocular air and discontinuity of the sclera. MR is also sensitive in diagnosing retinal and choroidal detachments. The sequelae of previous globe trauma may be identified in the form of heterogeneous signal within the globes on T1- and T2-weighted imaging owing to repeated haemorrhage and calcifications.

Hints and tips

MR imaging is of proven efficacy in delineating orbital soft tissue injury but can be dangerous if there is a chance that metallic foreign bodies have penetrated the globe.

Imaging in this region is prone to artefact including chemical shift and susceptibility artefacts as well as those due to motion. Fat-saturation and thin-section, small field-of-view (FOV) images are essential.

When evaluating choroidal detachments, MR can distinguish between haemorrhagic and serous variants, which can be significant as the former has a poorer prognosis.

Further reading

Dunkin JM, Crum AV, Swanger RS, Bokhari SA. Globe trauma. *Semin Ultrasound CT MR* 2011; **32**(1):51–6.

Case 7 Orbital trauma

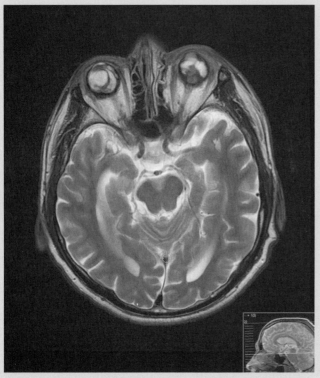

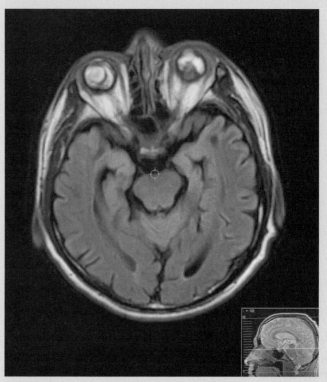

Case 7.1 T2-axial image at the level of the orbits demonstrates foci of abnormal signal within anterior and posterior chambers of both globes, in keeping with haemorrhage and calcification.

Case 7.2 T1-axial image demonstrating similar features. This patient had a history of psychosis and self-inflicted penetrating traumatic injury to both globes.

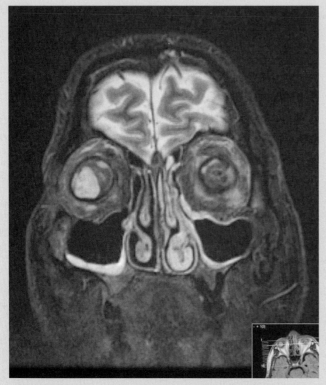

Case 7.3 T2-coronal image demonstrating similar features.

INDEX

Note: page numbers in **bold** refer to diagrams, page numbers in *italics* refer to information contained in tables and boxes.